*To Alice and Raffaella
my beloved daughters.*

*Never give up your dreams,
but believe in what you desire
and in what you do:
only thus will you find
the courage that is within you.*

M. M. Gulizia (Editor)

Emerging Pathologies in Cardiology

Proceedings of the
Mediterranean Cardiology Meeting

(Taormina, April 7-9, 2005)

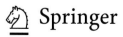 Springer

M. M. Gulizia, MD
Chief of Cardiology Division
S. Luigi - S. Currò Hospital
Catania, Italy

Library of Congress Control Number: 2005922178

ISBN 88-470-0311-3 Springer Milan Berlin Heidelberg New York

Springer is a part of Springer Science+Business Media
springeronline.com
© Springer-Verlag Italia 2005
Printed in Italy

Cover design: Simona Colombo, Milan, Italy
Typesetting: Graphostudio, Milan, Italy
Printing: Grafiche Porpora, Cernusco S/N, Italy

Preface

Clinical practice is evolving at a rapid pace, nowhere more so than in the field of cardiology. Acute Coronary Syndromes, Sudden Cardiac Death, Heart Failure, Atrial Fibrillation, Syncope, and Prevention of Global Cardiovascular Risk are the main *Emerging Pathologies* to which many investigators are addressing their researches. Less than 10 years ago, some of them were considered of relevance only to internists, and some others as a common benign arrhythmia or an ineluctable illness. Today, their prevalence amongst the population represents one of the major public health problems at the beginning of the third millennium.

The need to have *a state of the art overview* of the epidemiology, physiopathological and electrogenetic mechanisms, diagnosis, pharmacological or electrical treatment, prognosis, patient management in and out of hospital, organisational and economical implications of these emerging pathologies and the success of the previous edition inspired us to organise the second edition of this biannual International Meeting.

This book contains the Proceedings of the Mediterranean Cardiology Meeting held in Taormina, Italy, 7–9 April 2005. Like the previous volume, it boasts the participation of many nationally and internationally renowned speakers in the field of clinical and interventional cardiology who will interact actively with the delegates.

The book is divided into eight sections, each devoted to a different topic: *Emerging Concepts in the Assessment of Acute Coronary Syndromes and Global Cardiovascular Risk; Atrial Fibrillation: the Current Clinical Approach; Cardiac Resynchronisation Therapy: New Therapeutic and Diagnostic Perspectives in Heart Failure Management; Managing Sudden Death: Selection of Patients, Drugs, and Devices; New Trends in Physiological Pacing and Optimal Pacing Sites; Haemodynamic Sensing in the Control of Pacing Function; Syncope: Practical Issues of Diagnosis and Treatment; Latest Technologies in Cardiovascular Imaging: An Update for the Clinical Cardiologist.*

It aims to provide the latest information about the most recent and modern aspects of the above mentioned pathologies. It is intended not only for cardiologists, but also for those who are actively interested in the evidence-based approach to clinical care, such as internists, emergency and critical care clinicians, physicians of general medicine, fellows, students, nurses, and technicians. It may also be helpful for those engaged in the development and coordination of research strategies in biological engineering, industry, and regulatory affairs, who have a high interest in the overall management of these cardiac pathologies.

A Faculty, selected from leading Italian and foreign experts in the field, ensures the highest quality of this volume: the publications of many of them have contributed to the scientific development and influenced many of our professional considerations and decisions. I am really most indebted to all these authors, who have devoted the invaluable time and effort without which this book would not have been completed.

I also wish to thank the staff of Springer, and in particular Donatella Rizza, Executive Editor, who has facilitated the publication of this book since the first edition of the Mediterranean Cardiology Meeting, and who has kindly assisted me throughout. Special and deep words of thanks are addressed to Rita Reggiani, professional, tireless, and very kind Project Leader of Adria Congrex, who has helped and supported me in achieving the best possible organisation of this International Meeting, together with her staff members Silvana and Maristella.

I cannot forget to acknowledge the role of my two teachers Antonio Circo and Salvatore Mangiameli, who encouraged my passion for cardiology and particularly for arrhythmology and clinical management.

In addition, I would like to thank my co-workers Asmundo, Cacia, Compagnone, Francese, Portale, Raciti, Ragusa, Rubino, Vitale, and all the nursing staff of my division at the S. Luigi-S. Currò Hospital of Catania for their active collaboration and support during these years of work and for the organisation of this Meeting.

Finally, a special mention for my dear wife Luisa, my daughters Alice and Raffaella, and my parents Raffaele and Cettina. I am especially and deeply grateful to them. Without their love and patience I could not have spent so many nights and weekends preparing the Meeting and this volume.

Michele Gulizia

Table of Contents

NEW TRENDS IN PHYSIOLOGICAL PACING AND OPTIMAL PACING SITES

HAEMODYNAMIC SENSING IN THE CONTROL OF PACING FUNCTION

SYNCOPE: PRACTICAL ISSUES OF DIAGNOSIS AND TREATMENT

LATEST TECHNOLOGIES IN CARDIOVASCULAR IMAGING: AN UPDATE FOR
THE CLINICAL CARDIOLOGIST

List of Contributors

EMERGING CONCEPTS IN THE ASSESSMENT OF ACUTE CORONARY SYNDROMES AND GLOBAL CARDIOVASCULAR RISK

Pathogenetic and Immunological Paradigm of Atherosclerotic Plaque

G. Calcara, C. Corno

Atherosclerosis is the 'mother' of ischaemic cardiopathy, of cerebrovascular disease, and of peripheral vasculopathy, and consequently is the indirect cause of the majority of deaths and disability in the world. The general view of the atherosclerotic process has changed; attention to the chronic degenerative aspects has been replaced by the dominant hypothesis that considers atherosclerosis to be an inflammatory process of the arterial vascular wall [1, 2]. Atherosclerotic plaque thus represents a specific inflammatory response of the arterial wall to various damaging phlogogenic stimuli identified in the classical risk factors, such as hypercholesterolaemia, arterial hypertension, diabetes mellitus, cigarette smoking, obesity, being male (men are more at risk than women), insufficient physical activity, a history of atherosclerosis in the family, and ageing.

The 25% of patients who suffer cardiovascular problems during youth show none of the classical risk factors. Clinical research has identified at least a hundred additional conditions that may better indicate a tendency to future cardiovascular events. Among the well known and highly studied are homocysteine, lipoprotein (a), oxidative stress, fibrinogen, factor VII, protein C–reactive (PCR), adhesion molecules, and advanced glycation end-products.

Endothelial anatomical injury is not necessary for the start-up of the atherosclerotic plaque, but it is a consequence of functional alteration of the endothelium (endothelial dysfunction) [3]. The endothelium represents the critical cellular interface that governs the homoeostasis of the arterial wall. Under physiological conditions the effect of the paracrine endothelial substances consists in:

Divisione di Medicina Interna Ospedaliera, Garibaldi Hospital, Catania, Italy

- Maintenance of blood fluidity (function: anti-aggregation and anticoagulant)
- Maintenance of normal vascular tone
- Control of vascular inflammatory process and smooth muscle cell proliferation (function: antiphlogistic)

The endothelial activation involves a pro-coagulant effect due to a major synthesis of tissue factor that, associated with a reduced synthesis of thrombomodulin, heparin, and heparan sulphate, reduces the anticoagulant potential. The reduced synthesis of tissue plasminogen activator (tPA) and the increased level of PAI-1 reduces the fibrinolytic potential of the endothelium.

The functional control alteration of the vascular tone is due to reduced production of nitric oxide and of PGI_2. The immunophlogistic effect is due to:

- Production of endothelial chemotactic factors (M-CSF, GM-CSF), a higher expression of adhesion molecules (ELAM, ICAM, E-selectin) that facilitate the migration from the lumen to the vessel wall of inflammatory cells (leucocytes) [4]
- Production of inflammatory cytokines (IL-1, TNF-α)
- Production of growth factors (PDGF, TGF-β, PGF-basic)

The onset, progression, and consequent clinical manifestation of atherosclerotic plaque represents the inflammatory process of the arterial wall activated by risk factors.

Take the low-density lipoproteins (LDL), one of the classical risk factors. The early events of the atherosclerotic process are characterised by the migration of monocytes from the lumen to the arterial wall [5], helped by the endothelial expression of adhesion molecules and by the risk factors, in this case the oxidated LDL. The involvement of the adhesion molecules in the migration happens in three phases. The first phase is facilitated by the interaction between the E-selectin of the endothelium and the glycosidic ligand cells of the monocyte membrane. It is characterised by monocyte rolling. The second phase is facilitated by the interaction between MCP1 of the endothelium and the monocyte serpentine receptors that cause some modifications facilitating the interaction among the monocyte LFA-1, Mac-1, and VLA-4 and ICAM, VCAM, and PECAM of the endothelium that is the basis of the stop, flattening, and diapedesis of the monocytes (third phase).

Migrated into the vessel wall, the macrophage–monocytes express the scavenger receptors that interact with the modified LDL, becoming transformed into foam cells [6] that, activating themselves, produce proinflammatory cytokine and growth factors. These interact accordingly with the endothelial receptors and the smooth muscle cells that migrate to the intima and are able to secrete collagen fibres. The progression of the plaque is characterised by the migration of subsets of Th1 lymphocytes assisted by adhesion molecules whose increased expression is induced by cytokines (IL-1, TNF-α) produced by the activated macrophages (Fig. 1).

Still to be clarified is the simultaneous appearance of the adhesion and endothelial molecules that diffuse and represent traffic signals for the migration of the leucocytes from the lumen to the vessel walls. Since each gene synthesises a single protein molecule, their 'coordinated' activation must be due to the involvement of one or a few transcription factors (NF). The NF-kB system [7] is made of heterodimeric proteins caught in the cytoplasm, linked to a kB inhibitor (IkB), and it has been documented that the various risk factors that increase the production of the adhesion molecules act to start the oxidative stress, producing reactive species of the O_2 superoxide anion and peroxide H. The reactive oxygen species (H_2O_2, O_2) cause degradation of the NF inhibitors, making them available to interaction with the promoter region of the genes for adhesion molecule synthesis (Fig. 2) [8].

The subsequent interaction between macrophage and Th1 lymphocyte causes the lymphocyte production of IFN-γ that has an important role in the instability of the plaque.

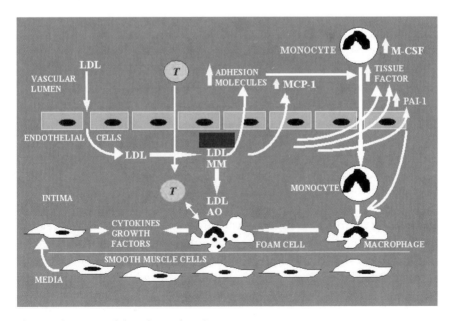

Fig. 1. Early events of the atherosclerotic process

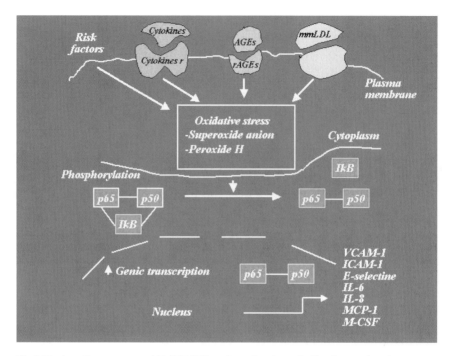

Fig. 2. Nuclear factor system kB (NF-kB) and production of adhesion molecules

The biological effect of the IFN-γ is to attach to the macrophage and to the smooth muscle cells, causing increased production of matrix metalloproteinase and inhibition of the proliferation of CML with consequently reduced production of collagen and amorphous fundamental substance [9].

Enhanced MMP9 production by macrophages in symptomatic plaques is caused by the enhancement in PGE2 synthesis as a result of the induction of the functionally coupled COX2/mPGES–1. This causes early degradation of the fibrous component which, associated with reduced production of the fibrotic component, causes degradation of the fibrous cap and thus a fissuring or rupture of the plaque (Fig. 3).

The physiopathological events responsible for transforming a fissured plaque into a clinical manifestation are characterised by an interaction between the tissutal factor (TF) of macrophagic source and factor VIIa, which through the activation of factor X causes the formation of the 'activator complex of prothrombin' (Xa, Va, platelet membrane phospholipids, Ca^{2+}), with production of thrombin and consequently of fibrin and formation of thrombus. Furthermore, the increased endothelial production of PAI-1 reduces the spontaneous fibrinolytic activity.

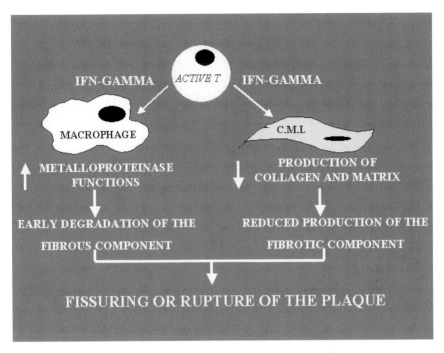

Fig. 3. Role of IFN-γ in plaque instability

The role of the platelets in the progression to and during the course of atherosclerotic disease has recently been emphasised. The interaction between the CD40L of platelet production and the CD40 expressed on the endothelial cells and on the macrophages is involved in the pathogenesis of atherosclerosis, provoking a complex of inflammatory reactions with endothelial production of VCAM-1, ICAM-1, E-selectin, MCP1 and production of reactive oxygen species from macrophage activation, legitimating the role of CD40L inflammatory marker as predictive criteria risk for cardiovascular events [10]. The platelet activation is preceded by recruitment and activation of polymorphonuclear neutrophils (PMNs), despite their apparent insignificance in coronary atherogenesis, has been shown an increased degranulation within the coronary circulation in acute coronary syndrome.

One of the principal mediators secreted on PMN activation is myeloperoxidase, which displays potent pro-atherogenic properties [11]. Myeloperoxidase can oxidise LDL cholesterol, amplifying and perpetuating foam cell formation, activate metalloproteinase, and consume endothelium-derived nitric oxide.

Conclusions

Inflammation plays a key role in atherosclerosis. A number of different bio-markers of inflammation are measurable in blood. These include cytokines, chemokines, soluble adhesion molecules, and acute-phase reactants. The first three of these groups of molecules are not routinely available in clinical laboratories. In contrast, however, C-reactive protein is readily measurable, and numerous clinical studies have demonstrated its usefulness as a marker of atherosclerotic risk [12, 13]. Other independent predictive risk factors of cardiovascular events are: myeloperoxidase, serum CD40L (sCD40L), adiponectin, and vWF.

Given its pro-inflammatory properties, myeloperoxidase, produced by the activated PMNs, could be utilised as a marker and mediator of vascular inflammation, confirming the importance of activated PMNs in the physiopathology of the acute coronary syndrome.

The different combinations of immunocompetent cells (macrophage--monocytes and T lymphocytes), of the vascular wall cells, of atheronecrotic material, and of fibrous material regulated by cytokines and growth factors produced by the same cells, allow us to say that every plaque is different from the next. This combination is responsible for the clinical manifestations of coronary atherosclerosis that affect only 5–10% of the individuals who have these lesions.

This hypothesised physiopathological and pathogenetic paradigm is a useful reference point for therapeutic strategies and prevention.

References

1. Moneta I, De Caterine R (1996) Aspetti infiammatori delle fasi iniziali dell'atero-sclerosi. G Ital Cardiol 25:225–239
2. Glass CK, Witztum JL (2001) Atherosclerosis: the road ahead. Cell 104:503–516
3. Gimbrone MA Jr, Kume N, Cybulsky M (1993) Vascular endothelial dysfunction and the pathogenesis of atherosclerosis. In: Weber P, Leaf A (eds) Atherosclerosis reviews. New York, Raven Press
4. Cybulsky M, Gimbrone MA Jr (1992) Endothelial leukocyte adhesion molecules in acute inflammation and atherogenesis. In: Simionescu N, Simionescu M (eds) Endothelial cell dysfuctions. New York, Plenum Press, pp 129–140
5. Libby P, Clinton S (1993) The role of macrophages in atherogenesis. Curr Opin Lipidol 4:355–363
6. Gerrity R (1981) The role of monocyte in atherogenesis I. Transition of blood from monocytes into foam cells in fatty lesions. Am J Pathol 103:181–190
7. Collins T (1993) Endothelial nuclear factor-kB and initiation of the atherosclerotic lesion. Lab Invest 68:499–508
8. Jander S, Sitzer M, Schumann R et al (1998) Inflammation in light grade carotid stenosis: a possible role for macrophages and T cells in plaque destabilisation, Stroke 29:1625–1630

9. Shankaravan UT, Lai WC, Netzel-Arnett S et al (2001) Monocyte membrane type 1-matrix metalloproteinase. Prostaglandin dependent regulation and role in metallo-proteinase-2 activation. J Biol Chem 276:1907–1032

10. Cipollone F, Ferri C, Desideri G et al (2003) Preprocedural level of soluble CD40L is predictive of enhanced inflammatory response and restenosis after coronary angioplasty. Circulation 108:2776–2782

11. Baldus S, Heeschen C, Meinertz T et al (2003) Myeloperoxidase serum levels predict risk in patients with acute coronary syndromes. Circulation 108:1440–1445

12. Paul A, Ko KW, Li L et al (2004) C-reactive protein accelerates the progression of atherosclerosis in apolipoprotein E-deficient mice. Circulation 109:647–655

13. Ridker PM, Rifai N, Rose L et al (2002) Comparison of C-reactive protein and low-density lipoprotein cholesterol levels in the prediction of first cardiovascular events. N Engl J Med 347:1557–1565

Are a Single Measurement of Troponin-I and C-Reactive Protein of Clinical Significance in Patients with Acute Coronary Syndromes?

L. Oltrona, R. Pirola

Clinicians have become increasingly sophisticated in their application of cardiac biomarkers in the management of acute coronary syndromes. In the 1950s, clinical investigators first reported that proteins released from necrotic cardiac myocytes could be detected in the serum and could aid in the diagnosis of acute myocardial infarction. The ensuing 40 years witnessed progressive improvement in the cardiac tissue-specificity of biomarkers of myocardial necrosis and a corresponding enhancement in the clinical sensitivity and specificity of their use for establishing the diagnosis of acute myocardial infarction.

In recent years, novel biochemical markers have been demonstrated to play a pivotal role in diagnosis, risk stratification, and guidance of treatment of acute coronary syndromes, complex clinical conditions with multiple causes: as such, treatment is likely to be most effective when directed at the underlying cause of the disease. Five principal causes of acute coronary syndromes have been described: (1) plaque rupture with acute thrombosis, (2) progressive mechanical obstruction, (3) inflammation, (4) secondary unstable angina, and (5) dynamic obstruction (coronary vasoconstriction) [1]. It is rare that any of these contributors exists in isolation. However, patients with acute coronary syndromes may vary substantially with respect to the mixture of contributions from each of these major mechanisms and are likely to benefit from different therapeutic strategies [1]. Moreover, the risk of subsequent death and/or recurrent ischaemic events among patients with acute coronary syndromes also varies widely, depending on the presence or absence of irreversible myocyte injury, the haemodynamic consequences of ischaemia and/or infarction, and the extent and tempo of atherosclerotic

Dipartimento CardioVascolare De Gasperis, Niguarda Hospital, Milan, Italy

vascular disease. With the emergence of novel, sensitive biomarkers of inflammation, myocyte necrosis, vascular damage, and haemodynamic stress, it is becoming possible to characterise non-invasively the participation of different contributors in any individual patient.

There is solid evidence from numerous studies that the unstable patient with elevated troponins has a nine-fold increased risk for myocardial infarction or death in the next 30 days [2]. Consequently, the American College of Cardiology/American Heart Association guidelines [3] as well as the European Society of Cardiology Task Force Report [4] incorporated troponin measurements into their diagnostic algorithms for patients with acute coronary syndromes.

Over the past decade, the emergence of convincing evidence for the value of cardiac troponin in guiding therapy has dramatically accelerated the integration of cardiac biomarkers into clinical decision making for patients with acute coronary syndromes. Concurrently, advances in our understanding of the pathogenesis and consequences of acute coronary atherothrombosis have stimulated the development of new biomarkers and created the opportunity for an expanded role of multiple biomarkers, some old and others new, in the classification and individualisation of treatment for acute coronary syndromes [5–7]. For example, detection of cardiac troponin in the blood of patients with non-ST-elevation acute coronary syndromes is not only indicative of myocardial necrosis, but is also associated with the presence of intracoronary thrombus and distal embolisation of platelet microaggregates [8]. These pathobiological links to elevated levels of cardiac troponin are likely to underlie, at least in part, the value of this biomarker in targeting potent antithrombin and antiplatelet therapy.

Inflammation has an essential role in the pathogenesis of atherosclerosis [9] and is also a consequence of myocardial damage. Elevated markers of inflammatory activity are associated with an increased risk of future cardiovascular events in healthy individuals [10, 11] and in patients with stable [12] and unstable coronary artery disease [13–16]. High-sensitivity testing for C-reactive protein (CRP) has emerged as a convenient tool for detecting low-level systemic inflammation that portends a higher risk of developing atherothrombotic vascular disease [17] and poor short- and long-term prognosis in patients after acute coronary syndromes [14, 16]. Although the precise mechanistic links between inflammation and risk in acute coronary syndromes are not conclusively established, it is plausible that elevated levels of circulating markers of inflammation reflect an intensification of focal inflammatory processes that destabilise vulnerable plaques [17]. Moreover, growing evidence implicates CRP as a mediator, in addition to a marker, of atherothrombosis [18].

However, many practical aspects of optimising the sampling protocols in the emergency unit and combining troponin measurements with other markers in the clinical routine setting still need to be clarified. There is general consent that a single test for troponins on the arrival of the patient to the hospital is insufficient because a single test can miss 10–15% of at-risk patients. The timing of the second test has not yet been clearly defined. The European Society of Cardiology (ESC) recommends repeating troponin testing 6–12 h after arrival in the emergency unit [4]. The American version asks for a repeat test 8–12 h after the onset of pain – a minor, but sometimes decisive difference in perception in the work-up of the individual patient [3]. Previous studies before the era of troponins had suggested a 12-h rule-out strategy [19]. Troponins have helped to shorten and to improve the diagnostic work-up. A prospective study using troponin T and troponin I bedside tests proposed an interval of 6 h to identify high-risk patients [20].

The World Health Organization (WHO) has traditionally defined myocardial infarction as requiring the presence of at least two out of three diagnostic criteria, namely, an appropriate clinical presentation, typical changes in the electrocardiogram (ECG), and raised 'cardiac' enzymes, essentially total CK or its MB iso-enzyme (CK-MB) activities [21]. In 2000, the ESC and American College of Cardiology (ACC) committee published its consensus recommendations for a new definition of myocardial infarction [22]. In particular, the ESC/ACC definition of acute myocardial infarction requires the rise and fall of the biochemical marker of myocardial necrosis together with other criteria, comprising ischaemic symptoms, the development of pathological Q waves, ischaemic ECG changes, or a coronary artery intervention [22]. Thus, according to the WHO definition, an acute myocardial infarction could be diagnosed without biochemical evidence of myocardial necrosis, while the ESC/ACC criteria stipulate that the biomarkers be elevated and subsequently be shown to fall in the appropriate clinical context. Quite simultaneously with the ESC/ACC re-definition of myocardial infarction, other expert committees published companion documents, according to which, in patients with no ST-segment elevation at ECG, but with ischaemic symptoms, a positive cardiac troponin result identifies those who have non-ST-segment elevation myocardial infarction (NSTEMI) and who could benefit from aggressive medical therapy [3, 4]. The new consensus documents have therefore based the new definition of myocardial infarction on biochemical grounds – a choice that was guided by the advent of new markers of myocardial necrosis, such as cardiac troponins [23–25]. The superior clinical value of troponin comes from its higher sensitivity to smaller myocardial injury and its virtually total specificity for cardiac damage [26]. Despite the ability to detect quantitatively smaller degrees of myocardial necrosis, cardiac troponins need 4–10 h after symptom onset to appear in serum, at about the same time as CKMB elevations become detectable, and peak at

12–48 h, then remaining abnormal for several days [27]. In applying the results of cardiac troponin testing to the defining of myocardial infarction, one should keep in mind that these markers actually reflect myocardial necrosis but do not indicate its mechanism. Thus, an elevated value in the absence of clinical evidence of ischaemia should prompt a search for other causes of cardiac damage. Many non-ischaemic pathophysiological conditions can cause myocardial necrosis and therefore elevations in cardiac troponin concentrations Strictly speaking, even in the 'troponin era', the diagnosis of myocardial infarction remains clinical. Measurement of cardiac troponin provides a valuable diagnostic test for myocardial infarction only when used together with other clinical information. Ideally, three measurements of cardiac troponin are suggested, with a sampling frequency of hospital admission, 6 and 12 h later, to demonstrate changing values.

From the point of view of risk definition, too, troponin measurements can be used less than optimally [28–30]. The data are clear and have shown for many years that the predictive accuracy of troponin measurements requires more than one measurement [2, 24, 31]. Thus, markers that rise earlier than troponin might be more predictive than a solitary admission troponin value, but not more predictive if an additional troponin value is included in the analysis. In some situations where immediate events are the outcomes of interest, such a strategy might be reasonable [7].

References

1. Braunwald E (1998) Unstable angina: an etiologic approach to management. Circulation 98:2219–2222
2. Ottani F, Galvani M, Nicolini FA et al (2000) Elevated cardiac troponin levels predict the risk of adverse outcome in patients with acute coronary syndromes. Am Heart J 140:917–927
3. Braunwald E, Antman EM, Beasley JW et al (2000) ACC/AHA guidelines for the management of patients with unstable angina and non-ST-segment elevation myocardial infarction: executive summary and recommendations. Circulation 102:1193–1209
4. Bertrand ME, Simoons ML, Fox KAA et al (2000) Management of acute coronary syndromes: acute coronary syndromes without persistent ST segment elevation. Recommendations of the Task Force of the European Society of Cardiology. Eur Heart J 21:1406–1432
5. Sabatine MS, Morrow DA, de Lemos JA et al (2002) Multimarker approach to risk stratification in non-ST elevation acute coronary syndromes: simultaneous assessment of troponin I, C-reactive protein, and B-type natriuretic peptide. Circulation 105:1760–1763
6. Galvani M, Ottani F, Oltrona L et al (2004) N-terminal pro-brain natriuretic peptide on admission has prognostic value across the whole spectrum of acute coronary syndromes. Circulation 110:128–134

7. Oltrona L, Ottani F, Galvani M (2004) Clinical significance of a single measurement of troponin-I and C-reactive protein at admission in 1773 consecutive patients with acute coronary syndromes. Am Heart J 148:405–415

8. Morrow DA (2001) Troponins in patients with acute coronary syndromes: biologic, diagnostic, and therapeutic implications. Cardiovascular Toxicology 1:105–110

9. Ross R (1999) Atherosclerosis – an inflammatory disease. N Engl J Med 340:115–126

10. Ridker PM, Cushman M, Stampfer MJ et al (1997) Inflammation, aspirin, and the risk of cardiovascular disease in apparently healthy men. N Engl J Med 336:973–979

11. Ridker PM, Hennekens CH, Buring JE et al (2000) C-reactive protein and other markers of inflammation in the prediction of cardiovascular disease in women. N Engl J Med 342:836–843

12. Haverkate F, Thompson SG, Pyke SD et al (1997) The European Concerted Action on Thrombosis and Disabilities Angina Pectoris Study Group. Production of C-reactive protein and risk of coronary events in stable and unstable angina. Lancet 349:462–466

13. Toss H, Lindahl B, Siegbahn A et al (1997) the FRagmin during InStability in Coronary artery disease (FRISC) Study Group. Prognostic influence of increased fibrinogen and C-reactive protein levels in unstable coronary artery disease. Circulation 96:4204–4210

14. Lindahl B, Toss H, Siegbahn A et al (2000) the FRagmin during InStability in Coronary artery disease (FRISC) Study Group. Markers of myocardial damage and inflammation in relation to long-term mortality in unstable coronary artery disease. N Engl J Med 343:1139–1147

15. Heeschen C, Hamm CW, Bruemmer J et al (2000) The Chimeric c7E3 AntiPlatelet Therapy in Unstable angina REfractory to standard treatment (CAPTURE) Investigators. Predictive value of C-reactive protein and troponin T in patients with unstable angina: a comparative analysis. J Am Coll Cardiol 35:1535–1542

16. Morrow DA, Rifai N, Antman EM et al (1998) C-reactive protein is a potent predictor of mortality independently of and in combination with troponin T in acute coronary syndromes: a Thrombolysis In Myocardial Infarction (TIMI-11A) substudy. J Am Coll Cardiol 31:1460–1465

17. Libby P, Ridker PM, Maseri A (2002) Inflammation and atherosclerosis. Circulation 105:1135–1143

18. Pasceri V, Willerson JT, Yeh ET (2000) Direct proinflammatory effect of C-reactive protein on human endothelial cells. Circulation 102:2165–2168

19. Lee TH, Juarez G, Cook EF et al (1991) Ruling out acute myocardial infarction: a prospective multicenter validation of a 12-hour strategy for patients at low risk. N Engl J Med 324:1239–1246

20. Hamm CW, Goldmann B, Heeschen C et al (1997) Emergency room triage of patients with acute chest pain based on rapid testing for troponin T or troponin I. N Engl J Med 337:1648–1653

21. Anonymous (1979) Nomenclature and criteria for diagnosis of ischemic heart disease. Report of the Joint International Society and Federation of Cardiology/World Health Organization Task Force on Standardization of Clinical Nomenclature. Circulation 59:607–608

22. Alpert J, Thygesen K for the Joint European Society of Cardiology/American College of Cardiology Committee (2000) Myocardial infarction redefined – a consensus document of the Joint European Society of Cardiology/American College of

Cardiology Committee for the Redefinition of Myocardial Infarction. Eur Heart J 21:1502–1513

23. Panteghini M, Apple FS, Christenson RH et al (1999) Use of biochemical markers in acute coronary syndromes. Clin Chem Lab Med 37:687–693

24. Jaffe AS, Ravkilde J, Roberts R et al (2000) It's time for a change to a troponin standard. Circulation 102:1216–1220

25. Hamm CW (2001) Acute coronary syndromes. The diagnostic role of troponins. Thromb Res 103:S63–S69

26. Panteghini M, Pagani F, Bonetti G (1999) The sensitivity of cardiac markers: an evidence-based approach. Clin Chem Lab Med 37:1097–1106

27. Panteghini M, Cuccia C, Pagani F et al (2002) Coronary angiographic findings in patients with clinical unstable angina according to cardiac troponin I and T concentrations in serum. Arch Pathol Lab Med 126:448–451

28. Morrow DA, Cannon CP, Rifai N et al (2001) Ability of minor elevations of troponins I and T to predict benefit from an early invasive strategy in patients with unstable angina and non-ST elevation myocardial infarction: results from a randomized trial. JAMA 286:2405–2412

29. Baldus S, Heeschen C, Meinertz T et al (2003) Myeloperoxidase serum levels predict risk in patients with acute coronary syndromes. Circulation 108:1440–1445

30. Heeschen C, Dimmeler S, Fichtlscherer S et al (2004) Prognostic value of placental growth factor in patients with acute chest pain. JAMA 291:435–441

31. James S, Armstrong P, Califf R et al (2003) Troponin T levels and risk of 30-day outcomes in patients with the acute coronary syndrome: prospective verification in the GUSTO-IV trial. Am J Med 115:178–184

New Strategies for Treating Myocardial Infarctions

F. Chiarella, A. Nicolino, K. Paonessa, F. Rossi

Sudden occlusion of the epicardial artery due to plaque rupture leads to ST elevation myocardial infarction (STEMI). STEMI is associated with a high rate of mortality, morbidity, and heart failure.

The past 10 years have seen a great fight against infarctions. Historically, the weapon of choice to battle infarctions is thrombolysis, which, in the first 12 h after the onset of symptoms, has demonstrated improvement in survival; the first trials to show this were ISIS 2 and GISSI 2 [1, 2]. After streptokinase (SK), the first drug used, new drugs were developed that are more fibrinospecific. Alteplase (co-administered with aspirin and heparin) [3, 4] demonstrated better performance in safety and effectiveness [5] than SK, whereas others (e.g. lanoteplase) did not show a relevant benefit. Randomised studies give us important information about better medical therapy, and also about pathophysiology and picking new research directions. For example, GUSTO 1 and GISSI 1 sub-analyses demonstrated the importance of 'time to treatment' (1% increase in mortality for every 1 h delay), and the angiographic GUSTO 1 sub-study demonstrated the importance of patency of the infarction-related artery (IRA) for survival. The importance of time led to the development of tenecteplase (TNK), which is more rapid, more fibrinospecific, and, due to its resistance to PAI-1, has a longer half-life and is thus easier to use (single bolus). In ASSENT 2 these drugs demonstrated no difference in 30-day mortality versus alteplase, with fewer non-cerebral haemorrhagic complications [6]. TNK can also be used in association with enoxaparin (no detrimental effect versus intravenous heparin in patients less than 75 years in age). However, data collected from registries from 1990 to 1998 show that 30% of patients eligible for thrombolysis do not receive this important treatment. The reasons for this are late

U.O. Cardiologia, Santa Corona Hospital, Pietra Ligure (Savona), Italy arrival, misdiagnosis, and the concern of the physician about the adverse effects of thrombolysis. In addition, pharmacological therapy showed failure to achieve complete restoration of coronary flow in 45–50% of patients [7]. An increasingly used intervention for revascularisation in STEMI is angioplasty (percutaneous coronary intervention, PCI), called primary when done in first 12 h from symptom onset. Primary PCI, done by a skilled and high-volume team, can achieve thrombolysis in myocardial infarction (TIMI) flow grade (TFG) 3 in more than 80% of patients. In a recent meta-analysis, fibrinolytic therapy (all drugs together) has been shown to be inferior to catheter-based intervention in reducing death, non-fatal reinfarction, or stroke [8]. But not all authors agree with these results, and these data need confirmation with new controlled studies [9, 10]. The war between fibrinolysis (which is available everywhere) and PCI (which is available in a few centres) led to the design of studies that compared the two therapies in several strategies: on-site medical therapy versus transfer for PCI (PRAGUE2, DANAMI 2), and prehospital thrombolysis versus PCI (CAPTIM). Result from these trials gave a new importance to time from onset of symptoms to treatment. In the first hours after MI (2 h for the CAPTIM analysis and 3 h for the PRAGUE2 analysis) medical therapy is at least as effective as PCI (same effect on mortality), whereas in patients who present later PCI is better. The importance of time is supported by the recent 2004 ACC/AHA Guidelines [11], where the invasive strategy is preferred if the onset of symptoms was more than 3 h before the patient presented.

Paradoxically, fibrinolytic agents may systemically activate platelets. Fibrinolysis generates plasmin, which degrades the fibrin component of the clot and exposes a highly active platelet-rich core. Thus, studies were done on the association between fibrinolytic drugs and platelet inhibitors to enhance clot lysis and prevent additional platelet aggregation on the surface of the clot [12]. This association showed a little more IRA patency in early angiographic follow-up, a reduction of in-hospital reinfarction, and a need for early PCI. However, this association did not show a beneficial effect on mortality, and bleeding complications increased in older people [13, 14].

The aim of successful reperfusion strategies – medical or mechanical or both together – is to quickly restore the oxygen supply of the myocytes. To do this in the best way, restoring IRA patency is very important but is not sufficient. Data from trials have demonstrated that mortality at 1 month is related to IRA patency on arrival in the catheterisation laboratory. Studies by Braunwald et al. [15] demonstrated that both improved epicardial flow, TIMI flow grade (TFG 2/3), and tissue-level perfusion [TIMI myocardial perfusion grade (TMPG 2/3)] at 90 min after thrombolysis are independent predictors of survival at 2 years. Another important study by Braunwald et al. [16]

showed that, after thrombolysis, impaired TMPG is a strong predictor of high mortality regardless of epicardial coronary flow. Patients with both normal epicardial flow (TGF3) and normal tissue-level perfusion (TMPG 3) have an extremely low risk of mortality, but in patients with TFG 3 an impaired TMPG is associated with the worst prognosis. The same group [17] found that TGF, TMPG, and ST segment resolution 90 min after administration of TNK (half dose) and eptifibatide is a powerful prognostic tool even after PCI on the remaining stenosis. In the same study, adjunctive PCI can achieve not only TGF 3 but also TMPG 3 in patients who have not tissue perfusion before PCI. However, Percutaneous transluminal coronary angioplasty (PTCA) and stent placement carry the risk of mobilising thrombotic and thrombogenic material, causing distal embolisation and microcirculatory impairment, which may limit the myocardial salvage gained by these techniques. Percutaneous revascularisation techniques are being developed with interesting tools [18]. For example, during primary PCI, pretreatment with the X-sizer catheter system demonstrated, in a small number of patients, improved epicardial flow and accelerated ST segment resolution compared with conventional PCI alone [18]. Another device, PercuSurge demonstrated a substantially higher rate of immediate final TFG 3 flow in epicardial vessels and increased the integrity of the microvasculature [19].

A good way to restore flow in the infarct area (epicardial vessels and microvessels) is a combined pharmaco-invasive approach that starts pharmacological reperfusion as soon as possible, followed by PCI to consolidate the results and prevent reinfarction [20]. An important subject for study will be the correct pharmacological therapy (TNK, platelet inhibitor, or both?) for every class of risk (TIMI risk and haemorrhagic risk). The ongoing trials on combined PCI will give important information on how to improve flow restoration. These trials are:

- ADVANCE-MI (epfitibatide vs epfitibatide + TNK; both treatments randomised to enoxaparin vs unfractionated heparin)
- FINESSE (placebo vs abciximab vs abciximab + reteplase and then angiography)
- TIGER (enoxaparin vs epfitibatideparin)
- CARESS (reteplase + abciximab and then randomisation to immediate PCI vs rescue PCI)
- ASSENT-4 PCI (ASA + unfractionated heparin vs ASA + unfractionated heparin + TNK and then immediate PCI)

We can save time and myocytes not only with powerful and fast drugs but also with good logistical organisation and a prehospital and interhospital net. Good organisation for prehospital thrombolysis allows fibrinolytic drugs to be given earlier; meta-analysis showed a 17% reduction in mortality

[21]. As a high-volume, full-time catheterisation laboratory cannot be developed in every hospital, an interhospital net would be useful for sending high-risk patients (high TIMI risk score) to a centre that has one.

In conclusion, the new challenge is to find the right treatment (combined treatment, fibrinolysis alone, or PCI alone) for every STEMI patient on the basis of time from onset of angina to treatment, haemorrhagic risk, response to treatment, and the availability of resources.

References

1. Gruppo Italiano per lo Studio della Streptochinasi nell'Infarto Miocardico (GISSI) (1986) Effectiveness of intravenous thrombolytic treatment in acute myocardial infarction. Lancet 22:397–402
2. ISIS-2 (Second International Study of Infarct Survival) Collaborative Group (1988) Randomised trial of intravenous streptokinase, oral aspirin, both, or neither among 17,187 cases of suspected acute myocardial infarction: ISIS-2. Lancet 2:349–360
3. GISSI-2 (1990) A factorial randomised trial of alteplase versus streptokinase and heparin versus no heparin among 12490 patients with acute myocardial infarction. Lancet 336:65–71
4. The GUSTO Investigators (1993) An international randomised trial comparing four thrombolytic strategies for acute myocardial infarction. N Engl J Med 329:673–682
5. Every NR, Parsons LS, Hlatky M et al for the TIMI Study Group (1985) The Thrombolysis in Myocardial Infarction (TIMI) trial: phase I findings. N Engl J Med 312:932–936
6. Assessment of the Safety and Efficacy of a New Thrombolytic (ASSENT-2) Investigators (1999) Single-bolus tenecteplase compared with front-loaded alteplase in acute myocardial infarction: the ASSENT-2 double-blind randomised trial. Lancet 354:716–722
7. Topol EJ (1998) Toward a new frontier in myocardial reperfusion therapy. Circulation 97:211–218
8. Keeley EC, Boura JA, Grines CL (2003) Primary angioplasty versus intravenous thrombolytic therapy for acute myocardial infarction: a quantitative review of 23 randomised trials. Lancet 361:13–20
9. Auer J, Berent R, Weber T et al (2003) Primary angioplasty or thrombolysis for acute myocardial infarction? (Letter to the editor). Lancet 361:965–966
10. Melandri G (2003) Primary angioplasty or thrombolysis for acute myocardial infarction? (Letter to the editor). Lancet 361:966
11. Management of Patients With ST-Elevation Myocardial Infarction ACC/AHA Pocket Guideline Based on the ACC/AHA Guidelines for the Management of Patients With ST-Elevation Myocardial Infarction, from American Heart Association website, July 2004
12. Gibson CM, Jennings LK, Murphy SA for the INTEGRITI Study Group (2004) Association between platelet receptor occupancy after eptifibatide (integrilin) therapy and patency, myocardial perfusion, and ST-segment resolution among patients with ST-segment-elevation myocardial infarction: an INTEGRITI

(Integrilin and Tenecteplase in Acute Myocardial Infarction) substudy. Circulation 110:679–684

13. Savonitto S, Armstrong PW, Lincoff AM et al (2003) Risk of intracranial hae-morrhage with combined fibrinolytic and glycoprotein IIb/IIIa inhibitor therapy in acute myocardial infarction. Dichotomous response as a function of age in the GUSTO V trial. Eur Heart J 20:1807–1814

14. Lincoff AM, Califf RM, Van de Werf F et al for the Global Use of Strategies To Open Coronary Arteries Investigators (GUSTO) (2002) Mortality at 1 year with combina-tion platelet glycoprotein IIb/IIIa inhibition and reduced-dose fibrinolytic therapy vs conventional fibrinolytic therapy for acute myocardial infarction: GUSTO V ran-domized trial. JAMA 288:2130–2135

15. Gibson CM, Cannon CP, Murphy SA et al for the TIMI Study Group (2002) Relationship of the TIMI myocardial perfusion grades, flow grades, frame count, and percutaneous coronary intervention to long-term outcomes after thrombolytic administration in acute myocardial infarction. Circulation 105:1909–1913

16. Gibson CM, Cannon CP, Murphy SA et al for the TIMI (Thrombolysis In Myocardial Infarction) Study Group (2000) Relationship of TIMI myocardial per-fusion grade to mortality after administration of thrombolytic drugs. Circulation 101:125–130

17. Giugliano RP, Sabatine MS, Gibson CM et al (2004) Combined assessment of thrombolysis in myocardial infarction flow grade, myocardial perfusion grade, and ST-segment resolution to evaluate epicardial and myocardial reperfusion. Am J Cardiol 93:1362–1367, A5–A6

18. Beran G, Lang I, Schreiber W et al (2002) Intracoronary thrombectomy with the X-Sizer catheter system improves epicardial flow and accelerates ST-segment resolu-tion in patients with acute coronary syndrome: a prospective, randomized, control-led study. Circulation 105:2355–2360

19. Wu CJ, Yang CH, Fang CY et al (2004) Six-month angiographic results of primary angioplasty with adjunctive PercuSurge GuardWire device support: evaluation of the restenotic rate of the target lesion and the fate of the distal balloon occlusion site. Catheter Cardiovasc Interv 64:35–42

20. Antman EM, Van de Werf F (2004) Pharmacoinvasive therapy: the future of treat-ment for ST-elevation myocardial infarction. Circulation 109:2480–2486

21. Morrison JL, Verbeek PR, McDonald AC et al (2000) Mortality and pre-hospital thrombolysis for acute myocardial infarction: a meta-analysis. JAMA 283:2686–2692

Tirofiban and NSTE-ACS: The Current Perspective

C. Cavallini

Acute coronary syndromes without persistent ST segment elevation (NSTE-ACS) are common manifestations of coronary artery disease and represent one of the most important reasons for emergency medical care and hospital-isation, accounting for approximately 2.5 million hospital admissions annually worldwide [1]. Although conventional antithrombotic therapy (e.g. unfractionated heparin and aspirin) have proved to reduce the incidence of ischaemic complications, a substantial burden of death and (re-)infarction still remains.

Considerable progress has been made recently in the optimal management of these patients, particularly with regard to (1) the introduction of new powerful antiplatelet drugs (mainly the IIb/IIIa platelet receptor inhibitors) and (2) the demonstration that, in selected cases, an aggressive approach with early coronary angiography and percutaneous coronary interventions (PCI) can be safely performed with low risk of procedural complications and with improved in-hospital and long-term outcome.

IIb/IIIa Platelet Receptor Inhibitors

It has recently been shown that the addition of glycoprotein (GP) IIb/IIIa receptor inhibitors to unfractionated heparin and aspirin further improves the clinical outcome of patients with NSTE-ACS [2]. From basic research on the congenital platelet defect involved in Glanzmann thrombasthenia and the identification of the mechanisms responsible for fibrinogen binding to GP IIb/IIIa receptors, a chimaeric monoclonal antibody was developed by Coller [3], tested in a randomised double-blind placebo-controlled study [4],

Division of Cardiology, Cardiovascular Department, Regional Hospital, Treviso, Italy

and subsequently approved for clinical use. Shortly thereafter, peptide and non-peptide compounds mimicking the RGD or KGD amino acid sequence responsible for fibrinogen binding to the GP IIb/IIIa receptor were synthesised. The three GP IIb/IIIa antagonists developed for parenteral use and extensively examined in clinical studies include the monoclonal antibody abciximab, the cyclic peptide eptifibatide, and the non-peptide tirofiban.

Several clinical trials have demonstrated a clear benefit from the use of GP IIb/IIIa inhibitors in reducing ischaemic complications in patients undergoing PCI and in patients with medically managed NSTE-ACS. Boersma et al. carried out a meta-analysis of all six large randomised place-bo-controlled trials of GP IIb/IIIa antagonists, which involved 31 402 patients with unstable angina or non-ST-elevation myocardial infarction (UA/NSTEMI) not routinely scheduled to undergo coronary revascularisa-tion [5]. A small reduction in the odds of death or myocardial infarction (MI) in the active treatment arm was observed (11.8% vs 10.8%, OR = 0.91, 95% CI 0.84 to 0.98, P = 0.015).

Although not scheduled for coronary revascularisation procedures, 11 965 of the 31 402 patients (38%) actually underwent PCI or coronary artery bypass graft (CABG) within 30 days, and in this subgroup the OR for death or MI in the patients assigned to GP IIb/IIIa antagonist treatment was 0.89 (95% CI 0.80 to 0.98). In the other 19 416 patients who did not undergo coronary revascularisation, the OR for death or MI in the GP IIb/IIIa group was 0.95 (95% CI 0.86 to 1.05, NS). Thus, GP IIb/IIIa inhibitors are of sub-stantial benefit in patients with NSTE-ACS who undergo PCI, whereas they are of questionable benefit in patients who do not undergo PCI. Hence the international guidelines recommend that a GP IIb/IIIa inhibitor be adminis-tered, along with acetylsalicylic acid (aspirin) and unfractioned heparin (UFH), to all of the patients with NSTE-ACS and high-risk features who are scheduled to undergo early catheterisation [6, 7].

Among the available GP IIb/IIIa antagonists, small molecules have been approved for medical treatment of patients with UA/NSTEMI, whereas abcix-imab is recommended in the setting of PCI. Small molecules are the drugs of choice for the 'upstream' or 'upfront' treatment of patients with NSTE-ACS during the waiting time for the scheduled coronary angiography. Abciximab is the preferred drug of this class to be used in the catheterisation laboratory for the 'downstream' treatment (i.e. immediately before and in the few hours after PCI). With contemporary trials favouring an early invasive strategy in the management NSTE-ACS, controversy has arisen regarding whether GP IIb/IIIa inhibitors should be started upstream for all patients or be reserved for use only for patients selected to undergo PCI. Multiple trials have shown that the benefit of upstream GP IIb/IIIa inhibitor therapy in NSTE-ACS is derived very early, during the period of medical management that precedes revascularisation procedures – a key observation when considering strategies to optimise procedural outcomes in this high-risk patient population. A meta-analysis of the PRISM-PLUS, PURSUIT, and CAPTURE trials demonstrated a 34% reduction in the rate of death or MI with GP IIb/IIIa inhibition during the period of initial medical stabilisation that preceded revascularisation (2.5% vs 3.8%; $P = 0.001$), with further benefit seen following PCI [2].

The use of tirofiban for the medical management of higher risk patients with NSTE-ACS was explored by the Platelet Receptor Inhibition in Ischemic Syndrome Management in Patients Limited by Unstable Signs and Symptoms (PRISM-PLUS) trial, [8] in which 1915 NSTE-ACS patients were randomised to receive either tirofiban/aspirin/heparin or aspirin/heparin. Patients were treated in a medical stabilisation phase for a minimum of 48 h before possible angiography. The results of PRISM-PLUS demonstrate significant reductions in death/MI, with benefits evident as early as 48 h (during the medical stabilisation phase) and persisting for at least 6 months.

The benefits of tirofiban in higher risk patients from PRISM-PLUS were observed in several subgroups, notably including patients with diabetes [9], patients with impaired renal function [10], and in the elderly [11]. In general, the higher the level of risk of the patients, the greater the benefits from the use of the drug, as shown in the study by Morrow et al. [12].

Similar to studies with other GP IIb/IIIa antagonists, 19 strong benefits of tirofiban were noted among patients treated with early PCI, with a 42% reduction in death/MI noted in these patients, compared to 23% among patients revascularised 72 h after randomisation [13].

Despite the data supporting GP IIb/IIIa inhibitors for high risk patients with NSTE-ACS and the consensus guidelines recommending their use, recent surveys suggest that there continues to be a low rate of use of these agents for eligible patients. This may be related to clinician confusion about which patients should receive GP IIb/IIIa inhibitors as well as the most appropriate timing for the initiation of treatment with these agents. The European guidelines suggest that in all of the patients with NSTE-ACS and high risk features the administration of IIb/IIIa inhibitors should start as soon as possible, in order to gain the higher benefit from the treatment [6].

Invasive Strategy

Patients with ACS undergoing early PCI are at increased risk of early ischaemic complications. This early hazard appears to be the result of a thrombin-mediated and platelet-dependent process that is initiated by mechanical plaque disruption and culminates in thrombus formation at the site of vessel injury. Distal embolisation of atherothrombotic debris into the coronary microcirculation may also occur as a complication of the unstable plaque. For these reasons, early randomised trials such as the TIMI IIIB [14, 15] and VANQWISH trials [16] failed to demonstrate that routine use of an early invasive strategy improves the outcome compared to a conservative strategy. Furthermore, the VANQWISH trial showed a significant difference in favour of conservative treatment in the composite end-point of death and MI at 1-month and 1-year follow-up. In contrast, the FRISC II study showed a significant and clinically relevant decrease in death and MI at 6-month [17] and 1-year [18] follow-up in patients randomised to an early invasive strategy. The TACTICS-TIMI 18 trial [19] confirmed these findings by showing that in patients with ACS receiving tirofiban, an early invasive strategy with stent implantation resulted in a significantly lower rate of the primary endpoint (death, non-fatal MI, and rehospitalisation for ACS), as well as a lower rate of death or non-fatal MI both at 30 days and at 6 months.

An invasive strategy appears to limit the increased risk conferred by raised levels of troponin (Tn). In both the FRISC II and the TACTICS-TIMI 18 trials, the benefit of the early invasive strategy was greater in high and intermediate risk patients with elevated levels of TnT.

More recently, the results of the third Randomised Intervention Trial of unstable Angina (RITA) study suggested that routine early invasive management was effective in reducing refractory or severe angina among patients at moderate risk of death after NSTE-ACS, but no reduction was seen in new MI [20].

In accordance with these studies two separate sets of guidelines, released by the European Society of Cardiology and by the American College of Cardiology/American Heart Association, respectively, recommended careful and prompt risk stratification in all patients with NSTE-ACS to identify those who will benefit more from an early invasive strategy [6, 7].

Risk Stratification

Patients with NSTE-ACS represent a heterogeneous population with a wide range of probability of cardiac events in the short and intermediate term. Identification of subsets of patients with different risk profiles is crucial in order to select the most appropriate therapy in each case. The patients considered to be at high risk on the basis of clinical, electrocardiographic, and biochemical characteristics benefit more from an aggressive strategy that includes powerful antithrombotic therapy and early angiography with revascularisation, if feasible. On the other hand, low risk patients need to be identified in order to avoid unnecessary resource use and the risks deriving from an unjustified aggressive approach. Risk stratification is a dynamic process that starts at the time of admission and is continuously updated with new information obtained during the subsequent hospital stay. However, immediate risk stratification is the most important step for the appropriate management of these patients, since the probability of events is highest in the very early phase of the disease and progressively decreases thereafter. Simple clinical data derived from the patient's medical history and physical examination, a standard 12-lead electrocardiogram (ECG), and measurements of biochemical markers of myocardial damage can be easily obtained in the emergency room and serve as a guide for deciding appropriate medical management and optimal use of available resources.

Two different models of risk stratification have been developed. The first is based on the simple, dichotomous description of a series of variables, whose presence, even when isolated, is sufficient to identify high risk patients. This method is currently suggested by the ESC guidelines. The second takes into account the prognostic information derived from a number of clinical, electrocardiographic, and biochemical parameters, analysed in a comprehensive manner [21]. These models have the advantage of allowing the identification of patients at the highest risk of events.

Timing of Intervention

The optimal time to intervene is not well defined as it was significantly different among clinical trials comparing invasive to conservative strategy in NSTE-ACS: this interval was 4–6 days in FRISC 2, while it was less than 48 h in TACTICS-TIMI 18 and in RITA 3. The ESC guidelines recommend that coronary angiography be performed within 48 h of admission, and earlier ('as soon as possible') for patients at very high risk such as those presenting with major arrhythmias, haemodynamic instability, a history of prior CABG, or early post-MI unstable angina.

Recently, the Intracoronary Stenting with Antithrombotic Regimen Cooling-off (ISAR-COOL) study [22] added further support to the combination of GP IIb/IIIa antagonism with early invasive management. ISAR-COOL compared routine invasive management among a high risk NSTE-ACS patient population treated either with prolonged medical stabilisation (with the combination of heparin, aspirin, clopidogrel, and tirofiban for a mean of 86 h) or by proceeding directly to the catheterisation laboratory within the first 24 h (mean 2.3 h) with the same medical therapy. The ISAR-COOL results suggested that expedited catheterisation with GP IIb/IIIa antagonism pretreatment was associated with a significant reduction in death/MI relative to the delayed invasive group (5.9% vs 11.6%, $P = 0.04$), due entirely to reductions in pre-PCI MI.

These results suggest that the benefits of early invasive therapy may outweigh those of prolonged pharmacological pretreatment. However, whether a strategy of immediate coronary angiography (within hours of presentation) leads to a significant clinical benefit in comparison with the overall accepted intervention within 48 h is unknown, and a larger randomised trial testing the two strategy will be needed.

Conclusions

The globality of current evidence strongly suggests that in high risk patients with ACS an early combined invasive strategy and treatment with GP IIb/IIIa antagonists considerably improves short- and long-term outcome.

As adjunctive therapies improve, lessening the risk associated with invasive cardiac procedures, we may well be moving to an era of rapid risk assessment and triage, initial medical stabilisation with very potent antithrombotic medications, and rapid transfer to cardiac centres of excellence for diagnostic and therapeutic procedures within 48 h of presentation. This should allow to patients admitted to peripheral hospitals to have access to the same type of care as those patients directly admitted to tertiary centres. A unified systematic approach to NSTE-ACS that incorporates all evidence-based therapies and interventions would be expected to maximise the positive impact of such strategies on long-term clinical outcome.

How best to incorporate this new knowledge into a better process of care for patients will need to be shown by prospective cohort studies showing how clinicians actually deliver care to their patients in 'real-life'.

References

1. Braunwald E, Antman EM, Beasley JW et al (2000) ACC/AHA guidelines for the management of patients with unstable angina and non-ST-segment elevation myocardial infarction: a report of the American College of Cardiology/American Heart Association Task Force on Practice Guidelines. Circulation 102:1193–1209
2. Boersma E, Akkerhuis KM, Theroux P et al (1999) Platelet glycoprotein IIb/IIIa receptor inhibition in non-ST-elevation acute coronary syndromes: early benefit during medical treatment only, with additional protection during percutaneous coronary intervention. Circulation 100:2045–2048
3. Coller BS (1995) Blockade of platelet GP IIb/IIIa receptors as an anti-thrombotic strategy. Circulation 92:2373–2380
4. The EPIC Investigators (1994) Use of a monoclonal antibody directed against the platelet glycoprotein IIb/IIIa receptor in high-risk coronary angioplasty. N Engl J Med 330:956–961
5. Boersma E, Harrington RA, Moliterno DJ et al (2002) Platelet glycoprotein IIb/IIIa

inhibitors in acute coronary syndromes: a meta-analysis of all major randomised clinical trials. Lancet 359:189–198

6. Bertrand ME, Simoons ML, Fox KAA et al (2002) Management of acute coronary syndromes in patients presenting without ST-segment elevation. Eur Heart J 23:1809–1840

7. Braunwald E, Antman EM, Beasley JW et al (2002) ACC/AHA guidelines for the management of patients with unstable angina and non-ST-segment elevation myocardial infarction: a report of the American College of Cardiology/American Heart Association Task Force on Practice Guidelines (Committee on the Management of Patients with Unstable Angina). J Am Coll Cardiol 106:1893–1900

8. Theroux P, Alexander J Jr, Pharand C et al (2000) Glycoprotein IIb/IIIa receptor blockade improves outcomes in diabetic patients presenting with unstable angina/non-ST-elevation myocardial infarction: results from the Platelet Receptor Inhibition in Ischemic Syndrome Management in Patients Limited by Unstable Signs and Symptoms (PRISM-PLUS) study. Circulation 102:2466–2472

9. Januzzi JL, Snapinn SM, DiBattiste PM et al (2002) Benefits and safety of tirofiban among acute coronary syndrome patients with mild to moderate renal insufficiency. Circulation 105:2359–2364

10. Januzzi JL Jr, Sabatine MS, Wan Y et al (2003) Interactions between age, outcome of acute coronary syndromes, and tirofiban therapy. Am J Cardiol 91:457–461

11. Morrow DA, Antman EM, Snapinn SM et al (2002) An integrated clinical approach to predicting the benefit of tirofiban in non-ST elevation acute coronary syndromes: application of the TIMI risk score for UA/NSTEMI in PRISM-PLUS. Eur Heart J 23:223–229

12. Morrow DA, Antman EM, Snapinn SM et al (2002) An integrated clinical approach to predicting the benefit of tirofiban in non-ST elevation acute coronary syndromes: application of the TIMI risk score for UA/NSTEMI in PRISM-PLUS. Eur Heart J 23:223–229

13. Roffi M, Chew D, Mukherjee D et al (2002) Platelet glycoprotein IIb/IIIa inhibition in acute coronary syndromes: gradient of benefit related to the revascularisation strategy. Eur Heart J 23:1441–1448

14. The TIMI IIIB Investigators (1994) Effects of tissue plasminogen activator and a comparison of early invasive and conservative strategies in unstable angina and non-Q-wave myocardial infarction: the results of TIMI IIIB trial. Circulation 89:1545–1556

15. Anderson HV, Cannon CP, Stone PH et al (1995) One year result of the TIMI IIIB clinical trial: a randomized comparison of tissue-type plasminogen activator versus placebo and early invasive versus early conservative strategies in unstable angina and non-Q-wave myocardial infarction. J Am Coll Cardiol 26:1643–1650

16. Boden WE, O'Rourke RA, Crawford MH et al (1998) Outcomes in patients with acute non-Q-wave MI randomly assigned to an invasive as compared with a conservative management strategy. Veterans Affairs Non-Q-Wave Infarction Strategies in Hospital (VANQWISH) Trial Investigators. N Engl J Med 338:1785–1792

17. Anonymous (1999) Invasive compared with non-invasive treatment in unstable coronary-artery disease: FRISC II prospective randomised multicentre study. FRagmin and Fast Revascularisation during InStability in Coronary artery disease Investigators. Lancet 354:708–715

18. Wallentin L, Lagerqvist B, Husted S et al (2000) Outcome at 1 year after an invasive compared with a non-invasive strategy in unstable coronary artery disease: The FRISC II invasive randomised trial. Lancet 356:9–16

19. Cannon CP, Weintraub W, Demopoulos LA et al (2001) Comparison of early invasi-
     ve and conservative strategies in patients with unstable coronary syndromes trea-
     ted with the glycoprotein IIb/IIIa inhibitor tirofiban. N Engl J Med 344:1879–1887
20. Fox KA, Poole-Wilson PA, Henderson RA et al (2002) Interventional versus conser-
     vative treatment for patients with unstable angina or non-ST-elevation myocardial
     infarction: the British Heart Foundation RITA 3 randomised trial. Randomized
     Intervention Trial of unstable Angina. Lancet 360:743–751
21. Antman EM, Cohen M, Bernink PJ et al (2000) The TIMI risk score for unstable
     angina/non-ST elevation MI: a method for prognostication and therapeutic deci-
     sion making. JAMA 284:835–842
22. Neumann FJ, Kastrati A, Murray GP et al (2003) Evaluation of prolonged antith-
     rombotic pretreatment ("cooling-off" strategy) before intervention in patients
     with unstable coronary syndromes. JAMA 290:1593–1599

Acute Coronary Syndromes and Diabetes: How Much Can We Intervene?

F. Bovenzi[1], L. De Luca[2], R. Adorisio[3]

Diabetes mellitus (DM) affects 150 million people worldwide. The prevalence of diabetes has increased by 40% in the past decade, and is expected to increase by 165% between 2000 and 2050 [1, 2]. Therefore, one-third of the population born in 2000 will develop DM, with the associated up to 30% reduction in life expectancy, mostly related to atherosclerosis, which is responsible for up to 80% of all deaths among North American diabetic patients [3, 4]. With increasing prevalence of DM, the burden of cardiovascular disease associated with this condition will increase dramatically [5].

Diabetic patients are at an increased risk of cardiovascular events as compared with non-diabetic patients. In a study by Haffner et al., patients with DM had a 20% risk of first myocardial infarction (MI) or death over a 7-year period, as compared to a risk of only 3.5% for non-diabetic patients [4]. A history of MI increased the rate of recurrent MI or cardiovascular death in both groups (45% in diabetics and 18.8% in non-diabetics). On the basis of these data, the risk of subsequent coronary events for patients with diabetes but without previous MI is the same as non-diabetic patients with previous MI [4].

In the setting of both ST-elevation MI and non-ST elevation acute coronary syndromes (ACS), diabetic patients suffer increased mortality as compared to non-diabetic patients. In a study of diabetic patients enrolled in the GUSTO-I (Global Utilisation of Streptokinase and t-PA for Occluded Coronary Arteries-I) trial, 30-day mortality was significantly higher among patients with diabetes [10.5% in diabetics versus 6.2% in non-diabetics; odds ratio (OR): 1.77; 95% confidence interval (CI): 1.61–1.95] [6]. In a pooled analysis of five randomised trials of thrombolytic therapy for acute MI, the

[1]Division of Cardiology, Campo di Marte Hospital, Lucca; [2]Department of Cardiovascular and Respiratory Sciences, La Sapienza University, Rome; [3]Department of Cardiology, Bambino Gesù Children's Hospital, Rome, Italy

30-day mortality was 11.7% in diabetics as compared with 7.1% in non-diabetics (OR: 1.71; 95% CI: 1.60–1.83) [6]. Similarly, in a combined analysis of the GUSTO-I, GUSTO-III, and GUSTO-V trials, diabetic patients, as compared to patients without diabetes, were at greater risk of in-hospital mortality (9.5% versus 5.5%, respectively; $P < 0.001$) and 30-day mortality (10.4% versus 6.0%, respectively; $P < 0.001$) [7].

Diabetes and Non-ST-Elevation Acute Coronary Syndromes

There is ample evidence that diabetic patients are at higher risk of subsequent cardiac events in the setting of non-ST-elevation ACS. In the OASIS (Organization to Assess Strategies for Ischemic Syndromes) Registry, which involved patients with unstable angina (UA) and non-Q wave MI, diabetes was an independent predictor of mortality at 2 years [18% in diabetics versus 10% in non-diabetics; adjusted relative risk (RR): 1.57; 95% CI: 1.38–1.81; $P < 0.001$] [8]. In a more recent analysis of four randomised trials of non-ST-elevation ACS, diabetes was again identified as an independent risk factor for mortality [9]. In this report, 30-day mortality was 5.5% among diabetic patients compared with 3.0% among non-diabetic patients ($P < 0.001$) [9]. Similarly, in the diabetic substudy of the FRISC-II (Fragmin and Fast Revascularization During Instability in Coronary Artery Disease) trial, which compared invasive versus conservative management of patients with non-ST-elevation ACS, diabetes remained an independent predictor of death (RR: 5.43; 95% CI: 2.09–14.1) and of death or MI (RR: 2.40; 95% CI: 1.47–3.91), even after controlling for revascularisation, extent of coronary artery disease, and signs of myocardial damage given by serum markers [10]. The TACTICS TIMI 18 trial, too, showed that diabetic patients had greater benefit than non-diabetics from the early invasive assessment both in terms of absolute (7.6% and 1.8%, respectively) and relative 6-month event reduction (27% and 13%, respectively) [11]. Therefore, an early invasive assessment and appropriate revascularisation should be considered the strategy of choice for diabetic patients with non-ST-elevation ACS. The question as to how early coronary angiography should be performed in this subset of patients has no definitive answer.

Diabetes and ST-Elevation Myocardial Infarction

In a major international trial involving more than 40 000 patients designed to evaluate four fibrinolytic strategies for the treatment of acute MI (AMI), 30-day mortality was 6.2% among patients without diabetes and 10.5% among patients with diabetes. Indeed, pooling the data from several large fibrinolytic trials with a total of more than 80 000 patients, 1-month mortality was increased by 1.7 times among diabetics [12]. Notably, mortality was highest among those treated with insulin. Undoubtedly less known is the fact that fibrinolysis saved 37 lives per 1000 patients with diabetes at 35 days, compared with 15 per 1000 patients without diabetes [13]. Thus, the absolute benefit of fibrinolytic therapy is more than doubled for diabetics.

Despite its tremendous benefit, however, patients with diabetes were less likely to receive fibrinolytic therapy [14], as evidenced in the Survival and Ventricular Enlargement (SAVE) Study [15]. In this trial, of the 2231 patients enrolled, fibrinolytic therapy was administered to 733 (32.9%) [15]. Diabetic patients undergoing a percutaneous coronary intervention (PCI) exhibited similar angiographic success rates to non-diabetic patients, but showed a trend toward higher in-hospital mortality rates, higher rates of urgent revascularisation, and greater incidence of acute coronary occlusions [15]. In a recent study, diabetes mellitus was associated with higher incidences of death, AMI, and repeated revascularisation at long-term follow-up after a primary PCI [16]. Therefore, the optimal strategy for coronary revascularisation in diabetic patients remains to be determined.

Re-stenosis and Platelet Function

The addition of stent implantation to balloon angioplasty in diabetic patients is feasible, with favourable procedural and in-hospital success rates. However, long-term outcomes after stenting remain worse because of a higher incidence of major adverse cardiac events and, above all, the re-stenosis rate compared with that in non-diabetic patients [17]. The increased risk of re-stenosis after angioplasty and/or stenting in diabetic patients is primarily due to exaggerated reactive intimal hyperplasia that causes increased late luminal loss and decreased vascular luminal area [18]. In a recent pooled analysis of several major recent stent trials, Cutlip et al. [19] found diabetes to be the strongest clinical predictor of re-stenosis, with an almost 50% increased risk for target lesion revascularisation (TLR) at 1-year follow-up. Considering the higher rate of re-stenosis and the current prevalence of diabetes among patients who undergo PCI (e.g. a prevalence of 18% to 30% in most series), a simple calculation would show that 30% to 40% of the patients who sustain clinical re-stenosis and eventually undergo target vessel revascularisation (TVR) are those with DM [20]. Thus, reduction of the re-stenosis rate among diabetic patients will have a major favourable impact on the global outcome of catheter-based coronary interventions.

There is ample evidence that platelets of diabetic patients are larger and hyper-reactive, showing increased adhesion and aggregation and increased platelet-dependent thrombin generation [21]. In fact, diabetes is characterised by elevated concentrations of procoagulant factors, including fibrinogen, von Willebrand factor, and factor VII, with decreased concentration of antithrombotic factors including antithrombin III and protein C [21]. Tissue factor, which is the most potent trigger of the coagulation cascade [22], is increased in patients with DM [23]. Recently, Sambola et al. [24] identified significant reductions in tissue factor activity and blood thrombogenicity in diabetic patients with improved glycaemic control. These observations highlight the concept of high-risk blood in the pathophysiology of diabetic atherosclerosis leading to coronary thrombosis.

Moreover, in patients with type 2 diabetes, there is an association between glycaemic control and blood thrombogenicity. Osende et al., using the Badimon ex vivo perfusion chamber, showed that improved glycaemic control, as indicated by $\geq$ 0.5% reduction in HbA$_{1c}$, resulted in a significant decrease in blood thrombogenicity [25].

Importance of Pre-procedural Glycaemic Control

Recently, a growing body of evidence has shown an association between optimal glycaemic control and improvement in major cardiovascular events [26]. In a meta-analysis of 95 783 patients who were observed for 12.4 years in order to explore the relationship between glucose levels and incident cardiovascular events, a fasting glucose of 110 mg/dl was associated with a relative cardiovascular event risk of 1.33 (95% CI, 1.06–1.67) [27]. In a study by Khaw et al. [28], a 1% increase in HbA$_{1c}$ was associated with a 38% increase in cardiovascular mortality and a 44% increase in risk of ischaemic mortality in diabetic patients. These findings are supported by the fact that pre-procedural hyperglycaemia is known to induce vascular endothelial cell damage, excessive extracellular matrix formation, and increased cellular proliferation [25, 29], which could progressively contribute to the adverse outcomes after stent implantation.

Conversely, recent studies identified poor glycaemic control as a significant predictor of angiographic re-stenosis without any impact on mortality [20, 30]. These results are in accordance with a study by Corpus et al. [31] which assessed the effect of glycaemic control on TVR at the time of coronary intervention among a group of 179 diabetic patients as compared with 60 non-diabetic control patients. Patients who had optimal diabetic control had a TVR rate of 15%, compared with 34% among counterparts with hyperglycaemia. By multivariate analysis, poor glycaemic control was a major independent predictor of TVR.

Interestingly, in all the above mentioned studies, the treatment with glycoprotein IIb/IIIa inhibitors was not specified and intracoronary stenting was performed only in a small percentage of diabetic patients.

Hyperglycaemia might be associated with impaired microvascular function after AMI, resulting in a larger infarct size and worse functional recovery [32]. A total of 146 consecutive patients with a first AMI were studied by intracoronary myocardial contrast echocardiography after successful reperfusion within 24 h after symptom onset. The no-reflow phenomenon was more often observed in the 75 patients with hyperglycaemia ($\geq$ 160 mg/dl) than in those without hyperglycaemia (52.0% vs. 14.1%; $P < 0.0001$) [32].

Antiplatelet Drugs in Diabetic Patients

A meta-analysis by Roffi et al., including the entire large-scale trial experience of intravenous platelet glycoprotein IIb/IIIa inhibitors for the medical management of non-ST-segment-elevation ACS, showed that these agents may significantly reduce mortality at 30 days in diabetic patients, especially patients undergoing PCI [33]. Another meta-analysis of three placebo-controlled abciximab trials, demonstrated a reduction of mortality (from 4.5% to 2.5%, $P = 0.099$) in diabetic patients treated with abciximab, with a mortality reduction particularly apparent among patients treated with stents [34]. A sub-study of the EPISTENT trial about the outcomes of 491 diabetic patients demonstrated that abciximab, irrespective of revascularisation strategy (stent or balloon angioplasty), resulted in a significant reduction in the 6-month death or MI rate: 12.7% for stent–placebo, 7.8% for balloon angioplasty–abciximab, and 6.2% for the stent–abciximab group ($P = 0.029$) [35]. Moreover, among the 346 patients with diabetes enrolled in the CADILLAC trial, TVR at 1 year was significantly reduced with routine stenting compared with balloon angioplasty (10.3% vs 22.4%, $P = 0.004$), with no differences in death, reinfarction, or stroke. Angiographic re-stenosis was also greatly reduced in diabetics randomised to stenting (21.1% vs 47.6%, $P = 0.009$) [35]. No beneficial effects were apparent with abciximab in diabetic patients at 1 year [36]. Despite the improved outcomes with stenting in patients with diabetes, 1-year mortality remained increased in diabetic patients who received stents compared with non-diabetics (8.2% vs 3.6%, $P = 0.005$) [37].

Thus, the combination of abciximab with stenting has been hypothesised to be the optimal percutaneous revascularisation strategy [38], not only for reducing TVR but also for improving survival to the level of placebo-treated non-diabetic patients in elective PCI [33, 38]. Anyway, published data on diabetic patient sub-sets from the various glycoprotein IIb/IIIa inhibitor trials have assessed different agents and forms of percutaneous revascularisation (stent versus non-stent) and used different end-points and durations of follow-up.

By contrast, the ISAR-SWEET study [39] randomised to abciximab or placebo 701 diabetic patients who underwent an elective PCI with bare metal stents after pre-treatment with a 600-mg loading dose of clopidogrel at least 2 h before the procedure. The incidence of death or MI at 1 year was 8.3% in the abciximab group and 8.6% in the placebo group $(P = 0.91)$ and the incidence of angiographic re-stenosis was 28.9% in the abciximab group and 37.8% in the placebo group $(P = 0.01)$.

In patients with DM, clopidogrel has been shown to be superior to aspirin in reducing recurrent ischaemic events [40]. The PCI-CURE study demonstrated that a strategy of clopidogrel pre-treatment followed by long-term therapy is beneficial in reducing cardiovascular events [41]. An analysis of the multi-centre, randomised, double-blind CAPRIE study showed that clopidogrel provided even greater reductions than aspirin in the risk of recurrent ischaemic events in diabetic patients [42]. Moreover, recent evidence demonstrates that a loading dose of 600 mg clopidogrel leads to more rapid platelet inhibition than a dose of 300 mg [43] and may obviate the need for abciximab during elective PCI in patients at low to intermediate risk [44].

Drug-Eluting Stents and Intracoronary Brachytherapy

The advent of drug-eluting stents (DES) is a remarkable improvement in preventing re-stenosis in coronary arteries after coronary angioplasty. The RAVEL study group [45] showed a significant reduction in re-stenosis with sirolimus-eluting stents compared with standard stents (27% vs 0%) among 238 patients with coronary artery disease. A sub-group analysis of patients with diabetes showed that among 19 patients who received sirolimus-eluting stents, the re-stenosis rate was 0% compared with 42% among 25 patients who received standard stents [45]. The more recent SIRIUS trial [46] focused on patients at higher risk of re-stenosis. Among the patients with diabetes, the re-stenosis rate was 18% in 131 patients who received sirolimus-eluting stents compared with 51% among 148 patients who received standard stents. Moreover, in the diabetic cohort of the TAXUS trial, target lesion revascularisation was reduced by approximately 66%, also using a polymer-based paclitaxel-eluting stent [47]. However, the use of DES in diabetic patients undergoing coronary stent placement cannot be considered standard of care until larger trials confirm its safety and efficacy in this patient population.

The mechanism by which brachytherapy reduces re-stenosis (reduction of intimal hyperplasia) could potentially be useful in diabetics treated with stent implantation. Recent studies demonstrate that the effectiveness of brachytherapy in reducing re-stenosis in the context of intra-stent re-stenosis is especially high in diabetics [48]. These results have inspired the design and execution of studies in which brachytherapy is applied with angioplasty in de novo lesions in diabetics.

Conclusions

Diabetes is a source of significant morbidity and mortality resulting from long-term micro- and macrovascular complications after coronary angioplasty in patients with ACS. Optimal pre-procedural glycaemic control and inhibition of intimal hyperplasia would reduce or impede re-stenosis, resulting in better clinical results.

References

1. Mokdad AH, Ford ES, Bowman BA et al (2000) Diabetes trends in the U.S.: 1990–1998. Diabetes Care 23:1278–1283
2. Mokdad AH, Bowman BA, Ford ES et al (2001) The continuing epidemics of obesity and diabetes in the United States. JAMA 286:1195–1200
3. Narayan KM, Boyle JP, Thompson TJ et al (2003) Lifetime risk for diabetes mellitus in the United States. JAMA 290:1884–1890
4. Haffner SM, Lehto S, Ronnemaa T et al (1998) Mortality from coronary heart disease in subjects with type 2 diabetes and in nondiabetic subjects with and without prior myocardial infarction. N Engl J Med 339:229–234
5. Beckman JA, Creager MA, Libby P (2002) Diabetes and atherosclerosis: epidemiology, pathophysiology, and management. JAMA 287:2570–2581
6. Mak KH, Moliterno DJ, Granger CB et al (1997) Influence of diabetes mellitus on clinical outcome in the thrombolytic era of acute myocardial infarction. J Am Coll Cardiol 30:171–179
7. Gurm HS, Tang WHW, Lee D et al (2002) Improving outcome of diabetics with ST-elevation myocardial infarction: insights from the GUSTO trials. J Am Coll Cardiol 39:292A
8. Malmberg K, Yusuf S, Gerstein HC et al (2000) Impact of diabetes on long-term prognosis in patients with unstable angina and non-Q-wave myocardial infarction: results of the OASIS (Organisation to Assess Strategies for Ischaemic Syndromes) Registry. Circulation 102:1014–1019
9. Roffi M, Cho L, Bhatt DL et al (2002) Dramatic increase in 30-day mortality in diabetic patients with non-ST segment elevation acute coronary syndromes. J Am Coll Cardiol 39:313A
10. Norhammar A, Malmberg K, Diderholm E et al (2001) Diabetes mellitus: the major risk factor in unstable CAD even after consideration of the extent of coronary lesions and benefits of revascularisation. J Am Coll Cardiol 43(4):585–591
11. Cannon CP, Weintraub WS, Demopoulos LA et al (2001) Comparison of early invasive and conservative strategies in patients with unstable coronary syndromes

treated with the glycoprotein IIb/IIIa inhibitor tirofiban. N Engl J Med 344:1879–1887

12. Mak KH, Topol EJ (2000) Emerging concepts in the management of acute myocardial infarction in patients with diabetes mellitus. J Am Coll Cardiol 35:563–568

13. Fibrinolytic Therapy Trialists' (FTT) Collaborative Group (1994) Indications for fibrinolytic therapy in suspected acute myocardial infarction: collaborative overview of early mortality and major morbidity results from all randomised trials of more than 1,000 patients. Lancet 343: 311–322

14. Bovenzi F, De Luca L, de Luca I (2004) Which is the best reperfusion strategy for patients with high-risk myocardial infarction? Ital Heart J 5:83–91

15. Pfeffer MA, Moye LA, Braunwald E et al (1991) Selection bias in the use of thrombolytic therapy in acute myocardial infarction. JAMA 266: 528–532

16. Bolognese L, Carrabba N, Santoro GM et al (2003) Angiographic findings, time course of regional and global left ventricular function, and clinical outcome in diabetic patients with acute myocardial infarction treated with primary percutaneous transluminal coronary angioplasty. Am J Cardiol 91:544–549

17. Elezi S, Kastrati A, Pache J et al (1998) Diabetes mellitus and the clinical and angiographic outcome after coronary stent placement. J Am Coll Cardiol 32:1866–1873

18. Kornowski R, Mintz GS, Kent KM et al (1997) Increased restenosis in diabetes mellitus after coronary interventions is due to exaggerated intimal hyperplasia. A serial intravascular study. Circulation 95:1366–1369

19. Cutlip DE, Chauhan MS, Baim DS et al (2002) Clinical restenosis after coronary stenting: perspectives from multicenter clinical trials. J Am Coll Cardiol 40:2082–2089

20. Kornowski R, Fuchs S (2004) Optimisation of glycemic control and restenosis prevention in diabetic patients undergoing percutaneous coronary interventions. J Am Coll Cardiol 43:15–17

21. Moreno PR, Fuster V (2004) New aspects in the pathogenesis of diabetic atherothrombosis. J Am Coll Cardiol 44:2293–1300

22. Nemerson Y (1988) Tissue factor and haemostasis. Blood 71:1–8

23. Zumbach M, Hofmann M, Borcea V et al (1997) Tissue factor antigen is elevated in patients with microvascular complications of diabetes mellitus. Exp Clin Endocrinol Diabetes 105:206–212

24. Sambola A, Fuster V, Badimon JJ (2003) Role of coronary risk factors in blood thrombogenicity and acute coronary syndromes. Rev Esp Cardiol 56:1001–1009

25. Osende JI, Badimon JJ, Fuster V et al (2001) Blood thrombogenicity in type 2 diabetes mellitus is associated with glycemic control. J Am Coll Cardiol 38:1307–1312

26. Muhlestein JB, Anderson JL, Horne BD et al (2003) Effect of fasting glucose levels on mortality rate in patients with and without diabetes mellitus and coronary artery disease undergoing percutaneous coronary intervention. Am Heart J 146:351–358

27. Coutinho M, Gerstein HC, Wang Y et al (1999) The relationship between glucose and incident cardiovascular events: a metaregression analysis of published data from 20 studies of 95,783 individuals followed for 12.4 years. Diabetes Care 22:233–240

28. Khaw KT, Wareham N, Luben R et al (2001) Glycated haemoglobin, diabetes, and mortality in men in Norfolk cohort of European Prospective Investigation of Cancer and Nutrition (EPIC-Norfolk). BMJ 322:15

29. Aronson D, Bloomgarden Z, Rayfield EJ (1996) Potential mechanisms promoting restenosis in diabetic patients. J Am Coll Cardiol 27:528–535

30. Mazeika P, Prasad N, Bui S et al (2003) Predictors of angiographic restenosis after coronary intervention in patients with diabetes mellitus. Am Heart J 145:1013–1021

31. Corpus RA, George PB, House JA et al (2004) Optimal glycemic control is associated with a lower rate of target vessel revascularisation in treated type II diabetic patients undergoing elective percutaneous coronary intervention. J Am Coll Cardiol 43:8–14

32. Iwakura K, Ito H, Ikushima M et al (2003) Association between hyperglycemia and the no-reflow phenomenon in patients with acute myocardial infarction. J Am Coll Cardiol 41:1–7

33. Roffi M, Chew DP, MukherjeeD et al (2001) Platelet glycoprotein IIb/IIIa inhibitors reduce mortality in diabetic patients with non-ST-segment-elevation acute coronary syndromes. Circulation 104:2767–2771

34. Bhatt DL, Marso SP, Lincoff AM et al (2000) Abciximab reduces mortality in diabetics following percutaneous coronary intervention. J Am Coll Cardiol 35:922–928

35. Marso SP, Lincoff AM, Ellis SG et al for the EPISTENT Investigators (1999) Optimizing the percutaneous interventional outcomes for patients with diabetes mellitus. Results of the EPISTENT (Evaluation of Platelet IIb/IIIa Inhibitor for Stenting Trial) diabetic study. Circulation 100:2477–2784

36. Stuckey TD, Stone GW, Cox DA et al (2005) Impact of stenting and abciximab in patients with diabetes mellitus undergoing primary angioplasty in acute myocardial infarction (the CADILLAC trial) Am J Cardiol 95(1):1–7

37. Lincoff AM, Califf RM, Moliterno DJ et al for the Evaluation of Platelet IIb/IIIa Inhibition in Stenting investigators (1999) Complementary clinical benefits of coronary-artery stenting and blockade of platelet glycoprotein IIb/IIIa receptors. N Engl J Med 341:319–327

38. Theroux P, Alexander J, Pharand C et al (2000) Glycoprotein IIb/IIIa receptor blockade improves outcomes in diabetic patients presenting with unstable angina/non-ST-elevation myocardial infarction. Circulation 102:2466–2472

39. Mehilli J, Kastrati A, Schühlen H et al for the Intracoronary Stenting and Antithrombotic Regimen: Is Abciximab a Superior Way to Eliminate Elevated Thrombotic Risk in Diabetics (ISAR-SWEET) Study Investigators (2004) Randomised clinical trial of abciximab in diabetic patients undergoing elective percutaneous coronary interventions after treatment with a high loading dose of clopidogrel. Circulation 110:3627–3635

40. Bhatt DL, Marso SP, Hirsch AT et al (2002) Amplified benefit of clopidogrel versus aspirin in patients with diabetes mellitus. Am J Cardiol 90:625–628

41. Mehta SR, Yusuf S, Peters RJ et al (2001) Effects of pretreatment with clopidogrel and aspirin followed by long-term therapy in patients undergoing percutaneous coronary intervention: the PCI-CURE study. Lancet 358:527–533

42. Jarvis B, Simpson K (2000) Clopidogrel: a review of its use in the prevention of atherothrombosis. Drugs 60:347–377

43. Müller I, Seyfarth M, Rüdiger S et al (2001) Effect of a high loading dose of clopidogrel on platelet function in patients undergoing coronary stent placement. Heart 85:92–93

44. Kastrati A, Mehilli J, Schühlen H et al (2004) A clinical trial of abciximab in elective percutaneous coronary intervention after pretreatment with clopidogrel. N Engl J Med 350:232–238

45. Morice MC, Serruys PW, Sousa JE et al (2002) A randomised comparison of a sirolimus-eluting stent with a standard stent for coronary revascularisation. N Engl J

Med 346:1773–1780

46. Moses JW, Leon MB, Popma JJ et al (2003) Sirolimus eluting stents versus standard stents in patients with stenosis in native coronary artery. N Engl J Med 349:1315–1323

47. Stone GW, Ellis SG, Cox DA et al (2004) One-year clinical results with the slow-release, polymer-based, paclitaxel-eluting TAXUS stent: the TAXUS-IV trial. Circulation 109:1942–1947

48. Williams DO (2001) Intracoronary brachytherapy. Past, present and future. Circulation 105:2699–2701

Spinal Cord Stimulation in Refractory Coronary Artery Disease: The Last Resort?

H. Theres[1], S. Eddicks[1], M. Schenk[2], K. Maier-Hauff[3], C. Spies[2], G. Baumann[1]

Major advances have been achieved during recent years in the treatment of coronary artery disease (CAD) by medication, catheter intervention, and surgery. Numerous improvements have expanded the spectrum of therapeutic options, e.g., with brachytherapy, drug-eluting stents, and the like. Despite such innovative procedures, however, it is not possible to effectively treat angina pectoris symptomatology for all patients.

If coronary revascularisation is not feasible – either by catheter intervention or by surgical placement of a bypass – and if the patient still suffers serious symptoms despite optimal anti-angina medication, the patient is said to suffer from refractory angina pectoris. Categorisation of the severity of an angina pectoris symptom complex normally takes place in accordance with the classification of the Canadian Cardiovascular Society (CCS) [1], which was developed on the basis of the NYHA classification of stages of heart failure. Severity classification CCS III, for example, describes appreciable restriction of normal bodily activity, e.g., climbing one flight of stairs at normal speed leads to angina pectoris. CCS IV characterises an inability to perform any type of bodily activity without discomfort. Patients with refractory angina pectoris (CCS III–IV) are highly symptomatic under everyday conditions, which results in massive restriction of physical functional activity. Many patients additionally report social isolation, since friends and family members consider frequently occurring angina pectoris attacks as particularly problematic, if not to say life-threatening. These chronically ill patients, on the whole, experience significant diminution of their quality of life. They

[1]Medizinische Klinik mit Schwerpunkt Kardiologie, Angiologie, Pneumologie, Universitätsklinikum Charité Campus Mitte, Berlin; [2]Klinik für Anästhesiologie und operative Intensivmedizin, Universitätsklinikum Charité Campus Mitte, Berlin; [3]Abteilung Neurochirurgie – Zentrum für Neuromodulation, Bundeswehrkrankenhaus Berlin, Germany

receive the impression that medical science has no additional therapeutic measures to offer them, and that they represent hopeless cases.

Since no exact epidemiological surveys have been conducted on this topic, it is difficult to estimate the number of patients suffering from refractory angina pectoris. On the basis of Scandinavian data [2], Mannheimer et al. [3] have estimated the incidence of refractory angina pectoris throughout to Europe to be approx. 30 000–50 000 patients. Mukherjee et al. even estimate the incidence at more than 100 000 patients annually in the USA: patients who on the basis of a hospital survey could be considered for alternative anti-angina therapy [4].

Various treatment concepts have by now been developed and introduced into clinical work: these include intermittent urokinase therapy [5], transmyocardial laser revascularisation [6–8], and external counterpulsation [9]. M.R. Chester, of Britain, has developed a highly promising interdisciplinary approach to pain therapy for patients suffering from refractory angina pectoris, and has published his results on the Internet (under www.angina.org). Only recently, the Working Group for Refractory Angina Pectoris of the European Cardiovascular Society has published an overview on refractory angina pectoris, in which it recommends neurostimulation as therapeutic alternative: two techniques are transcutaneous electrical nerve stimulation (TENS) and spinal cord stimulation (SCS) [3]. Numerous studies have demonstrated that this adjuvant therapy was associated with reduction in the frequency of attacks, and with increase in exercise capability.

The present article presents the procedure of neurostimulation for patients with refractory angina pectoris, with discussion on the indications, therapeutic mechanisms, and published results of studies concerning effectiveness and safety.

Indications

The indication for application of TENS or for implantation of a spinal cord stimulator may follow from interdisciplinary procedures, e.g., interventional cardiology, cardiosurgery, or pain therapy (including therapy by general practitioners and psychologists). As initial step, however, all necessary efforts should be undertaken to exclude secondary causes of angina pectoris (e.g. anaemia or uncontrolled arterial hypertension, as well as cardiac risk factors), by weight normalisation, cessation of smoking, and the like. In addition to optimisation of medical therapy, primary attention should be directed to the question of whether revascularisation by catheter intervention and/or by surgery is appropriate. For patients who have already undergone repeated cardiac catheter intervention procedures or bypass surgery, risk–benefit assessment will be necessary for continuation of invasive therapy. From the point of view of coronary anatomy, candidates for SCS implantation will primarily be found among those patients for whom diffuse alterations in coronary vessels that extend into the vascular periphery have rendered bypass surgery or catheter intervention inadvisable or impossible. Implantation of such a system may also prove worth considering among patients listed for heart transplantation in conjunction with ischaemic cardiomyopathy and refractory angina pectoris.

For cardiac syndrome X (myocardial microangiopathy as a result of arteriosclerosis and/or endothelial dysfunction), positive therapeutic experience has already been gained with neurostimulation [10]. Further experience could likewise be profitably gained here in the context of controlled studies.

As part of patient preparation, and on an intraoperative basis, investigation is also essential to determine the possibility of interference with already implanted pacemaker or cardioverter–defibrillator systems. One potential danger here is back-coupling of stimulation pulses from the neurostimulator to the sensing circuitry of the pacemaker system. This phenomenon can lead to inhibition of the pacemaker system and, in turn, to asystole among pacemaker users. Use of a pacemaker, however, does not automatically represent an absolute contraindication [11, 12].

Whatever the case, it is essential that the patient be sufficiently trained in the use of a neurostimulator. Since the system is controlled by the patient as needed, and is activated according to pre-set time sequences, a basic understanding of its functioning is necessary.

The TENS technique is used in patients who cannot immediately decide on implantation of a neurostimulator system. TENS therapy can be considered as a test phase for patients who demonstrate typical angina pectoris symptoms with the associated coronary findings, but for whom there is no definitive evidence of ischaemia. If these patients are identified as responders on the basis of reduction in their anginal symptom complex, definitive treatment with an SCS system is recommended.

The procedure for establishing the indication is shown in the flow diagram in Figure 1. The scope of this present article will not allow treatment of differential therapeutic application of other methods: e.g., general pain therapy or additional alternative procedures. Interested readers may consult the work of Chester (www.angina.org), Kim [13], and Mannheimer [3], for more details on these topics.

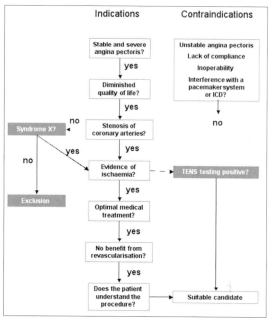

Fig. 1. Indication for neuromodulation for patients with the refractory angina pectoris complex

Therapeutic Mechanisms

Although neurostimulation has successfully been applied in specialised centres in Europe for more than 15 years now, the highly complex physiological and biochemical foundations of its therapeutic mechanisms have not yet been fully elucidated. The hypothesis currently considered most probable [14] is that, subsequent to diminution of pain, down-regulation of sympathicotonia, and consequently of myocardial oxygen demand, takes place in conjunction with optimisation of microcirculation (Fig. 2).

Anti-nociceptive Effect

In 1965 Melzack and Wall published their so-called gate control theory in the pioneering publication on this topic [15]. Since then, many standard works on pain therapy have cited their work. This theory postulated segmental pain inhibition induced by neurostimulation, under the assumption that selective activation of sensitive afferent fibres initially occurs as a result of regionally applied electrical stimuli, with slowly increasing intensity of stimulation below the threshold of pain [15, 16]. Melzack and Wall also postulated that this phenomenon leads in the dorsal horn of the spinal cord (the gate) to subsequent presynaptic inhibition of nociceptive afferents (A and C fibres), and consequently to local analgesia [15, 17]. The gate control theory has since undergone correction in many aspects, partly as a result of insights

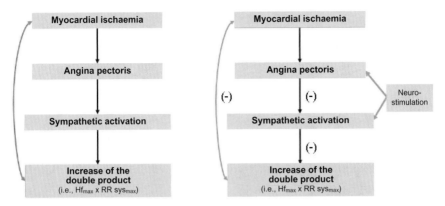

Fig. 2. Breakthrough of the chain of pain: neurostimulation leads to reduction in pain symptoms and, in turn, to diminution of sympathetic activity, accompanied by subsequent reduction in the frequency of occurrence of myocardial ischaemia episodes. Hf_{max}, maximum heart rate; $RRsys_{max}$, maximum systolic blood pressure

gained into the modulation of important neurotransmitters. According to these, neurostimulation elicits increased liberation of the inhibiting neurotransmitter γ-aminobutyric acid (GABA) in the dorsal horn and, in turn, effects a reduction of excitatorily acting amino acids (aspartate and glutamate) [18]. Eliasson et al. have reported an increase under SCS in β-endorphin, an endogenous agonist [19] to which a cardioprotective effect after myocardial ischaemia is attributed [20].

Effect on Sympathicotonia

In a human study, Norrsell et al. [21] simulated cardiac stress situations with the aid of tachycardial atrial stimulation. They reported noradrenaline liberation in the body that was diminished during stimulation in comparison to baseline. Important animal experiments conducted by Foreman et al. have shown that neurostimulation reduces the primarily sympathetically elicited responses to myocardial ischaemia [22]. Olgin et al. have recently attributed frequency-reducing (parasympathomimetic) effects to neurostimulation under conditions of sympathetic stress [23].

Effects on Myocardial Oxygen Demand

Several studies have reported the positive effects of neurostimulation on circulatory processes in the context of its application for peripheral vascular disease (PVD) [24, 25]. Kumar et al., for example, published a study on 46 patients with intractable PVD who underwent neurostimulation therapy [26]. This study revealed an increase in perfusion (pulse volume and maximum flow rate), as well as an increase in transcutaneously measured partial oxygen pressure. In the context of coronary circulation, evidence exists for homogenisation of myocardial blood supply. Using positron emission tomography, Hautvast et al. [27] revealed a redistribution of intramyocardial blood flow from non-ischaemic to ischaemic regions in patients under neurostimulation. Jessurun et al. [28] have published similar findings for administration of TENS. In addition to myocardial oxygen supply, oxygen consumption is of course of great significance for oxygen balance. Several studies have shown reductions in myocardial oxygen demand: Mannheimer et al., for example, have revealed a reduction in myocardial lactate production during neurostimulation [29].

Implantation Procedure

After local anaesthetic and under sterile conditions, the conscious patient, lying prone, undergoes puncture with a Tuohy 15-gauge needle of the peridural space, in the area of T8-10. A quadripole electrode is then advanced epidurally, under fluoroscopic guidance, to the level between C7 and T1. It is then positioned paramedially according to the side on which the area of pain is felt.

The exact electrode position is then determined during careful investigation of the zone of pain. The objective is to achieve as complete coverage as possible of the pain zone with electrically induced paraesthesia. Experience has shown that, under conditions of successful intraoperative testing, the response rate over the long term is sufficiently satisfactory to allow definitive implantation, during the same session, of the neurostimulator (subcutaneously, under the left costal arch) [30]. The time required for the implantation is approximately 45-60 min. After surgery, the stimulation parameters determined earlier can be transmitted to the neurostimulator by telemetry. After tuition, the patient can use his or her own programmer unit to switch the neurostimulator on and off, and can adjust the stimulation intensity through a range determined by the physician. Despite the severity of their heart disease, patients tolerate this implantation process well; no reports of perioperative myocardial infarction exist [30]. In the most favourable cases, discharge from hospital takes place on the same day as surgery, or the day after.

Complications worthy of report include pocket infections (5%) and lead fracture (3%) [31]. During the early years of this technology, slight lead dislocation made repositioning of the stimulation electrode necessary. Today, however, it is generally possible with the quadripole electrodes now available to solve this problem by reprogramming the stimulation poles. Although there has been widespread fear among patients of intraspinal bleeding complications, with paraplegia or intrathecal or intraspinal infections, no reports of any such occurrences have so far been published [30]. The neurostimulator battery will last 4–7 years, depending on intensity of use.

Study Results

Neurostimulation techniques have been used for many years as pain therapy for a variety of indications, e.g., chronic back pain, Buerger's disease, and PVD. Initial reports on the effects of neurostimulation for treatment of refractory angina pectoris were published in 1987 [32], when Murphy and Giles determined a marked reduction in pain severity in their patient cohorts, as well as in the number of angina attacks. In 1993 Harke et al. [33] described for two patients the long-term, positive anti-angina effects, as well as the appreciable enhancement of physical functional capacity. As early as 1985, Mannheimer et al. published reports on initial results gained with TENS [34]. A long-term study revealed a reduction in the frequency of angina pectoris attacks, increase in physical functional capacity, and reduction in stress-induced ST segment depression as a result of TENS therapy. In 1999 TenVaarweck published results of a course of therapy for 517 SCS patients [35]. A retrospective multi-centre study has also processed data from 14 implantation centres between 1987 and 1997. These patients had suffered from angina pectoris for an average of 8.1 years; 66% had already suffered at least one myocardial infarction, and 68% demonstrated coronary triple vessel disease. Follow-up care took place over a median period of 23 months, with the longest such care necessary for 12.5 years. On average, the angina pectoris class of these patients improved from 3.5 to 2.1 (Fig. 3) after implantation of a neurostimulation system.

The authors of the ESBY Study [36] pursued a more extensive approach. A team consisting of cardiosurgeons, cardiologists, and general practitioners (not all of whom took part in the study) identified patients with increased risk of surgical complications. They considered the following as risk factors in this context: cerebrovascular events experienced, complicated coronary anatomy, diabetes mellitus, reduced ejection fraction, peripheral arterial occlusion, previous coronary bypass operations, or renal insufficiency. A total of 104 patients either underwent bypass surgery or received a neurostimulator. Both of these patient groups experienced comparable reduction in their angina pectoris syndrome (Fig. 4). Ergometric stress testing revealed that the bypass patients enjoyed an advantage with respect to physical functional capacity. It must be noted here, however, that neurostimulation was deactivated during physical stress testing. Eight deaths took place

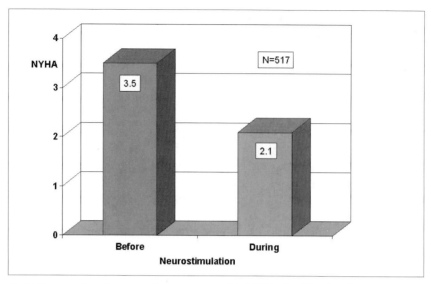

Fig. 3. Course of angina pectoris symptoms, with NYHA classification, for 517 patients (data from [35])

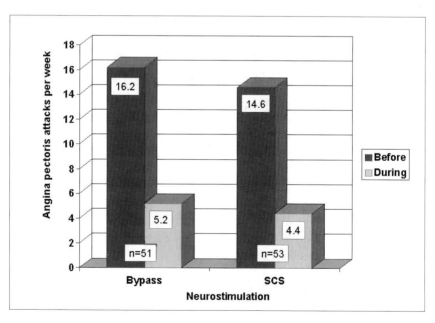

Fig. 4. Frequency of severe angina pectoris attacks among patients before and after surgical revascularisation, and before and after implantation of a spinal cord stimulation system, within the context of the ESBY Study (data from [29]). This study examined patients with increased risk of surgical complications

within the first 6 months: seven within the bypass group, and one in the SCS group. Follow-up data collected after 3 and 5 years revealed no significant difference in survival rate between the two groups. The authors concluded that neurostimulation therapy merited discussion as an alternative for patients with an increased risk of surgical complications.

Safety

Does neurostimulation suppress the angina pectoris syndrome to the extent that the patient no longer experiences the pain occurring even during a myocardial infarction? Anderson et al. addressed this crucial question as long ago as 1994 [37]. They monitored a total of 50 patients with implanted SCS systems over a period from 1 to 57 months. During this observation of patient progress, ten patients suffered acute myocardial infarctions. Nine of these ten patients reported the thoracic pain syndrome that typically accompanies myocardial infarction. One patient died acutely, with loss of the relevant information. Consequently, it may be stated that masking of infarction pain did not occur.

Another frequently posed question is: do these patients, with the aid of neuromodulation, achieve a higher level of physical functional capacity at the cost of no longer being able to sense dangerous myocardial ischaemia? Recently, a group working under Schwinger [38] published intermediate results of a controlled study of, so far, 15 patients who had suffered from refractory angina pectoris and undergone SCS. All patients demonstrated an increase in physical stress tolerance. Eight patients (53%) further experienced a reduction in myocardial ischaemia, proven by means of scintigraphy. The remaining seven patients showed no change. Even though these were only preliminary results, they may at least be taken as an indication that the clinical improvement of the patients was not at the cost of exacerbated but unperceived ischaemia. Other studies have provided further evidence by revealing a decrease in ST segment depression under physical stress [39, 40]. Data published by Eliasson et al. have also provided positive evidence of patient safety [41]. Their analysis of Holter ECGs revealed an increase in neither ischaemic episodes nor arrhythmias.

Risk–Benefit Analysis

Murray et al. have investigated the influence of SCS on the level of hospital admittance [42]. Their study compared the admittance rates of 19 patients after SCS implantation with rates before implantation. The results were 0.27

admittances per patient per year after SCS, in contrast to 0.97 before SCS implantation ($P = 0.02$). The mean bed-rest period was, analogously, 2.5 days after SCS vs 8.3 days before ($P = 0.04$). Patients with unstable angina pectoris or acute myocardial infarction reported for medical care without delay; silent myocardial ischaemia was not observed. Neuromodulation in the form of SCS therefore reduces the number of hospital admittances, without masking myocardial ischaemia or infarction. Cost savings achieved from fewer hospital admittances recover the cost of implantations after only 3 years.

References

1. Campeau L (1976) Letter. Grading of angina pectoris. Circulation 54:522–523
2. Brorsson B, Persson H, Landelius P et al (1998) Operation, ballongvidgning, medicinsk behandling. Statens beredning för utvärdering av medicinsk metodik, Stockholm, p 140
3. Mannheimer C, Camici P, Chester MR et al (2002) The problem of chronic refractory angina. Report from the ESC Joint Study Group on the Treatment of Refractory Angina. Eur Heart J 23:355–370
4. Mukherjee D, Bhatt DL, Roe MT et al (1999) Direct myocardial revascularization and angiogenesis – how many patients might be eligible? Am J Cardiol 84:598–600, A8
5. Leschke M, Schoebel FC, Jax TW et al (1997) Konservative Therapieansätze bei terminaler koronarer Herzkrankheit. Chronisch-intermittierende Urokinasetherapie. Herz 22:262–271
6. Grauhan O, Krabatsch T, Lieback E et al (2001) Transmyocardial laser revascularization in ischemic cardiomyopathy. J Heart Lung Transplant 20:687–691
7. Krabatsch T, Tambeur L, Lieback E (1998) Transmyocardial laser revascularization in the treatment of end-stage coronary artery disease. Ann Thorac Cardiovasc Surg 4:64–71
8. Schneider J, Diegeler A, Krakor R et al (2001) Transmyocardial laser revascularization with the holmium:YAG laser: loss of symptomatic improvement after 2 years. Eur J Cardiothorac Surg 19:164–169
9. Masuda D, Nohara R, Hirai T et al (2001) Enhanced external counterpulsation improved myocardial perfusion and coronary flow reserve in patients with chronic stable angina; evaluation by (13)N-ammonia positron emission tomography. Eur Heart J 22:1451–1458
10. Lanza GA, Sestito A, Sandric S et al (2001) Spinal cord stimulation in patients with refractory anginal pain and normal coronary arteries. Ital Heart J 2:25–30
11. Romano M, Brusa S, Grieco A et al (1998) Efficacy and safety of permanent cardiac DDD pacing with contemporaneous double spinal cord stimulation. Pacing Clin Electrophysiol 21:465–467
12. Romano M, Zucco F, Baldini MR et al (1993) Technical and clinical problems in patients with simultaneous implantation of a cardiac pacemaker and spinal cord stimulator. Pacing Clin Electrophysiol 16:1639–1644
13. Kim MC, Kini A, Sharma SK (2002) Refractory angina pectoris: mechanism and therapeutic options. J Am Coll Cardiol 39:923–934

14. Latif OA, Nedeljkovic SS, Stevenson LW (2001) Spinal cord stimulation for chronic intractable angina pectoris: a unified theory on its mechanism. Clin Cardiol 24:533–541

15. Melzack R, Wall PD (1965) Pain mechanisms: a new theory. Science 150:971–979

16. Koester J (1981) Functional consequences of passive electrical properties of the neuron. In: Kandel ER, Schwartz HJ (eds) Principles of neural science. Edward Arnold, London, p 44

17. Schmidt RF (1971) Presynaptic inhibition in the vertebrate central nervous system. Ergeb Physiol 63:20–101

18. Cui JG, O'Connor WT, Ungerstedt U et al (1997) Spinal cord stimulation attenuates augmented dorsal horn release of excitatory amino acids in mononeuropathy via a GABAergic mechanism. Pain 73:87–95

19. Eliasson T, Mannheimer C, Waagstein F et al (1998) Myocardial turnover of endogenous opioids and calcitonin-gene-related peptide in the human heart and the effects of spinal cord stimulation on pacing-induced angina pectoris. Cardiology 89:170–177

20. Oldroyd KG, Harvey K, Gray CE et al (1992) Beta endorphin release in patients after spontaneous and provoked acute myocardial ischaemia. Br Heart J 67:230–235

21. Norrsell H, Eliasson T, Mannheimer C et al (1997) Effects of pacing-induced myocardial stress and spinal cord stimulation on whole body and cardiac norepinephrine spillover. Eur Heart J 18:1890–1896

22. Foreman RD (2000) Integration of viscerosomatic sensory input at the spinal level. Prog Brain Res 122:209–221

23. Olgin JE, Takahashi T, Wilson E et al (2002) Effects of thoracic spinal cord stimulation on cardiac autonomic regulation of the sinus and atrioventricular nodes. J Cardiovasc Electrophysiol 13:475–481

24. Augustinsson LE, Carlsson CA, Holm J et al (1985) Epidural electrical stimulation in severe limb ischemia. Pain relief, increased blood flow, and a possible limb-saving effect. Ann Surg 202:104–110

25. Jacobs MJ, Jorning PJ, Beckers RC et al (1990) Foot salvage and improvement of microvascular blood flow as a result of epidural spinal cord electrical stimulation. J Vasc Surg 12:354–360

26. Kumar K, Toth C, Nath RK et al (1997) Improvement of limb circulation in peripheral vascular disease using epidural spinal cord stimulation: a prospective study. J Neurosurg 86:662–669

27. Hautvast RW, Blanksma PK, DeJongste MJ et al (1996) Effect of spinal cord stimulation on myocardial blood flow assessed by positron emission tomography in patients with refractory angina pectoris. Am J Cardiol 77:462–467

28. Jessurun GA, Tio RA, De Jongste MJ et al (1998) Coronary blood flow dynamics during transcutaneous electrical nerve stimulation for stable angina pectoris associated with severe narrowing of one major coronary artery. Am J Cardiol 82:921–926

29. Mannheimer C, Eliasson T, Andersson B et al (1993) Effects of spinal cord stimulation in angina pectoris induced by pacing and possible mechanisms of action. BMJ 307:477–480

30. Eliasson T, Augustinsson LE, Mannheimer C (1996) Spinal cord stimulation in severe angina pectoris – presentation of current studies, indications and clinical experience. Pain 65:169–179

31. Andersen C (1997) Complications in spinal cord stimulation for treatment of angi-

na pectoris. Differences in unipolar and multipolar percutaneous inserted electrodes. Acta Cardiol 52:325–333

32. Murphy DF, Giles KE (1987) Dorsal column stimulation for pain relief from intractable angina pectoris. Pain 28:365–368

33. Harke H, Ladleif HU, Rethage B et al (1993) Epidurale Rückenmarkstimulation bei therapieresistenter Angina pectoris. Anaesthesist 42:557–563

34. Mannheimer C, Carlsson CA, Emanuelsson H et al (1985) The effects of transcutaneous electrical nerve stimulation in patients with severe angina pectoris. Circulation 71:308–316

35. TenVaarwerk IA, Jessurun GA, DeJongste MJ et al (1999) Clinical outcome of patients treated with spinal cord stimulation for therapeutically refractory angina pectoris. The Working Group on Neurocardiology. Heart 82:82–88

36. Mannheimer C, Eliasson T, Augustinsson LE et al (1998) Electrical stimulation versus coronary artery bypass surgery in severe angina pectoris: the ESBY study. Circulation 97:1157–1163

37. Andersen C, Hole P, Oxhoj H (1994) Does pain relief with spinal cord stimulation for angina conceal myocardial infarction? Br Heart J 71:419–421

38. Diedrichs H, Zobel C, Voth E et al (2001) Spinal cord stimulation for intractable angina pectoris – a controlled study. Eur Heart J 22:172

39. De Jongste MJ, Hautvast RW, Hillege HL et al (1994) Efficacy of spinal cord stimulation as adjuvant therapy for intractable angina pectoris: a prospective, randomized clinical study. Working Group on Neurocardiology. J Am Coll Cardiol 23:1592–1597

40. Mannheimer C, Augustinsson LE, Carlsson CA et al (1988) Epidural spinal electrical stimulation in severe angina pectoris. Br Heart J 59:56–61

41. Eliasson T, Jern S, Augustinsson LE et al (1994) Safety aspects of spinal cord stimulation in severe angina pectoris. Coron Artery Dis 5:845–850

42. Murray S, Carson KG, Ewings PD et al (1999) Spinal cord stimulation significantly decreases the need for acute hospital admission for chest pain in patients with refractory angina pectoris. Heart 82:89–92

Guidelines for Antihypertensive Treatment: The Debate on the Choice of Antihypertensive Drugs

A. Salvetti, L. Ghiadoni, G. Salvetti

Introduction

Data from controlled clinical trials and above all their interpretation have strongly influenced guidelines on antihypertensive therapy, as shown by divergent recommendations on the choice of antihypertensive drugs in the three most widespread guidelines, namely the JNC-7 Report [1], ESH-ESC [2], and WHO-ISH [3] Guidelines.

According to the JNC-7 Report [1], for most patients with uncomplicated hypertension thiazide-type diuretics are the first-choice drug, either alone or combined with drugs from other classes, while the ESH-ESC Guidelines [2] state that the major classes of antihypertensive agents (diuretics, beta-blockers, calcium antagonists, ACE inhibitors, and Angiotensin-Receptor 1 (AT1) -receptor blockers) are suitable for initiation and maintenance of therapy. The ESH-ESC Guidelines [2] further suggest that alpha-blockers and central agents can also be considered, particularly for combination therapy, which need not necessarily include diuretics. Finally, the WHO-ISH Guidelines [3] recommend that for the majority of patients without compelling indication for another drug class, a low dose of diuretics should be considered as first choice of therapy.

Divergent Recommendations on the Choice of Antihypertensive Drugs: Why?

The JNC-7 Report [1] recommendation arose from the twofold recognition that thiazide-type diuretics have been the basis of antihypertensive therapy

Department of Internal Medicine, University of Pisa, Pisa, Italy

in most outcome trials and that in these trials, including the recently published Antihypertensive and Lipid-Lowering treatment to prevent Heart Attack Trial (ALLHAT) [4, 5], diuretics have been virtually unsurpassed in preventing the cardiovascular complications of hypertension. Moreover, diuretics can be useful in achieving blood pressure (BP) control as well as enhancing the antihypertensive efficacy of multidrug regimens, and they are more affordable than other antihypertensive agents.

The WHO-ISH Guidelines [3] acknowledge that the totality of trial evidence shows the major antihypertensive drug classes to be largely equivalent in efficacy and safety, the benefits deriving mainly from BP reduction. However, these Guidelines preferentially indicate a low dose of diuretics on the basis of greater availability and lower cost.

The ESH-ESC Guidelines [2] justify their liberal choice of antihypertensive drugs by noting that the main benefit of antihypertensive therapy is due to BP lowering *per se*. It is pointed out that drugs are not equal in terms of side effects, particularly in individual patients, and that drug choice will be influenced by many factors, including previous experience of patients with antihypertensive agents, patient's preference, patient's risk profile, presence or absence of subclinical target organ damage or of particular indications, and cost of drugs. Finally, the ESH-ESC Guidelines [2] clearly state that the emphasis on identifying the first class of drugs to be used is probably superseded by the need to use two or more drugs in combination in order to achieve goal BP.

Thus, the reasons why these Guidelines diverge as to recommended first-choice drug are, firstly, different interpretations of controlled clinical trials undertaken for drug class comparison and, secondly, drug cost considerations.

Data from Controlled Clinical Studies: Are Diuretics Really Unsurpassed?

Placebo-controlled clinical studies have shown that the benefit of antihypertensive therapy in preventing cardiovascular events with diuretics alone or combined with a beta-blocker [6] is similar to that achieved with ACE inhibitors and calcium antagonists [7]. Such a finding suggests that this benefit is due to BP lowering per se [6, 7].

The possibility that a particular drug class may have a BP-independent beneficial effect, thereby offering additional advantages in preventing cardiovascular morbidity and mortality, was evaluated in 11 controlled clinical trials for a total of 15 drug comparisons (Table 1). Overall, these studies showed no difference in primary endpoints among various drug classes, with the exception of two studies: the LIFE trial, in which treatment based on AT1-blockers significantly reduced cerebrovascular events compared to that based on a

Table 1. Controlled clinical studies on drug class comparison

Study	Drugs	Primary end-point	Relative risk (95% CI)
NORDIL	Diltiazem vs diuretics/ beta-blockers	Fatal and non-fatal stroke, MI, other CV death	1.00 (0.87–1.15)
CONVINCE	Verapamil vs atenolol/HCZ	First occurrence of stroke and MI, CV mortality	1.02 (0.88–1.18)
INVEST	Verapamil vs atenolol	CHD morbidity and mortality	1.02 (0.92–1.15)
INSIGHT	Nifedipine vs HCZ + amiloride	CV mortality, MI, CHF, stroke	1.10 (0.91–1.34)
ALLHAT	Chlorthalidone vs amlodipine	CHD morbidity and mortality	0.99 (0.91–1.08)
STOP-H 2	Diuretics/beta-blockers vs ACE-I/Ca-A	Fatal stroke, MI and other CV death	0.99 (0.84–1.16)
CAPPP	Captopril vs diuretics/ beta-blockers	CV mortality, MI, stroke	1.05 (0.90–1.22)
ALLHAT	Chlorthalidone vs lisinopril	CHD morbidity and mortality	0.98 (0.90–1.07)
ANBP-2	ACE-I vs diuretics	CV events and total mortality	0.89 (0.79–1.00) $P = 0.05$
ALLHAT	Chlorthalidone vs doxazosin	CHD morbidity and mortality	1.02 (0.92–1.15)
LIFE	Losartan vs atenolol	CV mortality, MI, stroke	0.87 (0.77–0.98) $P = 0.021$
SCOPE	Candesartan vs placebo (other drugs)	CV mortality, MI, stroke	0.89 (0.72–1.06)
VALUE	Valsartan vs amlodipine	CHD morbidity and mortality	1.04 (0.94–1.15)

MI, myocardial infarction; CV, cardiovascular; CHD, coronary heart disease; CHF, congestive heart failure; HCZ, hydrochlorothiazide; ACE-I, ACE inhibitors; Ca-A, calcium antagonists

NORDIL: NORrdic DILtiazem study; CONVINCE: Controlled ONset Verapamil INvestigation of Cardiovascular Endpoints; INVEST: International Verapamil–trandolapril STudy; ALLHAT: Antihypertensive and Lipid-Lowering Treatment to Prevent Heart Attack Trial; STOP-H2: Swedish Trial in Old Patients with Hypertension-2; CAPPP: CAPtopril Prevention Project; ANBP-2: Second Australian National Blood Pressure study; LIFE: Losartan Intervention For Endpoint reduction in hypertension; SCOPE: Study on Cognition and Prognosis in the Elderly; VALUE: Valsartan Antihypertensive Long-term Use Evaluation trial

beta-blocker [8], and the ANBP-2 trial, in which treatment based on an ACE inhibitor reduced a composite of all cardiovascular events (both initial and recurrent) as compared to thiazide diuretic-based treatment [9].

In seeking to comment on these data, the following lines of reasoning should be taken into consideration. First, the failure of these clinical trials to demonstrate BP-independent effects might be explained by study limitations. These studies may have been performed in patients at higher risk due to age, other risk factors, or known cardiovascular disease and therefore poorly representative of the hypertensive population [10]. Moreover, comparative drugs were often superimposed on other antihypertensive drugs in the attempt to achieve goal and similar BP values [10], a target which was not always reached as trial designs sometimes involved no-rational combination therapies and/or favoured the antihypertensive effect of a particular drug class as compared to others [11]. Since available data indicate that reduction in cardiovascular morbidity and mortality rates is dependent on BP reduction, lowering BP to optimal goal levels could attenuate the difference in outcomes resulting from specific effects of different antihypertensive drugs. Furthermore, differences in BP among treatments may explain some differences in secondary end-points [10, 11].

These hypotheses are in agreement with the following data. A recent meta-analysis [7] indicates a linear relationship between the change in systolic BP and reduction in morbidity and mortality for stroke, coronary heart disease, and cardiovascular disease, with the exception of heart failure. The analysis also makes it clear that larger reductions in BP produce larger reductions in risk of major cardiovascular events. Differences in systolic BP constitute a likely explanation for the greater incidence of stroke in the doxazosin [4] and lisinopril [5] arms of ALLHAT, in which the incidence of stroke in the lisinopril group is accounted for by a 40% greater incidence in black patients who showed the lowest degree of systolic BP reduction [11, 12]. Moreover, data from the VALUE trial indicate that early (within 6 months) control of systolic BP (< 140 mmHg) can significantly reduce the incidence of cardiovascular events and above all of stroke and congestive heart failure in high risk patients [13]. Finally, since in these trials a percentage of patients were either not on assigned comparative drugs or crossed over treatments, the intention-to-treat analysis of data might have favoured pseudo-equivalence.

The second line of reasoning to be taken into consideration is that the claimed superiority of diuretics derives from ALLHAT [4, 5] data and a network meta-analysis [14]. The strengths and limitations of ALLHAT have been already commented on [11] and can be summarised as follows. The main strength of this study is that with regard to primary outcomes (coronary mortality and non-fatal myocardial infarction) chlorthalidone-based treatment was equally as effective as treatment based on amlodipine or lisinopril or doxazosin, and with regard to some secondary end-points such as prevention of stroke it was superior when compared to doxazosin and lisinopril. It was also more effective in prevention of morbidity – but not mortality – from congestive heart failure when compared to the other three treatments [4, 5]. However, as stated above, the difference with regard to stroke could be due to a difference in systolic BP. In contrast, the difference with regard to congestive heart failure might be explained by poor accuracy and/or difficulty in diagnosis; alternatively, withdrawal of previous diuretic therapy may have unmasked congestive heart failure symptoms in patients with left ventricular dysfunction [11]. Thus ALLHAT confirmed and strengthened the clinical relevance of thiazide diuretics in the treatment of hypertension but did not prove the superiority of these drugs. This conclusion is in agreement with an expanded analysis of the ALLHAT data presented at the American Society of Hypertension Meeting 2004, which suggests the following interpretations [15]:

- The superiority of chlorthalidone versus lisinopril was detectable in black, but not in white patients. Therefore, it would be reasonable to state that, whereas diuretics remain the preferred first-line drugs for black patients, ACE inhibitors and diuretics could be regarded as co-equal recommendations for initiating therapy in whites.
- The primary coronary end-point was not different for amlodipine compared to the other two drugs, and the other major end-points of stroke and all-cause mortality tended slightly in its favour. Therefore, for many patients the excellent antihypertensive efficacy and tolerability of calcium antagonists continue to make them a popular and appropriate choice.

The latter interpretation can be reinforced by the VALUE trial data, in which amlodipine significantly reduced the incidence of fatal and non-fatal myocardial infarction when compared to the AT1-blocker [16]. It is further strengthened by a recent meta-analysis indicating that calcium antagonists, and above all dihydropiridine calcium antagonists, can reduce the risk of stroke when compared to other antihypertensive treatments [17]. Despite this, calcium antagonists did not decrease the risk of congestive heart failure when compared to placebo [7] and were inferior in this respect to active treatments based on diuretics, either alone or combined with beta-blockers [5, 7], or based on ACE inhibitors [7]. The meta-analysis [14], which claimed the superiority of diuretics versus all other antihypertensive drugs, not only included data from controlled clinical studies on drug class comparison, but also data from indirect comparative studies (active treatment versus placebo or no treatment). On the other hand, it did not take into account differences in BP, which can explain difference in outcomes [18].

The last issue to be discussed is whether all thiazide-like diuretics, when used at low and/or appropriate doses [19], offer similar beneficial effects. Attention focuses in particular on exploring whether positive results for chlorthalidone [5, 20] can be applied to thiazide diuretics in general and especially to hydrochlorothiazide [21]. The superiority of chlorthalidone versus hydrochlorothiazide is suggested by a post hoc analysis of the Multiple Risk Factor Intervention Trial (MRFIT) and by comparison of data from the ALLHAT and ANBP-2 studies. In MRFIT [22], which examined special intervention versus usual care groups, coronary heart disease and total mortality were reduced at clinics where special intervention clinicians used chlorthalidone and increased when hydrochlorothiazide was given. This latter pattern was reversed when clinicians switched patients from hydrochlorothiazide to chlorthalidone but at lower doses. At variance with the above described ALLHAT data, in which chlorthalidone was certainly not inferior to lisinopril [5], the ANBP-2 study [9] appeared to suggest that ACE-inhibitor-based treatment (enalapril recommended) offered greater protection from cardiovascular events than did diuretic-based treatment (hydrochlorothiazide recommended). However, a recent meta-analysis [23] of placebo-controlled trials of low-dose diuretics seemed to show that major cardiovascular outcomes resulting from chlorthalidone and other thiazide-like drugs were similar, indicating that the benefit of treatment with thiazide diuretics is a class effect. In conclusion, the overall data reported above do not point to a greater benefit of a particular drug class, beyond reduction in BP values, which is actually the more likely explanation of the benefit of antihypertensive therapy. In this setting thiazide-like diuretics can be viewed as efficient but not superior to other antihypertensive drugs. Therefore their preferential choice should be based principally on drug cost.

Cost-Benefit Analysis: Are Thiazide Diuretics Really Less Expensive?

Certainly thiazide-like diuretics are less expensive than newer types of antihypertensive agents, and are therefore favoured in terms of cost minimisation [21]. But cost is not the sole consideration, and further cost–benefit analyses, announced by the ALLHAT authors although not performed so far [21], are awaited. We believe that their analysis should also take into account the adverse metabolic effects of thiazide diuretics, consisting of an increase in cholesterol levels, blood glucose, new-onset diabetes, and hypokalaemia [5, 21]. While these metabolic effects did not translate to into a greater frequency of cardiovascular events in the relatively short-term follow-up of ALLHAT [5], they could have a major impact on the cost–benefit relationship, because in the long term they can reduce the benefit of treatment [24, 25] and increase the cost owing to the need for further pharmacological therapy designed to treat the metabolic abnormalities [11].

Is the Choice of First Drug Class Relevant in Clinical Practice?

The answer to this question is yes if the choice of antihypertensive drugs is based on the following considerations.

1. Efficacy in reducing BP and tolerability, the latter also including metabolic effects.
2. The benefit of particular drug classes in patients with compelling indications such as heart failure, previous myocardial infarction, high coronary disease risk, diabetes, chronic kidney disease, and previous stroke [1, 2].
3. Subclinical target organ damage, such as left ventricular hypertrophy [26] or ultrasound evidence of arterial wall thickening or atherosclerotic plaque of the carotid arteries [2] in which particular drug classes other than diuretics are suggested.
4. Other clinical conditions not causally but frequently associated with hypertension, such as headache, Raynaud's phenomenon, constipation, diarrhoea, gastrointestinal reflux, gout, renal stones, benign prostatic hyperplasia, chronic obstructive pulmonary disease, tremor, osteoporosis and psychiatric disorders, in which different antihypertensive drugs can have beneficial or detrimental effects.

However, we believe that the debate on the first-choice drug class has probably been emphasised since the above-mentioned clinical conditions frequently occur in hypertensive patients and in the majority of patients two or more drugs in combination are necessary in order to achieve goal BP [2].

Conclusions

Available data from controlled clinical trials comparing different drug classes seem to indicate a similar benefit in preventing cardiovascular morbidity and mortality in hypertensive patients. Although some differences in secondary end-points were detected, the overall benefit of various antihypertensive regimens seems to be linked to the extent of BP reduction. The cost of antihypertensive drugs (cost minimisation) is not an overwhelming consideration until cost–benefit analyses are correctly performed. Moreover, although the cost of drugs should be taken into account both for individual patients and for the health provider, cost considerations should not predominate over those of efficacy and tolerability in individual patients.

We therefore believe that liberality of choice among various antihypertensive drugs could offer an appropriate possibility of selecting the right drug for the right patient in order to achieve BP control, a goal which often requires rational combinations of antihypertensive drugs.

References

1. Chobanian AV, Bakris GL, Black HR et al (2003) The Seventh Report of the Joint National Committee on Prevention, Detection, Evaluation, and Treatment of High Blood Pressure: the JNC 7 report. JAMA 289:2560–2571

2. European Society of Hypertension-European Society of Cardiology Guidelines Committee (2003) 2003 European Society of Hypertension–European Society of Cardiology guidelines for the management of arterial hypertension. J Hypertens 21:1011–1053

3. Whitworth JA, World Health Organization, International Society of Hypertension Writing Group (2003) World Health Organization (WHO)/International Society of Hypertension (ISH) statement on management of hypertension. J Hypertens 21:1983–1992

4. Anonymous (2000) Major cardiovascular events in hypertensive patients randomized to doxazosin vs chlorthalidone: the antihypertensive and lipid-lowering treatment to prevent heart attack trial (ALLHAT) ALLHAT Collaborative Research Group. JAMA 283:1967–1975

5. Anonymous (2002) Major outcomes in high-risk hypertensive patients randomized to angiotensin-converting enzyme inhibitor or calcium channel blocker vs diuretic: The Antihypertensive and Lipid-Lowering Treatment to Prevent Heart Attack Trial (ALLHAT) ALLHAT Collaborative Research Group. JAMA 288:2981–2997

6. Collins R, Peto R, MacMahon S et al (1990) Blood pressure, stroke, and coronary heart disease. Part 2: Short-term reductions in blood pressure: overview of randomised drug trials in their epidemiological context. Lancet 335:827–838

7. Turnbull F (2003) Effects of different blood-pressure-lowering regimens on major cardiovascular events: results of prospectively designed overviews of randomised trials. Lancet 362:1527–1535

8. Dahlof B, Devereux RB, Kjeldsen SE et al (2002) Cardiovascular morbidity and mortality in the Losartan Intervention For Endpoint reduction in hypertension study (LIFE): a randomised trial against atenolol. Lancet 359:995–1003

9. Wing LM, Reid CM, Ryan P et al (2003) A comparison of outcomes with angiotensin-converting enzyme inhibitors and diuretics for hypertension in the elderly. N Engl J Med 348:583–592

10. Jones DW, Hall JE (2004) Seventh report of the Joint National Committee on Prevention, Detection, Evaluation, and Treatment of High Blood Pressure and evidence from new hypertension trials. Hypertension 43:1–3

11. Salvetti A, Ghiadoni L (2004) Guidelines for antihypertensive treatment: an update after the ALLHAT study. J Am Soc Nephrol 15:S51–S54

12. Ferdinand KC (2003) Recommendations for the management of special populations: racial and ethnic populations. Am J Hypertens 16:S50- S54

13. Weber MA, Julius S, Kjeldsen SE et al (2004) Blood pressure dependent and independent effects of antihypertensive treatment on clinical events in the VALUE Trial. Lancet 363:2049–2051

14. Psaty BM, Lumley T, Furberg CD et al (2003) Health outcomes associated with various antihypertensive therapies used as first-line agents: a network meta-analysis. JAMA 289:2534–2544

15. Weber MA (2004) New results and analyses expand and modify key interpretations of the ALLHAT Trial. Rev Cardiovasc Med 5:164–169

16. Julius S, Kjeldsen SE, Weber M et al (2004) Outcomes in hypertensive patients at high cardiovascular risk treated with regimens based on valsartan or amlodipine:

the VALUE randomised trial. Lancet 363:2022–2031

17. Angeli F, Verdecchia P, Reboldi GP et al (2004) Calcium channel blockade to prevent stroke in hypertension: a meta-analysis of 13 studies with 103,793 subjects. Am J Hypertens 17:817–822

18. Staessen JA, Wang JG, Thijs L (2003) Cardiovascular prevention and blood pressure reduction: a quantitative overview updated until 1 March 2003. J Hypertens 21:1055–1076

19. Psaty BM, Smith NL, Siscovick DS et al (1997) Health outcomes associated with antihypertensive therapies used as first-line agents. A systematic review and meta-analysis. JAMA 277:739–745

20. Anonymous (1991) Prevention of stroke by antihypertensive drug treatment in older persons with isolated systolic hypertension. Final results of the Systolic Hypertension in the Elderly Program (SHEP) SHEP Cooperative Research Group. JAMA 265:3255–3264

21. Davis BR, Furberg CD, Wright JT Jr et al (2004) ALLHAT: setting the record straight. Ann Intern Med 141:39–46

22. Anonymous (1990) Mortality after 10 1/2 years for hypertensive participants in the Multiple Risk Factor Intervention Trial. Circulation 82:1616–1628

23. Psaty BM, Lumley T, Furberg CD (2004) Meta-analysis of health outcomes of chlorthalidone-based vs nonchlorthalidone-based low-dose diuretic therapies. JAMA 292:43–44

24. Franse LV, Pahor M, Di Bari M et al (2000) Hypokalemia associated with diuretic use and cardiovascular events in the Systolic Hypertension in the Elderly Program. Hypertension 35:1025–1030

25. Verdecchia P, Reboldi G, Angeli F et al (2004) Adverse prognostic significance of new diabetes in treated hypertensive subjects. Hypertension 43:963–969

26. Klingbeil AU, Schneider M, Martus P (2003) A meta-analysis of the effects of treatment on left ventricular mass in essential hypertension. Am J Med 115:41–46

Aspirin and Cardiovascular Prevention in the Guidelines and in the Real World

G. Di Pasquale, P.C. Pavesi, G. Casella

Platelets play a pivotal role in the development and progress of atherosclerotic vascular disease, as well as in the pathogenesis of its unstable clinical manifestations (e.g., unstable angina, non-ST elevation myocardial infarction (MI), ST elevation MI, and stroke) [1].

Therefore, antiplatelet therapy is an integral component in the treatment of patients with atherosclerotic cardiovascular disease, which represents the leading cause of death and disability worldwide.

Aspirin is the cornerstone of oral antiplatelet therapy and is effective for the prevention and treatment of cardiovascular events [2].

The availability and cost-effectiveness of aspirin have made it the most widely employed antiplatelet agent for the prevention and treatment of vascular disease.

Mechanism of Action of Aspirin

Aspirin (acetylsalicylic acid) permanently inactivates by acetylation the activity of prostaglandin (PG) H synthase-1 and PGH synthase-2 (also referred to as COX-1 and COX-2) [3–6].

Platelet COX-1 inhibition leads to the prevention of thromboxane A2 (TXA2) synthesis and impairment of platelet secretion and aggregation. Moreover, since aspirin probably inactivates COX-1 in relatively mature megakaryocytes, and since only 10% of the platelet pool is replaced each day, a once-a-day dose of aspirin is able to maintain a virtually complete inhibition of platelet TXA2 production, despite aspirin's short half-life [7].

In addition, vascular endothelial cells process PGH2 to produce primarily

Division of Cardiology, Maggiore Hospital, Bologna, Italy

prostacyclin (i.e., PGI2), which inhibits platelet aggregation and induces vasodilation [5]. Vascular PGI2 derive both from COX-1, as short-term changes in response to agonist stimulation (e.g. bradykinin [8]), and to a greater extent from COX-2 [9] as long-term changes in response to laminar shear stress [10]. Also, vascular COX-1 is sensitive to transient aspirin inhibition at conventional antiplatelet doses, while vascular COX-2 is largely insensitive to aspirin inhibition at these doses. This may account for the substantial residual COX-2-dependent PGI2 biosynthesis in vivo at daily doses of aspirin between 30 and 100 mg, despite transient suppression of COX-1-dependent PGI2 release [8]. It has never been demonstrated that a more profound suppression of PGI2 formation by higher doses of aspirin may initiate or predispose to thrombosis.

Because aspirin is approximately 50- to 100-fold more potent in inhibiting platelet COX-1 than monocyte COX-2, the inhibition of COX-2-dependent pathophysiological processes (e.g. hyperalgesia and inflammation) requires larger doses of aspirin (because of decreased sensitivity of COX-2 to aspirin) and a much shorter dosing interval (because nucleated cells rapidly resynthesise the enzyme). Thus, there is an approximately 100-fold variation in the daily doses of aspirin when used as an anti-inflammatory rather than as an antiplatelet agent [7].

Aspirin in Secondary and Primary Prevention

The efficacy and safety of aspirin are documented from the analysis of approximately 70 randomised clinical trials that included 115 000 patients representing the whole spectrum of atherosclerosis, from apparently low-risk individuals to patients presenting with acute MI or acute ischaemic stroke.

The length of trials ranges from as short as a few weeks to as long as many years.

Long-term aspirin therapy confers a conclusive net benefit on the risk of subsequent MI, stroke, or vascular death among patients with chronic stable angina [11], patients with prior MI [12], patients with unstable angina [13–16], and patients with TIA or minor stroke [17-22], as well as other high-risk categories [12].

The effects of long-term aspirin therapy on vascular events in these different clinical settings are homogenous, ranging from a 20% to a 25% odds reduction of relative risk, based on an overview of all randomised trials [12].

In terms of absolute benefit, these protective effects of aspirin translate into avoidance of a major vascular event in 50 patients per 1000 patients with unstable angina who had been treated for 6 months, and in 36 patients per 1000 patients with prior MI, stroke, or TIA who had been treated for approximately 30 months [12].

Aspirin has been evaluated in five 'primary' prevention trials [23-28] in approximately 58 000 persons with different cardiovascular risk. All these studies, except the British Doctors' Trial, showed a reduction in the rates of cardiovascular events primarily driven by a reduction in the occurrence of MI [29]. Reductions in the relative risk ranged from 4 to 44%; reductions in the absolute risk ranged from 0.03 to 0.31% per year; and the number of patients who would need to be treated to prevent one MI during 5 years of treatment ranged from 65 to 667. None of the trials showed a reduction in the risk of death from any cause or stroke, although they were not statistically powered for such analyses.

These five primary prevention trials, and a larger number of randomised, controlled trials of secondary prevention, demonstrate that aspirin increases rates of major and minor bleeding. In particular, the rates of major gastrointestinal bleedings are approximately 2 to 4 per 1000 middle-aged persons (4 to 12 per 1000 for older persons) given aspirin for 5 years [30-32].

A meta-analysis of 16 placebo-controlled trials testing aspirin use for cardiac and other indications found that aspirin increased the absolute risk of cerebral haemorrhage by 12 events per 30 000 person-years of follow-up (95% confidence interval, 5 to 20) [33].

Furthermore, these controlled trials in primary and secondary prevention suggest that aspirin increases rates of haemorrhagic strokes by a small amount (0 to 2 per 1000 persons given aspirin for 5 years) [24, 25, 27].

However, such estimates are less reliable than those of gastrointestinal bleedings, because few strokes were reported in these trials.

If one compares the absolute benefits of aspirin in people without clinical manifestation of atherothrombosis (primary prevention), with those achieved in the prevention of MI in patients with chronic stable angina [11], it becomes apparent that the level of cardiovascular risk in the control population (i.e. those receiving placebo) is a major determinant of the absolute benefit of antiplatelet therapy. The results obtained in aspirin trials that have recruited high-risk male and female patients (e.g. the Thrombosis Prevention Trial, the Hypertension Optimal Treatment (HOT) trial [26], and the Primary Prevention Project [28]) clearly demonstrate that proper management of modifiable risk factors by current multifactorial strategies can reduce the actual risk of experiencing a major vascular event to a level at which the additional benefit of aspirin does not clearly outweigh the risk of major bleeding complications.

Additional data assessing the risk/benefit ratio of long-term aspirin prophylaxis in apparently healthy persons are currently being collected by the Women's Health Study, an ongoing trial of low-dose aspirin therapy (100 mg every other day) among 40 000 US female health-care professionals.

Dose of Aspirin in Prevention

Primary and secondary prevention trials have demonstrated benefits with a variety of regimens, including 75 mg/d, 100 mg/d, and 325 mg every other day. There has been no primary-prevention trial to date that has compared different doses of aspirin. However, studies of aspirin dosage and platelet function have suggested that, for the prevention of MI, low doses of aspirin (100 mg per day or less) are adequate. Furthermore, for other clinical purposes, such as the prevention of stroke, low-dose aspirin is just as effective as the high-dose therapy [7] and the risk/benefit profiles of the drug depend on the dose, since its gastrointestinal toxicity is dose-dependent.

Aspirin Resistance

Recently, the issue of aspirin resistance has become relevant in clinical practice. In fact, approximately 5–10% of patients with stable coronary disease do not have a decrease in platelet function when they are given aspirin; these patients with aspirin resistance tend to be older and are more often women and nonsmokers. However, clinical data on the real significance of such a resistance are still controversial; therefore, it is not known whether aspirin resistance predicts a worse overall prognosis or a lack of clinical benefit from aspirin therapy [34].

Current Guidelines

Long-term use of aspirin for the secondary prevention of all forms of coronary artery disease is recommended and consolidated in the guidelines [35], while the issue of primary prevention has been recently updated [36, 37].

National guidelines in the United States have recommended primary prevention with aspirin for patients with a 5-year cardiovascular risk above 3–5% [36, 38]. The risks, particularly for haemorrhagic stroke and gastrointestinal bleeding, may outweigh the benefits in people with a predicted cardiovascular risk below 3%.

Moreover, the prevalence of coronary heart disease varies widely, and is lower in many other countries than in the United States [39]. Therefore, at the population level, the absolute benefit of a preventive therapy in these countries would be less than the benefits observed in the United States [40].

For this reason, not only must the national guidelines consider the prevalence of coronary heart disease in the respective country, but also the likelihood of adverse events, because in some countries the incidence of haemorrhagic stroke may be higher that in the United States, and the risk/benefit ratio of preventive therapies may differ [41].

If a country has a higher prevalence of adverse effects with aspirin, in particular gastrointestinal bleeding or haemorrhagic stroke, the risk/benefit ratio of aspirin may become unfavourable, except in patients with a very high cardiovascular risk. The lack of epidemiological data about these events in many countries limits such comparisons. For example, most epidemiological studies comparing stroke incidence across countries have limited data that differentiate between ischaemic and haemorrhagic stroke [42].

The threshold to recommend aspirin for primary prevention in a country will depend on these risks and the relative prevalence of coronary heart disease. To recommend aspirin for primary prevention, national guidelines in countries with high rates of gastrointestinal bleeding or haemorrhagic stroke should probably modify the U.S. guidelines and use a higher threshold to obtain a favourable risk/benefit profile [40].

For this reason, recent guidelines from the Second Joint Task Force of European and Other Societies on Coronary Prevention emphasise the importance of estimating absolute coronary risk for designing primary-prevention regimens [43]. These guidelines recommend 75 mg of aspirin daily in patients with treated hypertension and in men who are particularly at risk for coronary heart disease [43].

Finally, 1999 guidelines for the management of hypertension from the British Hypertension Society recommend aspirin therapy for primary prevention in hypertensive patients 50 years of age or older who have satisfactory control of their blood pressure (<150/90 mm Hg) and either target-organ damage, diabetes, or a 10-year risk of coronary heart disease of at least 15% [44].

Although the risk/benefit ratio is most favourable in high-risk people (those with a 5-year risk ≥ 3%), certain subgroups could benefit from aspirin in primary prevention.

Hypertension

Although one of the trials on aspirin for the prevention of coronary disease specifically focused on patients with hypertension [26], concern has been expressed that aspirin may be less beneficial [24], or perhaps even dangerous, in patients with high blood pressure. According to a post hoc subgroup analysis [45] in the Thrombosis Prevention Trial [27], aspirin led to a significant reduction in the rate of coronary events among patients with baseline systolic blood pressure of less than 130 mm Hg, but not among those with a baseline systolic blood pressure of more than 145 mm Hg. Although this subgroup analysis must be interpreted cautiously, it suggests that adequate blood-pressure control is particularly critical among patients for whom aspirin is prescribed for the prevention of coronary disease [45].

Diabetes Mellitus

Diabetes mellitus is associated with a risk of fatal coronary heart disease that is as high as the risk associated with a history of MI in patients without diabetes [46]. Whether prophylactic aspirin therapy reduces the risk of coronary events in patients with diabetes has not been systematically studied. In the Physicians' Health Study, aspirin use reduced the risk of MI in patients with diabetes from 10% to 4% during 5 years of follow-up, and no interactions with treatments for diabetes were noted [24]. In the Early Treatment Diabetic Retinopathy Study, a randomised trial involving 3711 patients with diabetes and nonproliferative or early proliferative retinopathy, MI tended to be less frequent among subjects randomly assigned to receive 650 mg of aspirin per day than among those assigned to placebo [47]; aspirin had no effect on the progress of eye disease [48].

Elevated Levels of C-Reactive Protein

In addition to inhibiting thrombosis, aspirin is an anti-inflammatory drug. According to a subgroup analysis in the Physicians' Health Study, the benefit of aspirin was largely confined to men who had elevated levels of C-reactive protein [49]. Further study is needed to determine whether measurement of the level of C-reactive protein would be a better means of identifying appropriate candidates for aspirin therapy [50].

Aspirin Use in the Real World

The issue of aspirin use in the real world is strongly influenced by the clinical setting, which is where we treat the patient.

Of subjects hospitalised due to MI, between 60% [51] and 84% [52] receive aspirin. Similar rates of aspirin use during hospitalisation for unstable angina [53-59] have been noted. Aspirin use has increased over time, with a prominent increase associated [60-62] with the publication in 1988 of the results of the Second International Study of Infarct Survival [63].

After hospitalisation for coronary artery disease, relatively high rates of aspirin use were noted in the British Action on Secondary Prevention through Intervention to Reduce Events (ASPIRE) study (86%) [64] and the European Action on Secondary Prevention through Intervention to Reduce Events (EUROASPIRE) study (81%, which included other antiplatelet medications) [65]. Recently, the BLITZ survey, which enrolled patients with acute MI admitted to Italian Coronary Care Units, also confirmed the very high rate of aspirin use at discharge [52]. However, the Euro Heart Survey of

Acute Coronary Syndromes demonstrates that a substantial proportion of patients did not receive aspirin at discharge (11.5–16.9%), only partially explained by the widespread use of anticoagulation agents or the other antiplatelet agents, such as ticlopidine and clopidogrel [59].

On the other hand, aspirin use in outpatients is less likely than in hospitalised or recently hospitalised patients. In the Scandinavian Simvastatin Survival Study (4S), only 37% of randomised patients had been receiving aspirin [66]. In the Atherosclerosis Risk in Communities (ARIC) study, aspirin use was noted in 53% of patients with a history of MI and in 30% of those with a history of angina [67]. Among the patients of general practitioners in London, only 48% of those with coronary artery disease used aspirin [68]. Finally, aspirin use was noted in 63% of patients with coronary artery disease who were seen by Scottish general practitioners [69].

In the United States, aspirin use in outpatients increased from 1980 to 1996, but the magnitude of this increase was less than expected, and aspirin use in patients with coronary artery disease has not yet become a widely disseminated practice [70].

The results of these studies suggest that aspirin use in patients with coronary artery disease is less frequent than desirable, particularly in community settings. Because outpatients represent the majority of all patients with coronary artery disease, the overall impact of secondary prevention efforts are as yet suboptimal.

In primary prevention, the first steps in deciding whether to consider aspirin are the assessment of the 5-year risk for that individual of developing a cardiovascular event and the assessment of the relative potential harm. The decision to use aspirin should be based on the risk/benefit ratio at the patient level [38]. In the United States, the 5-year cardiovascular risk may be estimated through the Framingham risk score [50].

In countries outside the United States, where a lower prevalence of coronary heart disease is expected [71], cardiovascular risk assessment using the Framingham risk score may overestimate the risk. To overcome this problem, country-appropriate risk factor algorithms, like the new Italian risk prediction system, should be used (http://www.ministerosalute.it/).

Conclusions and Recommendations

Aspirin use in patients with coronary artery disease is less frequent than desirable, particularly in community settings. The low use of aspirin in these settings may result from the less-intense clinical attention received by outpatients as compared with hospitalised patients.

Practices in community settings, however, are likely to better represent the overall impact of secondary prevention efforts because hospitalised patients represent only a small proportion of all patients.

Therefore, despite substantial increases in aspirin use, patterns of use in secondary prevention remain suboptimal.

The decision to initiate aspirin therapy in primary prevention should be based on a careful assessment of absolute risk. Before advising aspirin for primary prevention, physicians must assess the patient's 5-year cardiovascular risk and compare it with the likelihood of adverse effects. The risk/benefit ratio should be re-assessed at least once every 3–5 years, since it might well increase to a point at which aspirin therapy would be appropriate.

References

1. Fuster V, Badimon L, Badimon JJ et al (1992) The pathogenesis of coronary artery disease and the acute coronary syndromes. N Engl J Med 326:242–250
2. Fuster V, Badimon L, Badimon JJ et al (1992) The pathogenesis of coronary artery disease and the acute coronary syndromes. N Engl J Med 326:310 –318
3. Roth GJ, Majerus PW (1975) The mechanism of the effect of aspirin on human platelets: I. Acetylation of a particulate fraction protein. J Clin Invest 56:624–632
4. Roth GJ, Stanford N, Majerus PW (1975) Acetylation of prostaglandin synthase by aspirin. Proc Natl Acad Sci USA 72:3073–3077
5. Majerus PW (1983) Arachidonate metabolism in vascular disorders. J Clin Invest 72:1521–1525
6. Smith WL, Garavito RM, DeWitt DL (1996) Prostaglandin endoperoxide H synthases (cyclooxygenases)-1 and -2. J Biol Chem 271:33157–33160
7. Cipollone F, Patrignani P, Greco A et al (1997) Differential suppression of thromboxane biosynthesis by indobufen and aspirin in patients with unstable angina. Circulation 96:1109–1116
8. Clarke RJ, Mayo G, Price P et al (1991) Suppression of thromboxane A2 but not systemic prostacyclin by controlled release aspirin. N Engl J Med 325:1137–1141
9. McAdam BF, Catella–Lawson F, Mardini IA et al (1999) Systemic biosynthesis of prostacyclin by cyclooxygenase (COX)–2: the human pharmacology of a selective inhibitor of COX–2. Proc Natl Acad Sci USA 96:272–277
10. Topper JN, Cai J, Falb D et al (1996) Identification of vascular endothelial genes differentially responsive to fluid mechanical stimuli: cyclooxygenase–2, manganese superoxide dismutase, and endothelial cell nitric oxide synthase are selectively up–regulated by steady laminar shear stress. Proc Natl Acad Sci USA 93:10417–10422
11. Juul–Moller S, Edvardsson N, Jahnmatz B et al (1992) Double–blind trial of aspirin in primary prevention of myocardial infarction in patients with stable chronic angina pectoris. Lancet 340:1421–1425
12. Antithrombotic Trialists Collaboration (2002) Collaborative metaanalysis of randomised trials of antiplatelet therapy for prevention of death, myocardial infarction, and stroke in high–risk patients. Br Med J 324:71–86
13. RISC Group (1990) Risk of myocardial infarction and death during treatment with low dose aspirin and intravenous heparin in men with unstable coronary artery disease. Lancet 336:827–830

14. Lewis HD, Davis JW, Archibald DG et al (1983) Protective effects of aspirin against acute myocardial infarction and death in men with unstable angina: results of a Veterans Administration cooperative study. N Engl J Med 309:396–403

15. Theroux P, Ouimet H, McCans J et al (1988) Aspirin, heparin, or both to treat acute unstable angina. N Engl J Med 319:1105–1111

16. Cairns JA, Gent M, Singer J et al (1985) Aspirin, sulfinpyrazone, or both in unstable angina. N Engl J Med 313:1369–1375

17. SALT Collaborative Group (1991) Swedish Aspirin Low–Dose Trial (SALT) of 75 mg aspirin as secondary prophylaxis after cerebrovascular ischaemic events. Lancet 338:1345–1491

18. Diener HC, Cunha L, Forbes C et al (1996) European Stroke Prevention Study: II. Dipyridamole and acetylsalicylic acid in the secondary prevention of stroke. J Neurol Sci 143:1–13

19. Farrel B, Godwin J, Richards S et al (1991) The United Kingdom transient ischae-mic attack (UK–TIA) aspirin trial: final results. J Neurol Neurosurg Psychiatry 54:1044–1054

20. Bousser MG, Eschwege E, Haugenau M et al (1983) 'AICLA' controlled trial of aspi-rin and dipyridamole in the secondary prevention of athero–thrombotic cerebral ischemia. Stroke 14:5–14

21. Canadian Cooperative Study Group (1978) A randomized trial of aspirin and sul-finpyrazone in threatened stroke. N Engl J Med 299:53–59

22. Fields WS, Lemak NA, Frankowski RF et al (1977) Controlled trial of aspirin in cerebral ischemia. Stroke 8:301–314

23. Juul–Moller S, Edvardsson N, Jahnmatz B et al (1992) Doubleblind trial of aspirin in primary prevention of myocardial infarction in patients with stable chronic angina pectoris. Lancet 340:1421–1425

24. Steering Committee of the Physicians' Health Study Research Group (1989) Final report on the aspirin component of the ongoing Physicians' Health Study. N Engl J Med 321:129–135

25. Peto R, Gray R, Collins R et al (1988) Randomised trial of prophylactic daily aspirin in British male doctors. Br Med J 296:313–316

26. Hansson L, Zanchetti A, Carruthers SG et al (1998) Effects of intensive blood–pres-sure lowering and low–dose aspirin in patients with hypertension: principal results of the Hypertension Optimal Treatment (HOT) randomised trial. Lancet 351:1755–1762

27. The Medical Research Council's General Practice Research Framework (1998) Thrombosis Prevention Trial: randomised trial of low–intensity oral anticoagula-tion with warfarin and lowdose aspirin in the primary prevention of ischemic heart disease in men at increased risk. Lancet 351:233–241

28. Collaborative Group of the Primary Prevention Project (PPP) (2001) Low–dose aspirin and vitamin E in people at cardiovascular risk: a randomised trial in gene-ral practice. Lancet 357:89–95

29. Sanmuganathan PS, Ghahramani P, Jackson PR et al (2001) Aspirin for primary prevention of coronary heart disease: safety and absolute benefit related to coro-nary risk derived from meta–analysis of randomised trials. Heart 85:265–271

30. Roderick PJ, Wilkes HC, Meade TW (1993) The gastrointestinal toxicity of aspirin: an overview of randomised controlled trials. Br J Clin Pharmacol 35: 219–226.

31. Dickinson JP, Prentice CR (1998) Aspirin: benefit and risk in thromboprophylaxis. QJM 91:523–538.

32. Stalnikowicz–Darvasi R (1995) Gastrointestinal bleeding during low–dose aspirin administration for prevention of arterial occlusive events. A critical analysis. J Clin

Gastroenterol 21:13–16

33. He J, Whelton PK, Vu B et al (1998) Aspirin and risk of hemorrhagic stroke: a meta–analysis of randomized controlled trials. JAMA 280:1930–1935

34. Patrono C (2003) Aspirin resistance: definition, mechanisms and clinical read–outs. J Thromb Haemost 1:1710–1713

35. Hennekens CH, Dyken ML, Fuster V (1997) Aspirin as a therapeutic agent in cardiovascular disease: a statement for healthcare professionals from the American Heart Association. Circulation 96: 2751–2753

36. Pearson TA, Blair SN, Daniels SR et al (2002) AHA guidelines for primary prevention of cardiovascular disease and stroke: 2002 update; consensus panel guide to comprehensive risk reduction for adult patients without coronary or other atherosclerotic vascular diseases. Circulation 106:388–391

37. Patrono C, Coller B, FitzGerald GA et al (2004) Platelet–Active Drugs: The Relationships Among Dose, Effectiveness, and Side Effects. The Seventh ACCP Conference on Antithrombotic and Thrombolytic Therapy. Chest 126:S234–S264

38. Aspirin for the primary prevention of cardiovascular events: recommendation and rationale. Ann Intern Med. 2002;136:157–160

39. Murray CJ, Lopez AD (1997) Mortality by cause for eight regions of the world: Global Burden of Disease Study. Lancet 349:1269– 1276

40. Morimoto T, Fukui T, Lee TH et al (2004) Application of U.S. Guidelines in Other Countries: Aspirin for the Primary Prevention of Cardiovascular Events in Japan. Am J Med 117:459–468

41. Rodondi N, Bauer DC (2004) Assessing the risk/benefit profile before recommending Aspirin for the primary prevention of cardiovascular events. Am J Med 117:528 –530

42. Thorvaldsen P, Asplund K, Kuulasmaa K et al (1995) Stroke incidence, case fatality, and mortality in the WHO MONICA project. World Health Organization Monitoring Trends and Determinants in Cardiovascular Disease. Stroke 26: 361–367

43. Wood D, De Backer G, Faergeman O et al (1998) Prevention of coronary heart disease in clinical practice: recommendations of the Second Joint Task Force of European and Other Societies on Coronary Prevention. Atherosclerosis 140:199–270

44. Ramsay LE, Williams B, Johnston GD et al (1999) British Hypertension Society guidelines for hypertension management 1999: summary. Br Med J 319:630–635

45. Meade TW, Brennan PJ (2000) Determination of who may derive most benefit from aspirin in primary prevention: subgroup results from a randomised controlled trial. Br Med J 321:13–17

46. Haffner SM, Lehto S, Rönnemaa T et al (1998) Mortality from coronary heart disease in subjects with type 2 diabetes and in nondiabetic subjects with and without prior myocardial infarction. N Engl J Med 339:229–234

47. Anonymous (1992) Aspirin effects on mortality and morbidity in patients with diabetes mellitus: Early Treatment Diabetic Retinopathy Study report 14. JAMA 268:1292–1300

48. Anonymous (1991) Effects of aspirin treatment on diabetic retinopathy: ETDRS report number 8. Ophthalmology 98(5 Suppl):757–765

49. Ridker PM, Cushman M, Stampfer MJ et al (1997) Inflammation, aspirin, and the risk of cardiovascular disease in apparently healthy men. N Engl J Med 336:973–979

50. Executive summary of the Third report of the National Cholesterol Education

Program (NCEP) (2001) Expert Panel on Detection, Evaluation, and Treatment of High Blood Cholesterol in Adults (Adult Treatment Panel III). JAMA 285:2486–2497

51. Ayanian JZ, Guadagnoli E, McNeil BJ et al (1997) Treatment and outcomes of acute myocardial infarction among patients of cardiologists and generalist physicians. Arch Intern Med 157: 2570 –2576

52. Di Chiara A, Chiarella F, Savonitto S et al. (2003) Epidemiology of acute myocardial infarction in the Italian CCU network. The BLITZ Study. Eur Heart J 24:1616–1629

53. Krumholz HM, Philbin DM Jr, Wang Y et al (1998) Trends in the quality of care for Medicare beneficiaries admitted to the hospital with unstable angina. J Am Coll Cardiol 31:957–963

54. Giugliano RP, Camargo CA Jr, Lloyd–Jones DM et al (1998) Elderly patients receive less aggressive medical and invasive management of unstable angina: potential impact of practice guidelines. Arch Intern Med 158:1113–1120

55. Maggioni AP, Schweiger C, Tavazzi L et al (2000) Epidemiologic study of use of resources in patients with unstable angina: the EARISA registry. On behalf on the EARISA Investigators (Epidemiologia dell'Assorbimento di Risorse nell'Ischemia, Scompenso e Angina). Am Heart J 140:253–263

56. RIKS–HIA (Register of Information and Knowledge about Swedish Heart Intensive care Admissions) a national quality register. (http://www.riks–hia.c.se/index.html). Accessed 4 January 2005

57. Fox KA, Cokkinos DV, Deckers J et al (2000) The ENACT study: a pan–European survey of acute coronary syndromes. European Network for Acute Coronary Treatment. Eur Heart J 21:1440–1449

58. Collinson J, Flather MD, Fox KA et al (2000) Clinical outcomes, risk stratification and practice patterns of unstable angina and myocardial infarction without ST elevation: Prospective Registry of Acute Ischaemic Syndromes in the UK (PRAIS–UK). Eur Heart J 21:1450–1457

59. Hasdai D, Behar S, Wallentin L et al (2002) A prospective survey of the characteristics, treatments and outcomes of patients with acute coronary syndromes in Europe and the Mediterranean basin; the Euro Heart Survey of Acute Coronary Syndromes (Euro Heart Survey ACS). Eur Heart J 23:1190–1201

60. Lamas GA, Pfeffer MA, Hamm P et al (1992) Do the results of randomized clinical trials of cardiovascular drugs influence medical practice? N Engl J Med 327:241–247

61. Pagley PR, Yarzebski J, Goldberg R et al (1993) Gender differences in the treatment of patients with acute myocardial infarction: a multihospital, community–based perspective. Arch Intern Med 153:625–629

62. Col NF, McLaughlin TJ, Soumerai SB et al (1996) The impact of clinical trials on the use of medications for acute myocardial infarction: results of a community–based study. Arch Intern Med 156:54–60

63. Second International Study of Infarct Survival (ISIS–2) Collaborative Group (1988) Randomised trial of intravenous streptokinase, oral aspirin, both, or neither among 17,187 cases of suspected acute myocardial infarction. Lancet 2:349–360

64. Bowker TJ, Clayton TC, Ingham J et al (1996) A British Cardiac Society survey of the potential for the secondary prevention of coronary disease: ASPIRE (Action on Secondary Prevention through Intervention to Reduce Events). Heart 75:334–342

65. EUROASPIRE Study Group (1997) A European Society of Cardiology survey of secondary prevention of coronary heart disease: principal results. Eur Heart J 18:1569–1582

66. Scandinavian Simvastatin Survival Study Group (1994) Randomised trial of cholesterol lowering in 4444 patients with coronary heart disease: the Scandinavian Simvastatin Survival Study (4S). Lancet 344:1383–1389

67. Shahar E, Folsom AR, Romm FJ et al (1996) Patterns of aspirin use in middle–aged adults: the Atherosclerosis Risk in Communities (ARIC) Study. Am Heart J 131:915–922

68. McCartney P, Macdowall W, Thorogood M (1997) A randomised controlled trial of feedback to general practitioners of their prophylactic aspirin prescribing. Br Med J 315:35–36

69. Campbell NC, Thain J, Deans HG et al (1998) Secondary prevention in coronary heart disease: baseline survey of provision in general practice. Br Med J 316:1430–1434

70. Stafford RS (2000) Aspirin use is low among United States outpatients with coronary artery disease. Circulation 101:1097–1101

71. Liu J, Hong Y, D'Agostino RB Sr et al (2004) Predictive value for the Chinese population of the Framingham CHD risk assessment tool compared with the Chinese Multi–provincial Cohort Study. JAMA 291:2591–2599

Serial Changes in Left Ventricular Mass in Hypertension: Prognostic Impact

P. Verdecchia, F. Angeli, M.G. Sardone, R. Gattobigio

Introduction

Among the several adverse changes in cardiovascular morphology and function that may occur in hypertension, increased left ventricular (LV) mass is of the utmost importance. Increased LV mass is a major predictor of cardiac and cerebrovascular events independently of the traditional cardiovascular risk factors such as blood pressure, diabetes, cholesterol levels, and smoking status [1–5]. The prevalence of ventricular arrhythmias is also substantially higher in hypertensive patients with LV hypertrophy than in those with no evidence of cardiac remodelling [6–8].

Although the mechanisms of the association between LV mass and prognosis are not completely clear, LV mass is generally considered a biological assay that reflects and integrates the long-term cumulative effect of several risk factors for cardiovascular disease.

LV hypertrophy can be schematically divided into three main types: concentric, eccentric, and asymmetric. Longitudinal studies have suggested that the definition of LV geometry may be used to refine cardiovascular risk stratification in hypertensive subjects [9–13]. Such studies have found that, overall, the risk of developing cardiovascular disease was greater in patients with concentric remodelling than in those with normal LV geometry, and greater in patients with concentric LV hypertrophy than in those with eccentric LV hypertrophy [10–13]. However, since LV mass was greater in subjects with concentric remodelling than in those with normal geometry, and also greater in subjects with concentric LV hypertrophy than in those with eccentric LV hypertrophy, the independent prognostic impact of LV geometry was reduced or abolished completely due to the overwhelming prognostic value of the LV mass itself [9–13].

Ospedale R. Silvestrini, Dipartimento Malattie Cardiovascolari, Perugia, Italy

Regression of LV Hypertrophy

The Framingham Heart Study [14] has shown that subjects with electrocardiographic (ECG) evidence of LV hypertrophy at entry and serial increase in the ECG voltages over time are twice as likely to suffer a major cardiovascular event over the subsequent years as are those with serial decrease in the voltages. Moreover, in the Heart Outcomes Prevention Evaluation (HOPE) study [15], the primary study end-point (cardiovascular death, myocardial infarction, or stroke) occurred in 12.3% of subjects with absence or regression of LV hypertrophy during the study, compared with 15.8% of subjects with new development or persistence of LV hypertrophy over the same time.

In the PIUMA study (Progetto Ipertensione Umbria Monitoraggio Ambulatoriale) [16], the rate of cardiovascular events was higher in patients who had not achieved regression of LV hypertrophy compared with those with persistently normal LV mass. Event rates did not differ between the group with regression of LV hypertrophy and the group with persistently normal LV mass.

The mechanisms by which serial changes in LV mass parallel the risk of major cardiovascular events in hypertensive subjects are still elusive. There is abundant evidence that several factors may induce parallel changes in LV mass and atherosclerotic lesions. Elevated blood pressure (BP) stimulates both LV hypertrophy [17, 18] and atherosclerosis [19]. In hypertensive subjects, LV mass and intima–media thickness seem to progress in parallel, generally in association with BP [20, 21]. Several non-haemodynamic factors may influence LV mass and atherosclerosis, such as insulin and insulin growth factors [22–27]. Furthermore, angiotensin II promotes the activation of intracellular reactions, which may lead both to cardiac hypertrophy [28–30] and progression of atherosclerotic lesions [31] through proliferation of vascular smooth muscle cells and production of extracellular matrix protein [31]. AT1-receptor activation also play a well-established role in the pathogenesis of atherosclerosis [32, 33]. Endothelin, a potent vasoconstrictor, stimulates both vascular cell migration and growth [34, 35] and cardiac muscle hypertrophy [36]. Studies have also reported that HDL cholesterol, a powerful determinant of atherosclerosis, shows an inverse association, independent of BP, with LV mass [37, 38]. In hypertensive subjects, plasma viscosity has been associated with both LV hypertrophy [39] and increased intima–media thickness [40].

The above considerations support the hypothesis that serial changes in LV mass in treated hypertensive subjects may reflect the long-term level of activity of several haemodynamic and non-haemodynamic factors potentially active on atherosclerosis. On the one hand, the favourable prognostic impact of regression of LV hypertrophy might reflect slower progression of atherosclerosis because of blunting of a variety of mechanisms not limited to BP overload. On the other hand, lack of regression of LV hypertrophy may be a marker of more advanced progression of atherosclerosis.

Serial Changes in LV Mass and Antihypertensive Treatment

Experimental studies [41, 42] suggested that afterload reduction is the main mechanism leading to a reduction in myocyte volume, while inhibition of the renin–angiotensin–aldosterone system is most effective in reducing interstitial enlargement and improving diastolic filling.

In patients with hypertensive LV hypertrophy, regression of hypertrophy is usually associated with reduction in BP [43, 44]. In clinical trials, as in everyday practice, it is difficult to establish whether a given antihypertensive drug is superior to another in inducing regression of LV hypertrophy. This is because hypertensive subjects often have to combine several drugs with different mechanisms of action in order to achieve adequate BP control. Subjects with LV hypertrophy, who generally have higher BP than those without, also frequently need treatment with multiple drugs. As a result, the merit of LV hypertrophy regression cannot really be attributed with any certainty to any specific drug class in clinical trials [45]. However, whatever the differences between antihypertensive drugs in the degree of regression of LV hypertrophy, systolic BP is the major determinant of the development and regression of LV hypertrophy in subjects with essential hypertension.

A recent analysis of the PIUMA study [46] showed that the degree of reduction in LV mass during treatment is associated more closely with the reduction in 24-h ambulatory systolic BP than with that in clinical BP, probably because 24-h ambulatory systolic BP better reflects the BP load to which the left ventricle is chronically exposed. The fundamental role of systolic BP in the basic mechanisms leading to LV hypertrophy is supported by several experimental data. The immediate cardiac consequence of a rise in SBP is an increase in end-systolic wall stress that triggers cellular reactions, ultimately leading to an increase in the volume of each cardiac myocyte. This process is mostly due to addition of sarcomeres in parallel, and the resulting increase in the cardiac mass tends to progressively normalise end-systolic wall stress. This pattern is typical of prevalent or near-pure pressure overload states such as hypertension and aortic stenosis.

Overview

A recent meta-analysis [47] of studies which were quite small in size, but similar in their design and experimental procedures, investigated the prognostic impact of serial changes in LV mass. In all these studies, hypertensive subjects were examined by echocardiography before and during antihypertensive treatment, before occurrence of major cardiovascular events. Patients were subsequently followed up for a further period of several years in order to establish the association between prior changes in LV mass and subsequent events. Overall, these studies included 1064 hypertensive subjects (41% women) aged 45–51 years, and 106 cardiovascular events. The echocardiographic study was carried out before the beginning of treatment and after 3–10 years of follow-up. Compared to subjects with lack of regression or new development of LV hypertrophy, those who achieved regression of LV hypertrophy showed a 59% lower risk of subsequent cardiovascular disease [95% confidence interval (CI): 22–79; $P = 0.007$]. The lower risk of events associated with regression of LV hypertrophy was consistent across the individual studies. Compared to subjects with regression of LV hypertrophy, those with persistently normal LV mass showed a similar risk of subsequent events (odds ratio 0.64, 95% CI: 0.31–1.30; $P = 0.21$). Since the event risk was 36% lower among the subjects who never experienced LV hypertrophy compared to those with regression and the confidence intervals were wide, our study could not provide conclusive evidence that regression of LV hypertrophy reduces the risk of subsequent events to the same level as that of subjects who never experienced LV hypertrophy (Fig. 1).

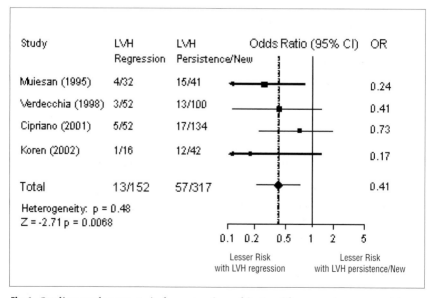

Fig. 1. Cardiovascular events in hypertensive subjects with regression vs. persistence or new development of left ventricular hypertrophy (data from [47])

References

1. Levy D, Garrison RJ, Savage DD et al (1990) Prognostic implications of echocardiographically determined left ventricular mass in the Framingham Heart Study. N Engl J Med 322:1561–1566
2. Verdecchia P, Porcellati C, Reboldi G et al (2001) Left ventricular hypertrophy as an independent predictor of acute cerebrovascular events in essential hypertension. Circulation 104:2039–2044
3. Kannel WB (1983) Prevalence and natural history of electrocardiographic left ventricular hypertrophy. Am J Med 75:4–11
4. Ghali JK, Liao Y, Simmons B (1992) The prognostic role of left ventricular hypertrophy in patients with or without coronary artery disease. Ann Intern Med 117:831–836
5. Koren MJ, Devereux RB, Casale PN et al (1991) Relation of left ventricular mass and geometry to morbidity and mortality in uncomplicated essential hypertension. Ann Intern Med 114:345–352
6. Messerli FH, Ventura HO, Elizardi DJ et al (1984) Hypertension and sudden death. Increased ventricular ectopic activity in left ventricular hypertrophy. Am J Med 77:18–22
7. McLenachan JM, Henderson E, Morris KI et al (1987) Ventricular arrhythmias in patients with hypertensive left ventricular hypertrophy. N Engl J Med 317:787–792
8. Haider AW, Larson MG, Benjamin EJ et al (1998) Increased left ventricular mass and hypertrophy are associated with increased risk for sudden death. J Am Coll Cardiol 32:1454–1459
9. Koren MJ, Devereux RB, Casale PN et al (1991) Relation of left ventricular mass and geometry to morbidity and mortality in uncomplicated essential hypertension. Ann Intern Med 114:345–352
10. Verdecchia P, Schillaci G, Borgioni C et al (1995) Adverse prognostic significance of concentric remodeling of the left ventricle in hypertensive subjects with normal left ventricular mass. J Am Coll Cardiol 25:871–878
11. Verdecchia P, Schillaci G, Borgioni C et al (1996) Prognostic value of left ventricular mass and geometry in systemic hypertension with left ventricular hypertrophy. Am J Cardiol 78:197–202
12. Krumholz HM, Larson M, Levy D (1995) Prognosis of left ventricular geometric patterns in the Framingham Heart Study. J Am Coll Cardiol 25:879–884
13. Ghali JK, Liao Y, Cooper RS (1998) Influence of left ventricular geometric patterns on prognosis in patients with or without coronary artery disease. J Am Coll Cardiol 31:1635–1640
14. Levy D, Salomon M, D'Agostino RB et al (1994) Prognostic implications of baseline electrocardiographic features and their serial changes in subjects with left ventricular hypertrophy. Circulation 90:1786–1793
15. Mathew J, Sleight P, Lonn E et al (2001) Reduction of cardiovascular risk by regression of electrocardiographic markers of left ventricular hypertrophy by the angiotensin-converting enzyme inhibitor ramipril. Circulation 104:1615–1621
16. Verdecchia P, Schillaci G, Borgioni C et al (1998) Prognostic significance of serial changes in left ventricular mass in essential hypertension. Circulation 97:48–54
17. Grossman W, Jones D, McLaurin LP (1975) Wall stress and patterns of hypertrophy in the human left ventricle. J Clin Invest 56:56–64
18. Ganau A, Devereux RB, Pickering TG et al (1990) Relation of left ventricular hemodynamic load and contractile performance to left ventricular mass in hyper-

tension. Circulation 81:25–36

19. Young W, Gofman JW, Tandy R (1960) The quantitation of atherosclerosis. Quantitative aspects of the relationship of blood pressure and atherosclerosis. Am J Cardiol 6:294–299

20. Roman MJ, Saba PS, Pini R et al (1992) Parallel cardiac and vascular adaptation in hypertension. Circulation 86:1909–1918

21. Khattar RS, Senior R, Swales JD et al (1999) Value of ambulatory intra-arterial blood pressure monitoring in the long-term prediction of left ventricular hypertrophy and carotid atherosclerosis in essential hypertension. J Hum Hypertens 13:111–116

22. Ito H, Hiroe M, Hirata Y et al (1993) Insulin-like growth factor-I induces cardiac hypertrophy with enhanced expression of muscle-specific genes in cultured rat cardiomyocytes. Circulation 87:1715–1721

23. Diez J, Laviades C, Martinez E et al (1995) Insulin-like growth factor binding proteins in arterial hypertension: relationship to left ventricular hypertrophy. J Hypertens 13:349–355

24. Verdecchia P, Reboldi G, Schillaci G et al (1999) Circulating insulin and insulin growth factor-1 are independent determinants of left ventricular mass and geometry in essential hypertension. Circulation 100:1802–1807

25. Rajala U, Laakso M, Paivansalo M et al (2002) Low insulin sensitivity measured by both quantitative insulin sensitivity check index and homeostasis model assessment method as a risk factor of increased intima-media thickness of the carotid artery. J Clin Endocrinol Metab 87:5092–5097

26. Urbina EM, Srinivasan SR, Tang R et al for The Bogalusa Heart Study (2002) Impact of multiple coronary risk factors on the intima-media thickness of different segments of carotid artery in healthy young adults (The Bogalusa Heart Study). Am J Cardiol 90:953–958

27. Watanabe S, Okura T, Kitami Y et al (2002) Carotid hemodynamic alterations in hypertensive patients with insulin resistance. Am J Hypertens 15:851–856

28. Dzau, VJ (1993) Tissue renin-angiotensin system in myocardial hypertrophy and failure. Arch Intern Med 153:937–942

29. Sadoshima J, Xu Y, Slayter HS et al (1993) Autocrine release of angiotensin II mediates stretch-induced hypertrophy of cardiac muscle in vitro. Cell 75:977–984

30. Sadoshima J, Izumo S (1993) Molecular characterization of angiotensin II-induced hypertrophy of cardiac myocytes and hyperplasia of cardiac fibroblasts. Critical role of the AT1 receptor subtype. Circ Res 73:413–423

31. Daugherty A, Manning MW, Cassis LA (2000) Angiotensin II promotes atherosclerotic lesions and aneurysms in apolipoprotein E-deficient mice. J Clin Invest 105:1605–1612

32. Nickenig G (2002) Central role of the AT(1)-receptor in atherosclerosis. J Hum Hypertens 16 (suppl 3):S26–S33

33. Weiss D, Kools JJ, Taylor WR (2001) Angiotensin II-induced hypertension accelerates the development of atherosclerosis in apoE-deficient mice. Circulation 103:448–454

34. Lerman A, Edwards BS, Hallett JW et al (1991) Circulating and tissue endothelin immunoreactivity in advanced atherosclerosis. N Engl J Med 325:997–1001

35. Ihling C, Szombathy T, Bohrmann B et al (2001) Coexpression of endothelin-converting enzyme-1 and endothelin-1 in different stages of human atherosclerosis. Circulation 104:864–869

36. Ichikawa KI, Hidai C, Okuda C et al (1996) Endogenous endothelin-1 mediates car-

diac hypertrophy and switching of myosin heavy chain gene expression in rat ventricular myocardium. J Am Coll Cardiol 27:1286–1291

37. Jullien V, Gosse P, Ansoborlo P et al (1998) Relationship between left ventricular mass and serum cholesterol level in the untreated hypertensive. J Hypertens 16:1043–1047

38. Schillaci G, Vaudo G, Reboldi G et al (2001) High-density lipoprotein cholesterol and left ventricular hypertrophy in essential hypertension. J Hypertens 19:2265–2270

39. Devereux RB, Drayer JI, Chien S et al (1984) Whole blood viscosity as a determinant of cardiac hypertrophy in systemic hypertension. Am J Cardiol 54:592–595

40. Levenson J, Gariepy J, Del-Pino M et al (2000) Association of plasma viscosity and carotid thickening in a French working cohort. Am J Hypertens 13:753–758

41. Brilla CG, Funck RC, Rupp H (2000) Lisinopril-mediated regression of myocardial fibrosis in patients with hypertensive heart disease. Circulation 102:1388–1393

42. Böcker W, Hupf H, Grimm D (2000) Effects of indapamide on regression of pressure overload hypertrophy in rat hearts. J Hypertens 18(suppl 4):S1–S8

43. Devereux RB, Palmieri V, Liu JE et al (2002) Progressive hypertrophy regression with sustained pressure reduction in hypertension: the Losartan Intervention For Endpoint Reduction study. J Hypertens 20:1445–1450

44. Fagard RH, Staessen JA, Thijs L (1997) Relationship between changes in left ventricular mass and in clinic and ambulatory pressure in response to antihypertensive therapy. J Hypertens 15:1493–1502

45. Devereux RB (1997) Do antihypertensive drugs differ in their ability to regress left ventricular hypertrophy? Circulation 95:1983–1985

46. Verdecchia P, Angeli F, Gattobigio R et al (2004) Does the reduction in systolic blood pressure alone explain the regression of left ventricular hypertrophy? J Hum Hypertens 1:1–6

47. Verdecchia P, Angeli F, Borgioni C et al (2003) Changes in cardiovascular risk by reduction of left ventricular mass in hypertension: a meta-analysis. Am J Hypertens 16:895–899

ATRIAL FIBRILLATION:
THE ACTUAL CLINICAL APPROACH

New Approach in the Prevention of Atrial Fibrillation: Role of Angiotensin II Antagonists

P. Verdecchia, F. Angeli, M. G. Sardone, R. Gattobigio

Introduction

Atrial fibrillation (AF) is a common cardiac disorder that may lead to significant morbidity and mortality. Its incidence in the general population is increasing; projections in the US population suggest that more than 5.6 million Americans (50% of whom will be 80 years of age or more) will have AF by the year 2050 [1, 2].

Although much remains to be known about the basic pathophysiological mechanisms underlying the disorder, several clinical factors have been identified as potential predictors of AF. The most important risk factors for AF are age, male sex, hypertension, thyrotoxicosis, smoking, diabetes, left ventricular (LV) hypertrophy, left atrial enlargement, valvular and coronary heart disease, congestive heart failure, and stroke. In the Framingham Heart Study, hypertension and diabetes were the sole cardiovascular risk factors to be predictive of AF after controlling for age and other predisposing conditions. The role of hypertension as risk factor for AF is established but still incompletely known. In the Manitoba follow-up study, the prevalence of hypertension was 53% and the risk of AF was 1.42 times higher in hypertensive subjects than in normotensives [2]. Because of its high prevalence in the population, hypertension independently accounts for more AF cases than any other risk factor. However, despite its leading importance as a highly prevalent and modifiable risk factor, few data are available regarding predictors and outcome of AF in large populations of subjects with essential hypertension free of coexisting valvular or coronary heart disease, congestive heart failure, hyperthyroidism, or other predisposing conditions.

Ospedale R. Silvestrini, Dipartimento Malattie Cardiovascolari, Perugia, Italy

Predictors and Outcome of Atrial Fibrillation

Among the general population, congestive heart failure and rheumatic heart disease are the most powerful predictive precursors of AF, with relative risks in excess of about six-fold [3–5]. Data from the Framingham Heart Study suggest that another predictor of AF is hypertensive heart disease, which usually is the most common antecedent disease, largely because of its frequency in the general population [4]. Among the common risk factors for cardiovascular disease, diabetes and ECG evidence of left ventricular hypertrophy (LVH) are related to the occurrence of AF [6].

Recently, an analysis of the PIUMA study (*Progetto Ipertensione Umbria Monitoraggio Ambulatoriale*) identified some predictors and outcome of AF in large populations of subjects with essential hypertension who were free of coexisting valvular or coronary heart disease, congestive heart failure, or hyperthyroidism at entry into the registry [7]. Overall, 2482 initially untreated subjects in sinus rhythm were followed for up to 16 years. Age and LV mass at echocardiography were the sole independent predictors of AF. Age, LV mass, and left atrial diameter were independent predictors of chronic AF (Fig. 1).

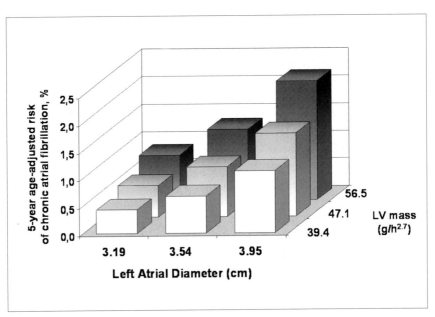

Fig. 1. Five-year age-adjusted risk of chronic atrial fibrillation in hypertension (data from the PIUMA study) according to left atrial diameter and left ventricular mass

One of the fundamental clinical complications of AF is thromboembolic stroke. In the PIUMA study, during a mean follow-up of 6 years an ischaemic stroke occurred in 12.1% of hypertensive subjects with paroxysmal and 30% of hypertensive subjects with chronic AF [7]. Notably, none of the subjects who were receiving warfarin experienced stroke during the course of the follow-up.

These data underline the clinical usefulness of LV mass and atrial diameter as detected by echocardiography to identify the subset of hypertensive subjects who are at increased risk of developing AF and its chronicisation. In agreement with data from randomised studies, the PIUMA results suggest a more liberal use of warfarin for prevention of stroke in hypertensive subjects with chronic and perhaps paroxysmal AF. Interestingly, recent evidence suggests that anticoagulation with warfarin is the only therapy with a proven efficacy in reducing mortality among patients with AF.

Furthermore, suppression of AF has not been shown to reduce the risk of stroke in high-risk patients [8], and recent data suggest that only 50–60% of the strokes in high-risk AF patients are cardioembolic when a high proportion of the patients are anticoagulated with warfarin (unpublished data, D. Sherman, 2004).

Atrial Fibrillation and Antihypertensive Treatment

The direct association between essential hypertension and AF suggests that blood pressure lowering treatment might contribute to reducing the incidence and complications of AF. A recent overview [8] described a hypothetical construct of the mechanisms whereby hypertension and vascular disease may increase the risk of stroke in patients with AF. Briefly, hypertension, LVH, and diastolic dysfunction may lead to atrial stretch and dilatation, with atrial electric remodelling and increased probability of AF and left atrial thrombus formation.

Figure 2 depicts some interrelationships in hypertension and the pathogenesis of stroke in AF. In this setting, interference with the renin–angiotensin system may be a novel approach to interrupt the vicious circle leading to AF. Indeed, emerging data from randomised controlled studies are providing new information about the prevention of AF in specific clinical contexts. For example, in the TRACE [9] and SOLVD studies [10] treatment with ACE inhibitors significantly reduced the incidence of AF in patients with left ventricular dysfunction.

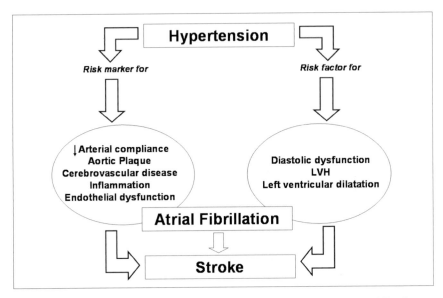

Fig. 2. Relationships between hypertension, pathogenesis of stroke, and atrial fibrillation (data from [8])

Angiotensin Receptor Blockers and Risk of Atrial Fibrillation

A relatively small study of 186 patients with paroxysmal AF showed that those treated with amiodarone and an angiotensin receptor blocker (ARB) had a lower 2-month recurrence rate and a longer time to first AF recurrence than did those treated with amiodarone alone [11].

In the Losartan Intervention For End-point reduction (LIFE) study [12], the hypothesis that the ARB losartan may be better than atenolol in reducing the risk of new-onset AF in hypertensive patients with ECG-documented LVH was tested. Briefly, 8804 patients with hypertension and ECG-documented LVH who did not have AF at enrolment were randomly assigned to once-daily losartan-based or atenolol-based antihypertensive therapy and followed for at least 4 (mean 4.9) years. During follow-up, new-onset AF occurred in 179 patients given losartan (8.2 per 1000 person-years of follow-up) and 252 patients treated with atenolol (11.7 per 1000 person-years of follow-up) [relative risk 0.75 (95% CI 0.58 to 0.85), $p < 0.001$] (Fig. 3). After adjustment for Framingham risk score and ECG LV mass by Sokolow-Lyon and Cornell voltage duration criteria, the relative risk of new-onset AF was 0.72 (95% CI 0.59 to 0.89; $p < 0.001$). An identical relative (0.72; 95% CI 0.59 to 0.89; $p = 0.003$) was found after adjustment for all potential predictors (age, male gender, potassium, creatinine, and log UACR). It remains to be clarified to what extent the reduction in the risk of stroke provided by losartan is mediated by prevention of AF.

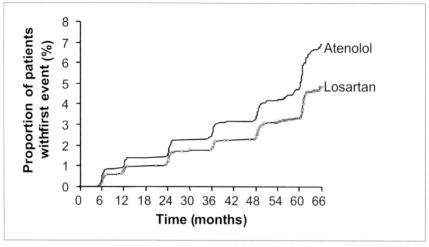

Fig. 3. Cumulative incidence of new-onset atrial fibrillation in the LIFE study among patients assigned to atenolol and losartan

Conclusions

Although lowering the blood pressure stands out as the fundamental mechanism for preventing any complication of hypertension, recent data suggest that ARBs might play an important and perhaps independent contribution in the prevention of AF. By inhibiting the effects of angiotensin II, ARBs reduce both blood pressure and myocardial fibrosis, with important potential implications for atrial and ventricular electric remodelling and atrial pressure and stretch. The LIFE study has shown the beneficial effect of losartan in reducing the risk of AF in hypertensive subjects in sinus rhythm. Further studies should clarify to what extent this effect applies to other ARBs.

References

1. Kannel WB, Abbott RD, Savage DD et al (1982) Epidemiologic features of chronic atrial fibrillation: the Framingham study. N Engl J Med 306:1018–1022
2. Psaty BM, Manolio TA, Kuller LH et al (1997) Incidence of and risk factors for atrial fibrillation in older adults. Circulation 96:2455–2461
3. Benjamin EJ, Wolf PA, D'Agostino RB et al (1998) Impact of atrial fibrillation on the risk of death: the Framingham Heart Study. Circulation 98:946–952
4. Kannel WB, Wolf PA, Benjamin EJ et al (1998) Prevalence, incidence, prognosis, and predisposing conditions for atrial fibrillation: population-based estimates. Am J Cardiol 82:2N–9N
5. Ciaroni S, Cuenoud L, Bloch A (2000) Clinical study to investigate the predictive parameters for the onset of atrial fibrillation in patients with essential hypertension. Am Heart J 139:814–819

6. WB Kannel, RD Abbott, DD Savage et al (2002) Epidemiologic features of chronic atrial fibrillation: the Framingham study. N Engl J Med 306:1018-1022
7. Verdecchia P, Reboldi GP, Gattobigio R et al (2003) Atrial fibrillation in hypertension: predictors and outcome. Hypertension 41:218-223
8. Wyse DG, Gersh BJ (2004) Atrial fibrillation: a perspective thinking inside and outside the box. Circulation109:3089-3095
9. Pedersen OD, Bagger H, Kober L et al (1999) Trandolapril reduces the incidence of atrial fibrillation after acute myocardial infarction in patients with left ventricular dysfunction. Circulation 100:376-380
10. Vermes E, Tardif JC, Bourassa MG et al (2003) Enalapril decreases the incidence of atrial fibrillation in patients with left ventricular dysfunction: insight from the Studies Of Left Ventricular Dysfunction (SOLVD) trials. Circulation 107:2926-2931
11. Madrid AH, Bueno MG, Rebollo JMG et al (2002) Use of irbesartan to maintain sinus rhythm in patients with long-lasting persistent atrial fibrillation: a prospective and randomized study. Circulation 106:331-336
12. Dahlöf B, Devereux RB, Kjeldsen SE for the LIFE study group (2002) Cardiovascular morbidity and mortality in the Losartan Intervention For Endpoint reduction in hypertension study (LIFE): a randomised trial against atenolol. Lancet 359:995–1003

Role of Echocardiography in the Management of Atrial Fibrillation Patients

F. Antonini-Canterin, G. Allocca, D. Rivaben, R. Korcova-Miertusova, R. Piazza, M. Brieda, E. Hrovatin, E. Dametto, F. Zardo, G.L. Nicolosi

Atrial fibrillation (AF) is the most common arrhythmia in adults, with a prevalence that increases from less than 1% in subjects aged below 60 years to more than 9% in those over 80 years old [1]. In recent years new and potentially curative therapeutic approaches have been developed [1]. Today, the role of echocardiography is very important in the assessment of the morphology and functionality of cardiac structures, risk stratification, and in guiding the management of AF. The guidelines consider two-dimensional transthoracic echocardiography (TTE) to be essential for the routine evaluation of patients with AF [2]. TTE should be performed in all AF patients to determine left atrial (LA) and left ventricular (LV) dimensions and LV wall thickness and function, and to recognise important underlying pathological conditions. TTE allows the identification of a possible aetiology of the FA, and the exclusion of occult valvular (particularly rheumatic mitral stenosis), myocardial, or pericardial disease. Lone AF, especially in young subjects, suggests a triggered mechanism that may be amenable to radiofrequency ablation. Abnormal myocardial LV relaxation is detectable from tissue Doppler imaging on the basis of reduced early diastolic mitral annular velocity or a reduced velocity of early mitral flow propagation [3].

The LA dimensions correlate with the probability of successful cardioversion and sinus rhythm maintenance. The anteroposterior LA dimension is usually calculated in the two-dimensional short axis view from M-mode imaging, while LA area or volume can be easily measured in four-chamber and two-chamber views from the apical approach. When the anteroposterior diameter of the left atrium is more than 45 mm, the likelihood of success in the maintenance of sinus rhythm after cardioversion is generally poor. It has

Unità Operativa di Cardiologia-ARC, A.O. S. Maria degli Angeli, Pordenone, Italy been suggested that LA volume measurement could be a stronger predictor of AF than LA dimension alone [4]. In the Stroke Prevention in Atrial Fibrillation (SPAF) III study, LA function and size on TTE were independent predictors of thromboembolism [5]. Furthermore, transoesophageal echocardiography (TEE) maintains an important role in identifying appropriate candidates for antithrombotic therapy and in guiding decisions regarding antiarrhythmic therapy. To evaluate the recovery of LA mechanical function after successful cardioversion, it is very important to detect the presence of LA stunning. Peak pulsed Doppler velocity of mitral inflow in late diastole produced by the atrial contraction wave (a-wave) was the initial parameter used to evaluate the LA function. An a-wave velocity above 50 cm/s is considered suggestive of atrial mechanical dysfunction. The mitral annular late diastolic velocity from tissue Doppler imaging can also be used as surrogate of LA function [6].

One of the most relevant sequelae of AF is its associations with thromboembolic disease and stroke. About 90% of LA thrombi are located in the left atrial appendage (LAA), and the TEE is the modality of choice for detecting LAA thrombi. Modern multiplanar TEE can detect thrombi with a sensitivity and specificity of around 95–100% [7, 8]. The search for cardiac sources of embolism is currently the leading indication for a TEE study in many centres (about 40% of the indications) [9]. The SPAF III study identified 'high risk' AF patients by TEE predictors of embolic events. These factors included: the presence of LAA thrombi, LAA flow velocities below 20 cm/s, spontaneous echo contrast (smoke), 'LAA sludge', and complex aortic atheroma [5]. LAA emptying velocities can be assessed by TEE using pulsed wave Doppler imaging with the sample volume placed about 1 cm into the appendage itself. LAA smoke, identified as swirling echo density in the LAA and LA, is a marker of blood stasis that is associated with later development of LAA thrombus and with systemic embolisation. LAA sludge is a particular, 'viscid' but not solid echodensity, and it represents a further stage along the continuum towards thrombus formation with a greater prognostic value than smoke. With the combination of a LA abnormalities and complex aortic atheromas among patients in AF (not on therapeutic warfarin doses), the annual incidence of embolic events was 20.8% as compared to 1.4% in absence of abnormal findings, while LAA emptying velocities above 40 cm/s predict a greater likelihood of sustained sinus rhythm 1 year after cardioversion [10].

In patients undergoing the pulmonary vein isolated procedure for AF ablation it is particularly important to perform TEE because it allows a more accurate assessment of systolic, diastolic, and atrial reversal flow velocities in pulmonary veins and can guide the catheter position [11].

Three-dimensional echocardiographic reconstruction enables excellent visualisation of LAA anatomy, dimensions, and function, with a high degree of accuracy in identifying a multilobed LAA (54% 3D vs 40% 2D), but there are no differences between two- and three-dimensional reconstruction in the detection of thrombi [12].

Atrial flutter has traditionally been considered an organised arrhythmia carrying a low or no risk of thromboembolic events [13, 14]. More recently, however, several studies have shown that atrial thrombi (prevalence of 4–27%) and atrial spontaneous echo contrast (prevalence of 8–34%) may be detected during TEE in patients with atrial flutter. The FLutter Atriale Società Italiana di Ecocardiografia Cardiovascolare (FLASIEC) multicentre study found that the prevalence of thrombi in LAA is 1–6% and that of LA spontaneous echo contrast is 13% [15]. The results of this study confirm the finding that atrial flutter may be associated with atrial thrombi, although in a smaller percentage of patients than in those with AF. Furthermore, in patients with atrial flutter, reversion to sinus rhythm may lead to thromboembolic complications, despite preliminary TEE results that are negative for thrombi, and this might be due to post-cardioversion atrial stunning.

Electrical cardioversion (EC) of patients with AF to sinus rhythm is frequently performed in symptomatic patients with elevated bleeding risk. In these patients EC offers the opportunity to relieve symptoms, improve cardiac performance rapidly, and possibly reduce cardioembolic risks and bleeding complications caused by prolonged anticoagulation. However, the EC procedure itself has an inherent risk of stroke due to possible embolisation of pre-existing thrombi in the LAA. In the 'conventional' approach, to avoid thromboembolic events, stable patients with AF of more than 48 h or of unknown origin must achieve a therapeutic anticoagulation range for at least 3 weeks prior to the procedure [2]. There are many disadvantages in this conventional approach. The 3-week period of anticoagulation prior to EC is based essentially on the theoretical assumption of thrombus stabilisation, but this interval is substantially empirical. In addition, with the conventional approach, extension of the interval until EC is attempted may reduce the initial success rate (about 86% of subjects) and the possibility of maintenance of sinus rhythm (about 50% at 1 year). Thus, conventional management necessitates a delay in the return of atrial function and increases the risk of post-cardioversion thrombus formation. The prolonged period of anticoagulation required by the conventional approach, which in routine clinical practice is often more than 6 weeks to reach a stable therapeutic INR level, can increase the risk of bleeding. The TTE-guided approach to EC with short-term anticoagulation offers some potential advantages over the conventional approach. TEE facilitates early EC without the need for prolonged anticoagulation in low risk patients and in those in whom the risk of bleeding is high. TEE identifies also high risk patients with LA thrombosis in whom EC should not be performed. TEE should be used to confirm thrombus resolution before EC is carried out in patients with previously documented thrombus. After 7 weeks of anticoagulation, up to 80% of LA thrombi are usually resolved. Finally, it has been postulated that earlier EC may increase the likelihood of successful return to and the maintenance of sinus rhythm [16].

The Assessment of Cardioversion Using Transoesophageal Echocardiography (ACUTE) multicentre study compared a TEE-guided strategy with short-term anticoagulation with the conventional anticoagulation approach [17]. There was no difference in the composite end-point of stroke, transient ischaemic attack, and peripheral embolism between the TEE-guided arm and the conventional arm (0.81% vs 0.50%; $p = 0.50$). However, there was a significant difference in the composite end-point of major and minor bleeding between the TEE-guided arm and the conventional arm (2.9% vs 5.5%; $p = 0.02$). There was no significant difference between the two arms in the 8-week maintenance of normal sinus rhythm, cardiac deaths, or cardioversion-related deaths. The results of this randomised study suggested that the TEE-guided approach with short-term anticoagulation may be considered as a clinical alternative to the conventional approach [17]. In combination with low-molecular-weight heparin, TEE-guided cardioversion may be considered a safe and clinically effective alternative to the conventional treatment strategy for the patients with AF, as recently demonstrated in the Anticoagulant in Cardioversion using Enoxaparin (ACE) trial [18]. Currently, the ACUTE II trial, a randomised study, is in progress evaluating the use of low-molecular-weight heparin in comparison with intravenous heparin as a bridge therapy to warfarin [19].

However, the decision to use one approach or the other is based on the individual characteristics of the patient, the experience of the physician and the centre, and the accessibility of the technique. These factors should be taken into consideration in choosing the best approach: (1) a severity of symptoms and haemodynamic effect of AF that require immediate EC; (2) level and chronicity of anticoagulation; (3) risk of bleeding; and (4) risk and likelihood of left atrial thrombi and risk of recurrence of AF, which require prolonged anticoagulation [16].

Intracardiac echocardiography (ICE) has been recently introduced in this setting. It is performed with a 6- to 12-MHz transducer placed into the right atrium via a 6–8F sheath in the right femoral vein. A high resolution multiple frequency transducer allows tissue penetration enhancement, thus allowing depth control. The ultrasound probes offer the same modalities as TEE, including colour, pulsed wave, and continuous wave Doppler, to allow assessment of the intracardiac flow. ICE has been used successfully to guide catheters during radiofrequency catheter ablation (RFCA) of the pulmonary veins or to visualise their ostia and to monitor the occurrence of acute pulmonary vein stenosis after RFCA at the site of the pulmonary veins, as well as, more recently, for percutaneous closure of the LAA [20, 21]. Continuous imaging with ICE can be performed during RFCA by the operator, and it facilitates trans-septal puncture and guides placement and optimal tissue contact of mapping and ablation catheters. In addition, it allows identification of LA thrombi before the procedure. ICE also facilitates instant detection of important potential complications such as pericardial effusion or tamponade, and may reduce the frequency of these complications. In up to 40% of patients an asymptomatic increase of peak systolic flow velocities in the pulmonary veins has been observed after RFCA. Progression to pulmonary vein stenosis after ablation is rare; more commonly, the degree of narrowing remains stable or even improves. Many patients with severe narrowing or complete occlusion of a single pulmonary vein are asymptomatic. Using TEE, the pulmonary vein ostia can be easily visualised for the evidence and assessment of stenosis [20, 21].

Percutaneous closure of the LAA is a new approach. It was initially performed in an early clinical experience with insertion of the device into the LAA, which was facilitated by ICE, allowing optimal positioning of the device itself [22]. The surgical Maze III procedure (excision or ligation of LAA, isolation of the pulmonary veins) abolishes AF in a significant number of patients. Intraoperative TEE can play a major role, with assessment of the efficacy of ligation by Doppler imaging [23].

In conclusion, echocardiography is a unique and very important technique in the management of AF patients, allowing a non-invasive and easily repeatable evaluation of cardiac anatomy and function. In addition, the TEE approach allows reliable exclusion of the presence of LA thrombosis, guiding the best clinical management of AF patients in different stages of the disease.

References

1. Peters NS, Schilling RJ, Kanagaratnam P et al (2002) Atrial fibrillation: strategies to control, combat, and cure. Lancet 359:593–603
2. Fuster V, Ryden LE, Asinger RW et al (2001) ACC/AHA/ESC guidelines for the management of patients with atrial fibrillation: executive summary. A report of the American College of Cardiology/American Heart Association task force on practice guidelines and the European Society of Cardiology committee for practice guidelines and policy conferences (committee to develop guidelines for the management of patients with atrial fibrillation) developed in collaboration with the North

American Society of Pacing and Electrophysiology. Circulation 104:2118–2150

3. Nagueh SF, Kopelen HA, Quinones MA (1996) Assessment of left ventricular filling pressures by Doppler in the presence of atrial fibrillation. Circulation 94:2138–2145

4. Mattioli AV, Tarabini Castellini B, Vovoli D et al (1996). Restoration of atrial function after atrial fibrillation of different etiological origins. Cardiology 87:205–211

5. SPAF III Investigators (1998) Transesophageal echocardiographic correlates of thromboembolism in high-risk patients with nonvalvular atrial fibrillation. The Stroke Prevention in Atrial Fibrillation Investigators Committee on Echocardiography. Ann Intern Med 128:639–647

6. Khan JA (2003) Atrial stunning: basics and clinical considerations. Int J Cardiol 92:113–128

7. Manning WJ, Weintraub RM et al (1995) Accuracy of transesophageal echocardiography for identifying left atrial thrombi. Ann Intern Med 123:817–822

8. Fatkin D, Scalia G, Jacobs N et al (1996) Accuracy of biplane transesophageal echocardiography in detecting left atrial thrombus. Am J Cardiol 77:321–323

9. Kühl HP, Hanrath P (2004) The impact of transesophageal echocardiography on daily clinical practice. Eur J Echocardiogr 5:455–468

10. Leung DY, Davidson PM, Cranney GB et al (1997) Thromboembolic risks of left atrial thrombus detected by transesophageal echocardiogram. Am J Cardiol 79:626–629

11. Marrouche NF, Martin DO, Wazni O et al (2003) Phased-array intracardiac echocardiography monitoring during pulmonary vein isolation in patients with atrial fibrillation: impact on outcome and complications. Circulation 107:2710–2716

12. Galzerano D, Tuccillo B, Tedeschi C et al (2002) Three and two-dimensional echocardiographic imaging of left atrial appendage: a comparative study. Ital Heart J 3(Suppl): 101(abstract no c118)

13. Arnold AZ, Mick MJ, Mazurek RP (1992) Role of prophylactic anticoagulation for direct current cardioversion in patients with atrial fibrillation or atrial flutter. J Am Coll Cardiol 19:851–855

14. Irani WN, Grayburn PA, Afridi I (1997) Prevalence of thrombus, spontaneous echocontrast, and atrial stunning in patients undergoing cardioversion of flutter atrial. A prospective study using transesophageal echocardiography. Circulation 95:962–966

15. Corrado G, Sgalambro A, Mantero A et al (2001) Thromboembolic risk in atrial flutter: the FLASIEC multicentre study. Eur Heart J 22:1042–1051

16. Klein AL, Murray RD, Grimm RA (2001) Role of transesophageal echocardiography-guided cardioversion of patients with atrial fibrillation. J Am Coll Cardiol 37:691–704

17. Klein AL, Grimm RA, Murray RD et al (2001) Use of transesophageal echocardiography to guide cardioversion in patients with atrial fibrillation. N Engl J Med 344:1411–1420

18. Stellbrink C, Nixdorff U, Hoffman T et al (2004) Safety and efficacy of enoxaparin compared with unfractionated heparin and oral anticoagulants for prevention of thromboembolic complication in cardioversion of non valvular atrial fibrillation (ACE study). Circulation 109:997–1003

19. Murray RD, Shah A, Jasper SE et al (2000) Transesophageal echocardiography guided enoxaparin antithrombotic strategy for cardioversion of atrial fibrillation: the ACUTE II pilot study. Am Heart J 139:1–7

20. Marrouche NF, Martin DO, Wazni O et al (2003) Phased-array intracardiac echocardiography monitoring during pulmonary vein isolation in patients with atrial fibrillation: impact on outcome and complications. Circulation 107:2710–2716
21. Cooper JM, Epstein LM (2001) Use of intracardiac echocardiography to guide ablation of atrial fibrillation. Circulation 104:3010–3013
22. Sievert H, Lesh M, Trepeles T et al (2002) Percutaneous left atrial appendage occlusion to prevent stroke in high-risk patients with atrial fibrillation: early clinical experience. Circulation 105:1887–1889
23. Gillinov AM, McCarthy PM (2002) Intraoperative bipolar radiofrequency clamp for intraoperative ablation of atrial fibrillation. Ann Thorac Surg 74:2165–2168

Pharmacological Prevention of Arrhythmic Recurrences

G. Chiarandà[1], M.L. Cavarra[1], C.L. Romeo[1], M. Chiarandà[1], T. Regolo[2]

Atrial fibrillation (AF) is the most common cardiac arrhythmia in the general population, with a prevalence ranging from 0.5% to 9% between the ages of 50 and 80 years. Literature data [1] suggest that the incidence of this arrhythmia increases dramatically in patients with heart failure. AF can cause a rise in morbidity and mortality due to the loss of atrial function and the consequent decrease in heart performance and increase in embolic risk Moreover, a persistently elevated ventricular rate during AF can produce dilated ventricular cardiomyopathy. For these reasons, recovery and maintenance of sinus rhythm is one of main objectives of treatment.

A series of anti-arrhythmic agents have been demonstrated to be highly effective in terminating recent-onset AF; however, the results obtained in preventing recurrences are scanty [2, 3]. The anti-arrhythmic agents most used in Europe are class IA disopyramide and quinidine, class IC flecainide and propafenone, and class III amiodarone and sotalol. Table 1 summarises reported data from the literature.

The percentage of patients who maintain sinus rhythm without arrhythmia recurrence under placebo treatment is around 30% after 6 months and 25% after 12 months. Anti-arrhythmic agents can may increase the percentage of patients in sinus rhythm, but the overall efficacy is limited. No more than 50% of treated patients are free from arrhythmia recurrences after 12 months; only for amiodarone do the efficacy rates range from 50% to 73% at 12 months. Of course, the final result may be influenced by the selection of the patient population, the types of AF, and the way in which anti-arrhythmic agents are begun.

[1]Coronary Care Unit, Muscatello Hospital, Augusta (Syracuse); [2]Coronary Care Unit, Ferrarotto University Hospital, Catania, Italy

Table 1. Drugs for prevention of atrial fibrillation recurrence: success in sinus rhythm maintenance following cardioversion of atrial fibrillation

Drugs	Sinus rhythm At 1 month (%)	At 3 months (%)	At 6 months (%)	At 12 months (%)
Placebo	58	15–56	19–35	0–43
Quinidine	65	44–75	27–58	23–51
Disopyramide	–	72	45–50	55
Propafenone	54	44	40	–
Flecainide	–	44	–	34–42
Dofetilide	–	58–44	51–71	40–66
Sotalol	–	49–50	46–50	37–46
Amiodarone	–	–	75–78.5	50–73

We should consider an increase in time to first recurrence or time in sinus rhythm as a good primary result in order to ameliorate the possible haemodynamic complications of AF. Many variables affect the maintenance of sinus rhythm and the efficacy or not of the anti-arrhythmia therapy:

- Duration of the arrhythmia (from the literature there appears a cut-off at between 6 months and 2 years)
- Left atrial size (from >45 mm to > 60 mm) (this variable is not yet accepted by everybody because the atrial enlargement could be a consequence rather than the cause of the arrhythmia)
- Early recurrence of the arrhythmia
- The presence of a severe valvular rheumatic disease
- Advanced NYHA functional class
- The presence of a cardiopathy (for example, a hypertensive cardiopathy)
- Advanced age
- Doppler echocardiographic index [A wave peak and integral velocity/time soon after electrical cardioversion (ECV), fibrillation wave peak during auricular filling and emptying before ECV; early left auricular end-diastolic or diastolic length] [4, 5].

Class I Anti-arrhythmic Agents

Class I anti-arrhythmic drugs have been shown to be superior to placebo, but there are contrasting data because they were often tested in small studies involving patients with different clinical features. On the whole, they are effective in preventing AF recurrences in about 40–50% of patients after 12 months.

Quinidine is effective in maintaining sinus rhythm (Table 1). However, its use is limited by the demonstrated high risk for torsades de pointes and the mortality rate (total mortality at 1 year with quinidine 2.9% vs. control group 0.8%) [6].

Two placebo-controlled studies supported the efficacy of flecainide in increasing time to first AF recurrence and reducing AF burden [7, 8]. Other randomised studies evidenced comparable efficacy to that of quinidine, coupled with fewer side effects [9, 10]. Flecainide (200 mg daily) was shown to be effective in postponing the first recurrence of AF, and superior to long-acting quinidine (1100 mg daily) without the occurrence of severe side effects or pro-arrhythmia [11].

Compared with placebo, propafenone also increased the overall time free from AF and the interval to first recurrence [6, 12]. In an open-label randomised study involving 100 patients with AF, propafenone and sotalol were similar in preventing AF episodes (30% vs 37%, respectively) [13].

Class IC drugs may be initiated out of hospital: in a selected risk-stratified population with recurrent AF, 'pill in the pocket' treatment is feasible and safe, with a high rate of patient compliance and low adverse event rate, and markedly reduces hospital admissions [14].

Class III Anti-arrhythmic Agents

Amiodarone and sotalol are the most frequently used class III drugs for maintaining sinus rhythm in patients with AF [15].

The efficacy of sotalol seems to be similar to that of class I drugs. The ventricular rate during AF recurrences is attenuated and the haemodynamic pattern of AF recurrences is better after sotalol treatment than without. The likelihood of remaining in sinus rhythm is higher in younger patients, with a smaller left atrial size and without concomitant heart disease. Patients treated with sotalol must initially be monitored with ECG (for 3 days) in hospital because of the potential pro-arrhythmic effect.

Amiodarone is the most effective anti-arrhythmic agent. A large randomised trial (CTAF) compared the effects of low-dose of amiodarone (200 mg daily) with conventional therapy (propafenone and sotalol) in maintenance of sinus rhythm during a follow-up of 1 year: 70% of patients assigned to amiodarone had no recurrence of AF and the amiodarone was superior to class I drugs [16].

In the randomised CHF-STAT trial amiodarone was used in order to evaluate its effects on mortality in patients with heart failure. The drug showed a significant potential to convert AF to sinus rhythm, and prevented the development of new-onset AF [6].

In a cohort of post-cardioversion patients the group treated with amiodarone showed a significantly lower incidence of AF relapses in comparison with quinidine and was coupled with fewer side effects [17].

The efficacy of amiodarone for maintenance of sinus rhythm has been supported by many studies, but the relatively high incidence of side effects [18] justifies its common use as a second-line or last-resort option, with the important exception of heart failure.

Other Drugs

Dofetilide, a new anti-arrhythmic agent approved for use in the USA but not in Europe, is effective in preventing AF and atrial flutter. Two large-scale and double-blind randomised studies have supported its efficacy: the SAFIRE-D and EMERALD studies [19, 20]. Sixty-six of patients in the SAFIRE and 71% of patients in the EMERALD study were free from AF relapses, compared with 21–25% in the placebo group and 60% in the sotalol group.

Beta-blockers are generally not included among the anti-arrhythmic agents; however, metoprolol has demonstrated a good rate of maintaining persistent sinus rhythm as compared with placebo (51% vs 40%; $P < 0.05$) and can be considered in some clinical situations, especially in the postoperative protocols of myocardial revascularisation for patients with no contraindications for its use [21, 22].

Dronedarone shares the electrophysiological properties of amiodarone: at 800 mg daily dose, it appears to be effective and safe for the prevention of AF relapses after cardioversion [23]. The absence of thyroid side effects and of pro-arrhythmia are important feature of the drug, but further studies are needed.

Role of Pharmacological Pre-treatment in Reducing AF Recurrences

The most relevant clinical problem after successful cardioversion is the risk of recurrences resulting from fibrillation-induced electrical remodelling of the atrium. The recurrences may occur acutely in the very early phase (minutes), or in the subacute phase, or they may be early recurrences (from 24–48 h to 7–14 days), or, in the weeks to months range, they may be late. The efficacy of pre-treatment with class I and III anti-arrhythmic drugs in preventing acute and subacute AF recurrences has been reported [24, 25].

Recently the role of the verapamil alone or combined with another anti-arrhythmic drugs has been investigated. The VERAF study clearly demonstrated that verapamil alone, in patients who were not taking anti-arrhythmic agents at the time of cardioversion, is highly effective in reducing very early and early recurrences of AF after successful cardioversion, but is ineffective in the long run [26]. The VEPARAF study suggested that oral verapamil administration, combined with a class IC or III anti-arrhythmic drug, is effective in reducing both primary and secondary recurrences after cardioversion [27].

Angiotensin Antagonist Receptors

A recent study has shown that irbesartan combined with amiodarone was more effective than amiodarone alone in the prevention of AF recurrences after ECV [28]. In our experience, candesartan combined with class IC drugs has reduced the numbers of relapses and the time to first relapse of AF after effective ECV [29].

Pro-arrhythmic Effects

Today there is major concern over the risk of potentially fatal ventricular pro-arrhythmic effects caused by drugs employed for a relatively benign arrhythmia such as AF.

Sotalol may cause torsades de pointes, but the risk is dose-dependent (1% for dosage between 160 and 240 mg daily and 4–5% for a dosage higher than 480 mg daily), and torsades de pointes may be precipitated by hypokalaemia, bradycardia, reduced creatinine clearance, and other drugs inducing CT prolongation.

The prevalence of torsades de pointes is lower with amiodarone (less than 1% despite frequently marked QT prolongations). However, the use of amiodarone is limited by other side effects (skin discoloration 4.5%, pulmonary fibrosis 3.6%, thyroid abnormalities 2.7%). The mortality rate associated with amiodarone treatment is around 0.6%, comparable to that of control patients.

Class IC drugs have a marked effect on conduction velocity and may organise and slow the rate of AF, converting it into atrial flutter. The pro-arrhythmic effect is favoured by adrenergic stimulation and has been reported in 3–5% of patients treated with flecainide or propafenone; patients with significant left ventricular dysfunction are potentially at higher risk.

Some categories of patients are at higher risk of pro-arrhythmia: those with previous myocardial infarction, overt or previous congestive heart failure, significant left ventricular dysfunction, previous conduction disease, or electrolyte impairment, or those of advanced age.

Choice of Anti-arrhythmic Drugs

The choice of one anti-arrhythmic drug rather than another one depends on the risk/benefit ratio relating to specific aspects: (a) underlying cardiopathy and degree of left ventricular systolic dysfunction; (b) pharmacokinetics, pharmacodynamics, electrophysiological characteristics, and mode of action; (c) possible haemodynamic effects; (d) pro-arrhythmic risks and side effects.

In general, in patients with no or minimal structural heart disease, class IC drugs or sotalol appear to be the first-line choice.

In patients with hypertension with no or minimal left ventricular hypertrophy, or in patients with a high resting sinus rate, or with adrenergically mediated AF, sotalol or other beta-blockers could represent the first-line choice. In patients with severe left ventricular hypertrophy or valvular heart disease the first-line choice is amiodarone.

In the presence of ischaemic heart disease, or left ventricular dysfunction, in patients with very frequent AF recurrences or large right or left atria, or with a long history of AF, amiodarone is the anti-arrhythmic drug of choice. In patients with vagally mediated AF, the use of drugs with vagolytic action such flecainide or disopyramide is suggested.

Finally, in some clinical situations there is no indication for any anti-arrhythmic drug: (a) after the first episode, unless there is significant haemodynamic impairment; (b) when AF is well-tolerated, short-lasting, and self-limited; (c) when AF occurs during acute myocardial infarction or other acute conditions; (d) when AF occurs just after cardiac surgery, unless there is a history of previous AF attacks.

References

1. Fuster V, Gibbons RJ (2001) ACC AHA/ESC: Guidelines for the management of patients with atrial fibrillation. Eur Heart J 22:1852–1923
2. Boriani G, Biffi M, Branzi A (1998) Pharmacological treatment of atrial fibrillation: a review of prevention of recurrences and control of ventricular response. Arch Gerontol Geriatr 27:127–139
3. Alessie MA (1998) Atrial electrophysiologic remodeling: another vicious circle. J Cardiovasc Elettrophysiol 9:1378–1393
4. Verhorst PMJ, Kamp O, Welling RC (2001) Transesophageal echocardiographic predictors for maintenance of sinus rhythm after electrical cardioversion of atrial fibrillation. Am J Cardiol 79:1235–1239
5. Mattioli AV, Vivoli D, Bastia E (1997) Doppler echocardiographic parameters predictive of recurrence of atrial fibrillation of different etiologic origins. J Ultrasound Med 16:695–698
6. Deedwania PC, Singh BN, Ellenbogen K et al (1998) Spontaneous conversion and maintenance of sinus rhythm by amiodarone in patients with heart failure and atrial fibrillation. Observation from the Veterans Affairs Congestive Heart Failure

Survival Trial of Anti-arrhythmic Therapy (CHF-STAT). Circulation 98:2574–2579

7. Anderson JL, Gilbert EM, Alpbert PL et al (1989) Prevention of symptomatic recurrences of paroxysmal atrial fibrillation in patients initially tolerating anti-arrhythmic therapy. A multicenter double-blind crossover study of flecainide and placebo with transtelephonic monitoring. Flecainide Supraventricular Tachycardia Study Group. Circulation 80:1557–1570

8. Pietersen H, Hellemann H (1991) Usefulness of flecainide for prevention of paroxysmal atrial fibrillation and flutter. Danish-Norwegian Flecainide Multicenter Study Group. Am J Cardiol 67:713–717

9. Carelli G, Dorian P (1996) Prospective comparison of flecainide versus quinidine for the treatment of paroxysmal atrial fibrillation/flutter. Am J Cardiol 77:53A–59A

10. Van Wijklm, Den Heijr P (1989) Flecainide versus quinidine in the prevention of paroxysms of atrial fibrillation. J Cardiovasc Pharmacol 13:32–36

11. Van Gelder IC, Crijnshj (1989) Efficacy and safety of flecainide acetate in the maintenance of sinus rhythm after electrical cardioversion of chronic atrial fibrillation or atrial flutter. Am J Cardiol 64:1317–1321

12. Lee Sh, Chen S, Chiang CE et al (1996) Comparison of oral propafenone and quinidine as an initial treatment option in patients with symptomatic paroxysmal atrial fibrillation: a double-blind, randomized trial. J Intern Med 239:253–260

13. Reinol SC, Cantillon CO (1993) Propafenone versus sotalol for suppression of recurrent symptomatic atrial fibrillation. Am J Cardiol 79:1198–1202

14. Alboni P, Botto GL (2005) Out of hospital treatment of recent onset atrial fibrillation with the "pill in the pocket" approach. N Engl J Med (in press)

15. Kochiadakis GE, Igoumenidis NE, Marketou ME et al (2000) Low dose amiodarone and sotalol in the treatment of recurrent symptomatic atrial fibrillation: comparative placebo controlled study. Heart 84:251–257

16. Roy D, Talajic M (2000) Amiodarone to prevent recurrence of atrial fibrillation. N Engl J Med 342:913–920

17. Vitolo E, Tronci M, La Rovere M (1981) Amiodarone versus quinidine in the prophylaxis of atrial fibrillation. Acta Cardiol 36: 431–434

18. Vorperian VR, Havighurst TC (1997) Adverse effects of low dose amiodarone: a meta-analysis. J Am Coll Cardiol 30:791–798

19. Sing S, Zoble RG (2000) Efficacy and safety of oral dofetilide in converting to and maintaining sinus rhythm in patients with chronic atrial fibrillation or atrial flutter: the Symptomatic Atrial Fibrillation Investigative Research on Dofetilide (SAFIRE-D) study. Circulation 102:2385–2390

20. Greenbaum RA, Campbell TJ (1998) Conversion of atrial fibrillation and maintenance of sinus rhythm by dofetilide: DE EMERALD (European and Australian Multicenter Evaluative Research on Atrial Fibrillation Dofetilide) study. Circulation 98:1663–1671

21. Kuhlkamp V, Schirdewan A, (2000) Use of metoprolol CR/XL to maintain sinus rhythm after conversion from persistent atrial fibrillation. A randomized double-blind placebo-controlled study. J Am Coll Cardiol 36:139–146

22. Lucio E, Flores A (2003) Effectiveness of metoprolol in prevention of atrial fibrillation and flutter in the postoperative period of coronary artery by-pass graft surgery. Arq Bras Cardiol 82:42–46

23. Toboul P, Brugada, Capucci A (2003) Dronedarone for prevention of atrial fibrillation: a dose-ranging study. Eur Heart J 24:1481–1487

24. Rossiem Lown B (1967) The use of quinidine in cardioversion. Am J Cardiol 19:234–238

25. Cappucci A, Villani GQ, Aschieri D (2000) Oral amiodarone increases the efficacy of direct current cardioversion in restoration of sinus rhythm in patients with chronic atrial fibrillation. Eur Heart J 21:66–73

26. Botto GL, Belotti G, Cirò A, on behalf of the VERAF study group (2002) Verapamil in prevention of early recurrence of atrial fibrillation: final results of the VERAF study. Eur Heart J 23:660

27. De Simone A, De Pasquale M, De Matteis C, on behalf of the VEPARAF study (2003) Verapamil class antiarrhythmic drugs reduce atrial fibrillation recurrences after an electrical cardioversion (VEPARAF Study). Eur Heart J 24: 1425–1429

28. Madrid AH, Bueno MG (2002) Use of irbesartan to maintain sinus rhythm in patients with long-lasting persistent atrial fibrillation. A prospective and randomized study. Circulation 106:16

29. Chiarandà G, Cavarra ML, Busacca G (2004) The role of candesartan in the maintenance of sinus rhythm in patient with atrial fibrillation lasting > 48 h, Italian Heart J, 5(Suppl 5):C108

Timing and Typology of Cardio-Embolic Prevention in Patients with Atrial Fibrillation

G. Di Pasquale, G. Casella, P.C. Pavesi

Atrial fibrillation (AF) is the most common cardiac arrhythmia detected by physicians, and its prevalence is projected to rise dramatically as the population ages [1]. In fact, the estimate of AF in Italy is about 500 000 subjects, with an incidence of 60 000 new cases per year. Furthermore, the real prevalence of AF is difficult to establish, because arrhythmia is often silent or paroxysmal, and even in patients with symptomatic paroxysmal AF, asymptomatic episodes are at least ten times more frequent than symptomatic ones. This high prevalence of AF places an increasing strain on healthcare resources needed to treat this disease and its complications, the most serious of them being ischaemic stroke. At least 15% of strokes are due to AF and this kind of arrhythmia accounts for almost half of all cardio-embolic strokes [2]. Several randomised clinical trials suggest that the yearly incidence of stroke for patients with non valvular AF is almost 4.5%, half of the strokes being disabling [3]. Interestingly, this risk is age-related, ranging from 1.5% in the younger ages (50-59 years) up to 23.5% in patients older than 80 years, according to the Framingham data [2]. Moreover, even in the absence of stroke, AF can lead to cognitive deficits, probably related to silent cerebral infarcts. Finally, today there is a clear evidence of which patients may be recognised as at risk for stroke, and well-defined factors separate a subset of subjects with a 8-10% yearly incidence of stroke from a moderate-to-low risk group (Table 1) [3].

Division of Cardiology, Maggiore Hospital, Bologna, Italy

Table 1. Risk factors for stroke in atrial fibrillation

High risk	Moderate risk
Prior stroke/Transient ischaemic attack	Age 65-75
Systemic embolus	Diabetes mellitus
(History of) hypertension	Coronary artery disease with preserved left ventricular systolic function
Poor left ventricular systolic function	
Age > 75 year	
Rheumatic mitral valve disease	
Prosthetic heart valve	

Oral Anticoagulation Therapy

During the last decades, several different treatments or strategies to prevent embolic complications in AF have been investigated. At present, oral anticoagulation therapy (OAT) is considered the gold standard, since several randomised clinical trials clearly demonstrated that the drug can reduce the relative risk of stroke by about 62% [3, 4]. Conversely, aspirin may reduce that risk only by 22% as compared to placebo [3]. Therefore, current guidelines recommend OAT for patients with AF at high risk for stroke and aspirin for low risk subjects, while in medium-risk subjects, treatment should be chosen on an individual basis [3, 5]. Despite this evidence, less than half of patients with AF eligible to OAT actually receive it, with the elderly patients the least likely [6]. Several factors may be involved in this under-use, the most noteworthy being the fear of bleeding [3, 6]. However, the management of OAT needs careful and regular monitoring of the international normalised ratio (INR) to maintain its values within the narrow therapeutic range (2.0-3.0) most of the time and precise adjustments of the daily dose. Unfortunately, many factors, such as interactions with different drugs or diseases, changes in dietary habits, poor patient or physician compliance, may influence the stability of the INR. Furthermore, other factors may increase the OAT-related risk of bleeding. These include advanced age, OAT intensity, recent initiation of this therapy, patients' own characteristics and compliance to OAT, as well as the administration of other interacting drugs.

The relationship between advanced age and OAT-associated bleeding is of particular concern, since the elderly have the highest risk of stroke; therefore, they would benefit most from an effective preventive therapy. The prospective Italian ISCOAT study evaluated the frequency of bleeding complications in AF outpatients treated with OAT according to an Anticoagulation Clinic model [7]. In this study, the rate of fatal, major and minor bleeding events was quite low (0.25, 1.1, and 6.2 per 100 patients-years of follow-up, respectively), but significantly higher in older patients or during the first 90 days from the beginning of OAT. Furthermore, a clear correlation between OAT intensity and risk of bleeding was observed. In fact, in the ISCOAT study patients over 75 years had an increased risk of bleeding when INR was above 3.0, and this risk became enormous for INR values above 4.5 [7]. On the other hand, about 20% of all bleedings occurred when the INR was below 2.0, indicating that sub-therapeutic INR values neither protect against bleedings nor prevent embolisms.

Furthermore, multiple drug therapies are quite common in elderly AF patients, and this increases the risk of adverse drug interactions with OAT. In a recent large study in patients treated with OAT for nonvalvular AF, subjects receiving more than 3 drugs had a 6-fold higher risk of bleeding or embolic complications as compared with patients receiving less than 3 drugs (24.4% per 100 patient-years versus 4.3%) [8].

All these limitations could partially explain why, even in the third millennium, not enough patients with AF at risk of stroke receive OAT, and the patients with the highest risk are the ones who receive it least [6].

The Seventh ACCP Consensus Conference on Antithrombotic Therapy deeply discussed this issue and recommended that the quality of care for OAT should be considered a key point and should be significantly improved in the real world [3]. These guidelines encourage clinicians to adopt a systematic and comprehensive system of care to improve the quality of OAT. According to this, patients treated with OAT should expect a well-informed provider, reliable monitoring devices and healthcare resources, an effective follow-up and careful education [9]. All these key points are effectively accomplished by a coordinated healthcare system, like the one provided by an Anticoagulation Clinic. Several studies had already demonstrated that such clinics are more effective than usual care in managing OAT, allow better results and consequently reduce the incidence of adverse events [10]. Even in our experience, where more than 800 patients with nonvalvular AF are managed every year according to an 'Anticoagulation Clinic' model (a computerised system to manage OAT, two specialised nurses and a referring physician), INR values fell within the therapeutic range in more than 70% of measurements with a low incidence of values above 3 (less than 13%).

New Antithrombotic Agents

To overcome the above limitations of OAT, several potential pharmacological or device-based alternatives have been investigated or are currently under evaluation (Table 2) [11]. In particular, fixed mini-doses of warfarin or the low-intensity anticoagulation regimen (INR 1.5-2.5) failed to meet expectations.

At present, the most promising strategies address new antithrombotic agents, more specific and stable than warfarin. The association between aspirin and clopidogrel looks very promising and is currently compared to dose-adjusted warfarin in the ongoing ACTIVE trial. Idraparinux, a pentasaccharides agent, has a favourable pharmacokinetic profile and is suitable for once-a-week, subcutaneous administration. The ongoing randomised AMADEUS trial compares idraparinux once-a-week to dose-adjusted OAT (INR 2-3) for stroke prevention in AF patients. Perhaps, the most practical and important alternative strategy for stroke prevention in AF patients involves direct thrombin inhibitors, like ximelagatran. This drug has a very favourable and stable pharmacokinetics and does not require coagulation monitoring [12]. Ximelagatran has been deeply investigated in the SPORTIF programme, a large series of different studies evaluating short- and long-term safety and efficacy of ximelagatran in patients with nonvalvular AF. The most important of these studies are the SPORTIF-III and SPORTIF-V, which enrolled patients with nonvalvular AF and risk factors for stroke to 36 mg ximelagatran or dose-adjusted warfarin (INR 2.0-3.0).

In the SPORTIF-III trial, an open-label, multicentre international study enrolling a medium-to-high risk population, ximelagatran reduced the incidence of stroke and systemic embolism by 29% at intention to treat analysis [13]. However, when only treated patients were evaluated, ximelagatran demonstrated a significant 43% reduction in the primary end point. Interestingly, there were no differences in relation to intracranial haemorrhages or major bleeding between the two drugs, whereas patients treated with ximelagatran demonstrated less incidence of major and minor bleedings when taken together. Notably, the quality of OAT was remarkable

Table 2. New strategies for stroke prevention in atrial fibrillation

Other antiplatelet agents	Indobufen (SIFA II)
	Clopidogrel plus aspirin (ACTIVE)
Synthetic pentasaccharide	Idraparinux (AMADEUS)
Direct thrombin inhibitors	Ximelagatran (SPORTIF Studies)
Device-based alternatives	PLAATO, Amplatzer occluder

throughout the study. The mean INR was 2.5, and INR values fell within the therapeutic range for 66% of the entire duration of exposure, a rate much better than that observed in previous studies or experienced in clinical practice.

The SPORTIF-V trial [14] included 3922 patients at moderate-to-high risk of stroke, and compared a 36 mg ximelagatran dose with dose-adjusted warfarin. Like the SPORTIF-III, the SPORTIF-V study was a non-inferiority trial and met its primary objective by demonstrating an incidence of stroke and other thrombo-embolic complications in the ximelagatran arm similar to that observed in patients treated with dose-adjusted warfarin. As already observed in SPORTIF-III, the quality of anticoagulation was excellent in SPORTIF-V also, and this could partially explain the lower-than-expected event rate of subjects treated with warfarin (1.2% per year). In the SPORTIF-V study, rates of intracranial haemorrhage were low with either treatment, neither was there a significant difference between the two groups in rates of major bleeding. When minor and major events were pooled, however, patients randomised to ximelagatran had significantly less bleeding then those given warfarin. The similar design of the two studies allowed their analysis to be combined, and taken together, the two trials showed that the effect of ximelagatran on prevention of stroke and systemic embolism was similar to warfarin (Table 3) [15]. However, in SPORTIF-V there was a 6% incidence of elevation of the alanine aminotransferase (ALT) levels to > 3 times the upper limit of normal. Similar elevation of ALT levels has been observed in all the previous ximelagatran trials. However, such elevations in ALT levels seem to be limited to the first 6 months of therapy, and reverse toward normal over time whether or not the drug was stopped.

Table 3. SPORTIF III/V: combined analysis. Modified from [15]

Events	Warfarin	Ximelagatran	P
Primary events (stroke and systemic embolism) (%/yr)	1.7	1.6	0.941
Secondary events (%/yr)	3.3	2.8	0.625
Major bleeding (%/yr)	2.5	1.9	0.054
Combined major plus minor bleeding (%/yr)	39	32	< 0.0001

New Device-Based Alternatives

Other potential device-based alternatives for stroke prevention in AF patients who are not candidates for OAT are under investigation. The most promising is the occlusion of the left atrial appendage (LAA), the most relevant source of embolism in patients with AF. This occlusion is accomplished by means of an implant, called the Percutaneous Left Atrial Appendage Transcatheter Occlusion (PLAATO) device, which is placed into the LAA to seal the LAA ostium so that cardiac emboli cannot migrate. The PLAATO, which consists of a self-expanding metal cage covered with a plastic membrane, is delivered percutaneously using a trans-septal approach. Preliminary clinical experiences with the PLAATO system are very favourable, with a high success rate and few device-related complications [16, 17]. Future studies are needed to assess long-term results.

Rhythm Control

The hypothesis that the persistence of sinus rhythm in patients with AF could effectively prevent embolic events was a secondary end point of several randomised trials comparing the two strategies of 'rate control' and 'rhythm control'.

In the AFFIRM trial [18], the study protocol allowed in the 'rhythm control' arm to discontinue OAT after sinus rhythm had been achieved and maintained for at least one month. Therefore, at an average 3.5 year follow-up, 85-90% of patients in the 'rate control' group were still being treated with OAT as compared to 70% of subjects in the 'rhythm control' arm. INR values below 2.0 were detected in 33% of patients in the 'rate control' arm and in 58% of those in the 'rhythm control' arm, respectively. At follow-up, 60% of patients in the 'rhythm control' arm were in sinus rhythm. Notably, ischaemic stroke occurred in 5.7% of patients enrolled in the 'rate control' arm as compared to 7.3% of subjects of the 'rhythm control' group. Likewise, in the RACE trial [19] in which the protocol allowed discontinuation of OAT in patients in whom sinus rhythm had been achieved and maintained for at least one month, patients in the 'rhythm control' group experienced more thrombo-embolic complications (7.5%) than those in the 'rate control' group (5.5%).

In addition, a meta-analysis of four studies comparing a 'rate control' with a 'rhythm control' strategy (AFFIRM, RACE, STAF, and PIAF), including 5034 patients with non valvular AF, demonstrates an unfavourable odds ratio of 1.36 (95% CI 1.03 - 1.78 ; $p = 0.04$) for ischaemic stroke with the 'rhythm control' strategy as compared to the 'rate control' policy [20]. The cumulative results of these studies clearly indicate that a strategy of vigorous 'rhythm control' by means of cardioversion and antiarrhythmic prophylaxis is not guarantee against thrombo-embolism. Only a policy of high-quality OAT, even after restoration of sinus rhythm, could effectively prevent embolic complications in most patients with AF at medium-to-high risk.

Conclusions

OAT currently represents the most effective therapy for cardio-embolic prevention in patients with non-valvular AF at moderate-to-high risk. Antiplatelet therapy may represent an alternative for low-risk patients or patients who are poor candidates for OAT, due to a high risk of bleeding or limited compliance. The hope for the future is the development of newer alternatives to OAT with a more convenient pharmacological profile, less risk of bleeding and easier management [21]. At present, oral direct thrombin inhibitors seem the most promising alternatives, but further studies are needed to confirm their safety.

References

1. Go AS, Hylek EM, Phillips KA et al (2001) Prevalence of diagnosed atrial fibrillation in adults. National implications for rhythm management and stroke prevention: the Anticoagulation and Risk Factors in Atrial Fibrillation (ATRIA) study. JAMA 285:2370-2375
2. Wolf PA, Abbott RD, Kannel WB (1991) Atrial fibrillation as an independent risk factor for stroke: the Framingham study. Stroke 22:983–988
3. Singer DE, Albers GW, Dalen JE et al (2004) Antithrombotic therapy in atrial fibrillation. The Seventh ACCP Conference on antithrombotic and thrombolytic therapy. Chest 126: S429-S456
4. Hart RG, Benavente O, McBride R et al (1999) Antithrombotic therapy to prevent stroke in patients with atrial fibrillation: a meta-analysis. Ann Intern Med 131:492–501
5. Fuster V, Rydén LE, Asinger RW et al (2001) ACC/AHA/ESC guidelines for the management of patients with atrial fibrillation. Eur Heart J 22:1852–1923
6. Di Pasquale G, Cerè E, Lombardi A et al (2003) Anticoagulation therapy of atrial fibrillation in the elderly. In: Gulizia M (Ed) New advances in heart failure and atrial fibrillation . Springer, Milan, pp 329-334
7. Palareti G, Leali N, Coccheri S et al (1996) Bleeding complications of oral anticoagulant treatment: an inception-cohort, prospective collaborative study (ISCOAT). Lancet 348:423-428
8. Wehinger C, Stollberger C, Langer T et al (2001) Evaluation of risk factors for stroke/embolism and of complications due to anticolagulant therapy in atrial fibrillation. Stroke 32:2246-2252
9. Ansell J, Hirsh J, Dalen J et al (2001) Managing oral anticoagulant therapy. Chest 119 (Suppl):S22-S38

10. Chiquette E, Amato MG, Bussey HI (1998) Comparison of an anticoagulation clinic with usual medical care: anticoagulation control, patients outcome and health care costs. Arch Intern Med 158:1641-1647
11. Weitz JI, Hirsh J, Samama MM (2004) New anticoagulant drugs. The seventh ACCP conference on antithrombotic and thrombolytic therapy. Chest 126:S265-S286
12. Eriksson UG, Bredberg U, Gislén K et al (2003) Pharmacokinetics and pharmacodynamics of ximelagatran, a novel oral direct thrombin inhibitor, in young healthy male subjects. Eur J Clin Pharmacol 59:35–43
13. Executive Steering Committee on behalf of the SPORTIF III investigators (2003) Stroke prevention with the oral direct thrombin inhibitor ximelagatran compared with warfarin in patients with non-valvular atrial fibrillation (SPORTIF III): randomised controlled trial. Lancet 362:1691-1698
14. SPORTIF Executive Steering Committee for the SPORTIF V Investigators (2005) Ximelagatran vs warfarin for stroke prevention in patients with non valvular atrial fibrillation: a randomized trial. JAMA, 293:690–698
15. Diener HC (2004) SPORTIF-III/V combined analysis. Cerebrovasc Dis 17(Suppl.5):16
16. Sievert H, Lesh MD, Trepels T et al (2002) Percutaneous left atrial appendage transcatheter occlusion to prevent stroke in high-risk patients with atrial fibrillation. Early clinical experience. Circulation 105:1887-1889
17. Barbato G, Carinci V, Pergolini F et al (2005) Percutaneous occlusion of the left appendage for systemic embolism prevention in patients with atrial fibrillation: state of the art and report of two cases. Ital Heart J (submitted)
18. The Atrial Fibrillation Follow-up Investigation of Rhythm Management (AFFIRM) Investigators. (2002) A comparison of rate control and rhythm control in patients with atrial fibrillation. N Engl J Med 347:1825-1833
19. Van Gelder IC, Hagens VE, Bosker HA et al (2002) A comparison of rate control and rhythm control in patients with recurrent persistent atrial fibrillation for the Rate Control versus Electrical Cardioversion for Persistent Atrial Fibrillation Study Group. N Engl J Med 347:1834-1840
20. Wyse DG (2004) Personal communication
21. Di Pasquale G, Casella G (2005) Antithrombotic strategies for atrial fibrillation: on the threshhold for a change? Yes. J Thromb Haemost (in press)

Non-Electric Treatment of Atrial Fibrillation: When Not to Treat?

R.F.E. PEDRETTI

Atrial fibrillation (AF) is the most common sustained dysrhythmia in clinical practice. Atrial fibrillation can be divided into three categories: paroxysmal, persistent, and permanent. Paroxysmal AF is AF that has occurred and resolves, then recurs. Persistent AF is AF that does not resolve spontaneously, but aggressive attempts to perform cardioversion have not yet been attempted. Permanent AF is AF that has been unresponsive to multiple attempts to cardiovert.

Approximately 30–45% of paroxysmal cases and 20–25% of persistent cases of AF occur in younger patients without demonstrable underlying disease (lone AF) [1]. In the other cases, AF is associated with several cardiopulmonary or systemic disease. Patients present with a range of symptoms: none, palpitations, systemic embolism or cardiovascular accident, syncope, angina, exercise intolerance, and congestive heart failure.

Haemodynamically unstable patients should undergo immediate cardioversion; the choice may be also relatively easy for a patient with symptomatic AF despite adequate ventricular rate control. Such a patient needs a rhythm control strategy to restore and maintain sinus rhythm to alleviate symptoms. One could also argue that every patient with an initial episode of AF should be offered at least one chance to have sinus rhythm restored by electrical cardioversion without long-term anti-arrhythmic drug therapy. But what about patients who tolerate AF with minimal or no symptoms?

For many years we assumed that rhythm control would be the best treatment approach for patients with AF. The presumed benefits of rhythm control are better relief of symptoms and a lower risk of stroke. In contrast, ventricular rate control was used more often as a secondary strategy when sinus

Divisione di Cardiologia, IRCCS Fondazione Salvatore Maugeri, Istituto Scientifico di Tradate (Varese), Italy

rhythm could not be restored and maintained despite the use of multiple anti-arrhythmic drugs and cardioversions. This approach generally involves the use of drugs that block the AV node, such as beta-blockers, calcium antagonists, and digoxin. Concerns about the rate control approach particularly involved the perceived risks of allowing AF to continue, e.g. thromboembolism and stroke, haemorrhagic complications from anticoagulation, atrial myopathy from long-standing atrial fibrillation, and increased mortality.

The dilemma for patients with asymptomatic or minimally symptomatic AF became magnified as data began to emerge about the risks of anti-arrhythmic drugs, particularly for patients with structural heart disease. These observations led to concern that the potential beneficial effects of restoring and maintaining sinus rhythm may be offset by the adverse effects of the treatment itself.

Several recent randomised studies would appear to support continuing ventricular rate control alone with appropriate anticoagulation for patients who tolerate AF after ventricular rate control is achieved. However, these studies had important limitations, and, as with any study, we must be cautious in interpreting the results and keep in mind what type of patients were studied, which treatment options were studied, and to which patients in your practice the results are applicable.

The Atrial Fibrillation Follow-up Investigation of Rhythm Management (AFFIRM), the largest of these studies, directly compared the two strategies, with total mortality as the primary end-point. A total of 4060 patients who were at least 65 years old or who had other risk factors for stroke were randomised to a strategy of rhythm control or rate control. The rhythm control group received anti-arrhythmic drugs and cardioversion as necessary to maintain sinus rhythm. Continuous anticoagulation was encouraged but could be stopped if sinus rhythm had apparently been maintained for at least 4 weeks. The rate control group received AV nodal-blocking agents and continuous anticoagulation, with the goal of a heart rate ≤ 80 bpm at rest and ≤ 110 bpm during a 6-min walking test. Catheter ablation of the AV node with pacemaker implantation could be used if ventricular rate control was not achieved with a combination of drugs. After 5 years of follow-up, more patients had died in the rhythm control group (24% vs 21%), but the difference was not statistically significant. More rhythm control patients were hospitalised or had adverse drug effects; ischaemic stroke occurred in about 1% of patients per year in each group, mostly those in whom warfarin had been stopped or whose international normalised ratio was subtherapeutic. Other studies comparing rate control vs rhythm control treatment strategies showed similar results [2–5].

These studies showed that a strategy of rhythm control was not superior to a strategy of ventricular rate control for older patients with AF. There were no significant differences in mortality or quality of life. The incidence of ischaemic stroke was not reduced by attempts to maintain sinus rhythm. Also, many patients with stroke (about 50% in the AFFIRM trial and 30% in the RACE trial) were in sinus rhythm at the time of the event. Some of the strokes in the rhythm control groups may have been due to subclinical episodes of AF, raising concern about the practice of stopping warfarin after a patient is presumed to be maintaining sinus rhythm on the basis of symptom reporting. This, along with the potential side effects of anti-arrhythmic drugs, could have negated the potential advantages of rhythm control.

The patient population in both studies was reasonably representative of patients with AF seen in clinical practice. However, there were two sources of possible inclusion bias:

- Only patients who were able and willing to tolerate AF after ventricular rate control had been achieved were included
- Patients were relatively old, and the conclusions of these studies may therefore not apply to younger patients
- Follow-up was relatively short. The effects of ongoing AF over long periods of time remain unclear, in particular concerning the consequences of the progression of the atrial myopathy in such patients
- Another important limitation of these studies is that they did not assess other, potentially curative treatments.

Therefore, one could argue that these trials compared two suboptimal strategies, and the most appropriate conclusion may be that a rhythm control strategy using anti-arrhythmic drugs is just as bad or worse than a ventricular rate control strategy. Interestingly, the AFFIRM trial investigators recently reported that sinus rhythm is associated with a lower risk of death. For these reasons, we cannot yet conclude that restoring sinus rhythm has been eliminated as a management strategy for many patients with AF. Further studies are required to determine the best strategy for younger patients and to investigate alternative treatment strategies.

Atrial fibrillation remains a common problem in medicine; its incidence is projected to increase significantly over the next few decades. The optimal treatment strategy has yet to be clarified, especially because of the large variance in presentation and degree of symptoms among different patients. Effective stroke prevention remains an important consideration. Recent trials suggest that patients with minimal symptoms may be better served with simple rate control and anticoagulation rather than aggressive attempts to restore sinus rhythm, particularly as attempts to maintain sinus rhythm are costly, time-intensive, and ineffective. For patients with problematic symptoms, anti-arrhythmic drug therapy is the first line of treatment, but newer, invasive procedures are being developed and refined. So far, these invasive therapies have shown efficacy only in limited patient populations. It is hoped that, as medical knowledge of the mechanisms of AF continues to progress and technologies continue to be refined, improved options will become available.

References

1. Lévy S, Maarek M, Coumel P et al (1999) College of French cardiologists. Characterization of different subsets of atrial fibrillation in general practice in France: the ALFA Study. Circulation 99:3028–3035
2. Wyse DG, Waldo AL, DiMarco JP et al (2002) A comparison of rate control and rhythm control in patients with atrial fibrillation. N Engl J Med 347:1825–1833
3. Hohnloser SH, Kuch KH, Lilienthal J (2000) Rhythm or rate control in atrial fibrillation – pharmacological intervention in atrial fibrillation (PIAF): a randomised trial. Lancet 356:1789–1794
4. Van Gelder IC, Hagens VE, Bosker HA et al (2002) A comparison of rate control and rhythm control in patients with persistent atrial fibrillation. N Engl J Med 347:1834–1840
5. Carlsson J, Miketic S, Windeler J et al (2003) Randomized trial of rate-control versus rhythm-control in persistent atrial fibrillation: the Strategies of Treatment of Atrial Fibrillation (STAF) study. J Am Coll Cardiol 41:1690–1696

The Role of Imaging in Catheter Ablation of Atrial Fibrillation

J. Kautzner, P. Peichl, H. Mlcochova

Catheter ablation of atrial fibrillation (AF) has become a real therapeutic option for symptomatic patients resistant to or intolerant of antiarrhythmic drugs. Since the first reports of curative catheter ablation a decade ago, several techniques have evolved [1–5]. Despite the fact that these techniques vary significantly, they all have something in common: the predominant target has become the left atrium and pulmonary veins (PVs). Underestimated by many operators, the variability of the anatomy makes the procedure complex and seems to explain most failures and/or complications. The aim of this review is to discuss the importance of imaging techniques for guidance of catheter ablation of AF.

Anatomy of the Left Atrium and Pulmonary Veins

Remarkably little attention was paid to PV anatomy before the era of catheter ablation of AF [6]. The first anatomical study that dealt with the arrangement and diameters of the PV ostia was published by Ho et al. [7]. This study reported no difference in PV ostial diameters. Variant anatomy (i.e. anything other than four distinct ostia) was observed in 23% of the hearts, the remaining specimens showing four distinct PVs. In another study by these authors, 2 of the 20 hearts had a common orifice of the right PVs and another 3 had a common vestibule of the left PVs (i.e. variant anatomy in 20% cases) [8]. Discounting the common ostia, the diameter of PV orifices ranged from 8 mm to 21 mm with a mean of 12.5 mm. Moubarak et al. described confluent PVs (i.e. common vestibules) in 25% of the specimens, more commonly on the left side [9]. Thus, for the first time, these studies suggested that PV arrangements could vary from patient to patient.

Department of Cardiology, Institute for Clinical and Experimental Medicine, Prague, Czech Republic

Pulmonary Venous Angiography

In the early days of experience, PV angiography was performed at the beginning of the ablation procedure in order to determine the position and the size of the PV ostia. Lin et al. were among the first to evaluate PV size in patients with AF using biplanar PV angiography [10]. They revealed that the superior PVs are greater in diameter than the inferior PVs, and that the mean ostial diameters of the superior PVs in patients with AF were significantly greater than in a control group. On average, the diameter of superior PVs at the ostia in controls was 10.9 mm, compared with 13.1–13.6 mm in AF patients. The corresponding diameters of the inferior PVs were 7.5 mm and 8.3 mm, respectively. The relatively small diameters of PV ostia suggest that tube-like portions of the PVs and not the ostia are usually measured by contrast PV angiography. This may result in a higher risk of PV stenosis after energy delivery within the PVs.

Wittkampf et al. published one of the first studies that clearly demonstrated how contrast angiography could be misleading [11]. Using magnetic resonance angiography (MRA), they showed that the majority of PV ostia are oval in shape, with a significantly shorter diameter in the anteroposterior direction (mean ratio between maximum and minimum diameter was 1.5 ± 0.4 for left PVs, a little less for right PVs). Maximum diameters of PVs ranged between 15.9 and 18.7 mm; left common ostia measured 27.3 mm on average. Therefore, this study emphasised for the first time that true ostial dimensions can only be measured using 3D imaging techniques.

A more recent study compared contrast PV angiography obtained in two perpendicular projections with MRA in 20 consecutive patients undergoing catheter ablation [12]. A PV ostium was angiographically defined as the junction of the PV with the left atrium and measured from both projections with a correction for the degree of magnification. Measurements were made at the end of ventricular systole. MRA images from 2D maximum intensity projections and multiplanar reformations were analysed. The study revealed excellent correlation between the PV ostial diameters obtained by these two techniques. The mean diameters measured by both of them ranged between 16.9 and 19.4 mm. Although these values appear to be more realistic than in the study by Lin et al., the two diameters measured from two PV angiographic projections for each vein were similar and thus did not exhibit the characteristic oval shape described above. This again suggests that PV angiography may not be an appropriate tool for the assessment of the true PV ostial anatomy. Despite this, many operators still use this technique alone to guide catheter ablation of AF.

MR Angiography

Since the time of Wittkampf´s study, several other studies have explored the potential of MRA for determining the anatomy of PVs and non-invasive assessment of PV stenosis after catheter ablation [13–17]. Unfortunately, they mostly used 2D data format for this purpose. Some studies compared AF subjects with controls and suggested that the former group had larger PV diameters, especially superior PVs. PV ostia were found to be oblong in shape with the anteroposterior dimension less than the superoinferior dimension. AF subjects also presented with complex branching patterns, especially in the inferior PVs [15]. Variant anatomy was observed in 38% of subjects and there was no difference between patients in the AF and control groups. A short common left trunk was observed in 15% and the remaining 18% of subjects presented with more marked anatomic variation. So far, the largest study using MRA to establish PV anatomy was published by Mansour et al., who analysed diameters and branching patterns of PVs in 105 patients undergoing PV isolation [17]. They concluded that 56% had four separate ostia, 29% presented with an additional PV, and 17% showed a common left trunk. The PV ostium was smaller than 10 mm in 26 (25%) subjects and larger than 25 mm in 15 (14%) patients.

After ablation, Kato et al. observed detectable PV narrowing in 24% of the veins [15]. However, severe PV stenosis was described in 1 PV (1.4%), moderate stenosis in 1 PV (1.4%), and mild stenosis in the remaining 15 PVs (21.1%). Dill et al. used MRA in 44 subjects before and after segmental PV isolation, and described a very good correlation between the diameters of PV ostia measured from contrast angiography and from MRA [14]. Mild or moderate diameter reduction after catheter ablation was observed in 18% of patients one day after, with a reversal in 5.8% and a progression in 7.2% during a 3-month period.

Our experience confirms the above observations that MRA is an excellent tool for detailed evaluation of PV anatomy [18]. However, our data vary to some extent from previous studies as we documented even higher variability in the arrangement of PV ostia. Analysis of 3D reconstructions documented clearly that variant anatomy of the PV ostia can be revealed in 80% of subjects (Fig. 1). This was mainly due to a relatively high occurrence of short left-sided common trunk. The explanation is that although previous studies claimed the use of 3D data, the analysis and measurements were definitely performed on 2D images. In a fair proportion of patients, the true pattern of the PV arrangement may be recognised only from 3D reconstructions and is easily underestimated from 2D maximum intensity projection images. The

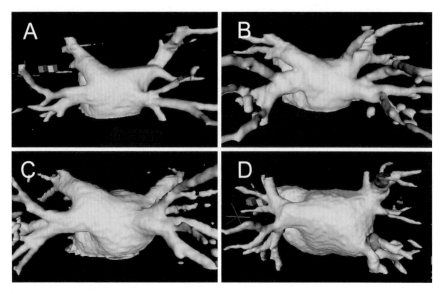

Fig. 1a-d. Four examples of MR angiographic 3D images of the left atrium and PVs in patients before catheter ablation of AF. Note the variable anatomy with a predominant pattern of a left-sided common vestibule

high frequency with which the common left-sided vestibule occurs suggests that this may be labelled as the 'normal' pattern of arrangement of the left-sided PVs. A detailed knowledge of anatomy may decrease the risk of development of PV stenosis.

Multidetector CT Angiography

Modern multidetector CT scanners (4-, 16-, or 64-slice) allow non-invasive CT angiography (CTA) of the majority of vascular beds after injection of the contrast agent into a peripheral vein. In addition, they provide an accurate 3D reconstruction of the recorded data using volume-rendering technique. One of the first studies of the PVs in humans using four-slice CT was published by Scharf et al. [19]. They found four separate PV ostia in 47 AF patients (81%). Using 2D maximum intensity projections, they observed a left common trunk in only 3% of subjects. AF patients had larger ostial diameters than control subjects, and superior PVs were larger than inferior PVs. Up to 60% stenosis was revealed after catheter ablation in 3% of 128 isolated PVs. Schwartzman et al. examined the dimensions and morphology of the left atrium and PVs in 70 patients with and 47 subjects without AF [20]. They correlated measurements obtained from 3D CT reconstructions with those obtained from intracardiac echocardiography. Variant anatomy was relatively more frequent than in the above study –more than 2 PVs were frequently observed on the right (18–25%), as well as PV ostial branching, and a common PV frequently occurred on the left (6–20%). PV ostia were neither circular nor planar. Left atrial and PV dimensions were significantly greater in the AF group. However, after correction for left atrial volume, all PV diameters were similar.

The largest population (201 patients), predominantly of subjects without AF, was evaluated by CT angiography and 2D images were analysed [21]. Right PV drainage patterns varied in 32% of subjects, most commonly due to the presence of a third PV draining directly into the left atrium. On the left side, 86% of subjects had two ostia for the upper and lower lobes, while a common trunk was observed in the remaining 14%. No association was found between any drainage pattern and the presence of AF.

Our pilot data suggest that there is excellent anatomical correlation between MRA and 16-slice CT angiography, once 3D reconstruction (volume-rendering technique) is used. Therefore, these methods can be used alternatively (Fig. 2), both for preoperative assessment of anatomy and for postoperative detection of PV stenosis.

Intracardiac Echocardiography

Recent advances in technology have allowed the design of catheter-based ultrasound transducers for imaging of intracardiac structures. Two types of catheter are currently in use. One is a mechanical catheter with a rotating transducer which results in a 360° view perpendicular to the catheter shaft.

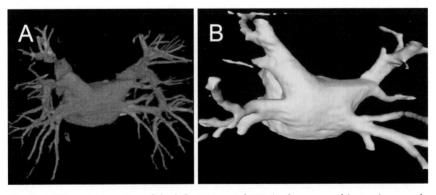

Fig. 2a, b. 3D reconstruction of the left atrium and PVs in the same subject using **a** multidetector CT angiography and **b** MRA. Note the perfect correspondence in anatomy

The other is a phased array echocardiographic catheter that employs electronically controlled multiple transducers close to the tip, which results in a wedge-shaped image sector similar to that of a transoesophageal probe. This second type of catheter offers a greater depth of penetration and the possibility of Doppler imaging, including colour-coded.

There is mounting evidence that intracardiac echocardiography (ICE) can facilitate catheter ablation of AF by increasing efficacy and reducing complications [22]. Compared to fluoroscopy, ICE provides multiple advantages. It allows: (1) real-time definition of cardiac anatomy, especially of PV ostia; (2) positioning of the catheter tip and assessment of its contact with atrial tissue; (3) visualisation of microbubble formation as a sign of tissue overheating; (4) assessment of PV flow and recognition of PV stenosis; and (5) early detection of thrombus and/or char formation.

The advantage of ICE in guiding AF catheter ablation starts to show during trans-septal puncture. An ICE catheter positioned in the middle of the right atrium provides clear images of the fossa ovalis and allow safe trans-septal puncture even in anticoagulated patients. The trans-septal sheath and the needle are visible as they tent the membranous part of the septum. This allows 'mapping' of the fossa ovalis and selection of a preferential puncture site posteriorly and lower, in order to have better access to the PVs. The penetration of the needle to the left atrium is then followed on the screen.

Given the enormous variability in PV ostial anatomy and arrangement of the PVs, ICE provides very accurate information about the catheter tip position around the PV ostia. Where required, ICE allows exact positioning of the circular mapping catheter (Lasso, Biosense Webster) at the very level of the ostium (Fig. 3a). It has been shown to visualise PV ostia better than angiography, and to ensure proper electrode alignment and contact [23]. Monitoring of microbubble formation can reveal tissue overheating before impedance rises, and thus before the pop phenomenon can occur [24]. Whether this approach could eliminate the risk of atrio-oesophageal fistula remains to be documented.

ICE carries additional potential for prevention of complications. It has been shown that monitoring of the catheter position decreases the risk of thromboembolic complications (Fig. 3b). In one recent study, thrombus formation was observed within the left atrium in 10% of cases, despite anticoagulation treatment with activated clotting time (ACT) above 250 s [25]. Another study suggested that ICE-guided power titration has an additive effect in terms of safety – i.e. it leads to a further decrease in the thromboembolic event rate as compared with ICE imaging only [24]. At the same time, ICE navigation minimises the risk of PV stenosis [26].

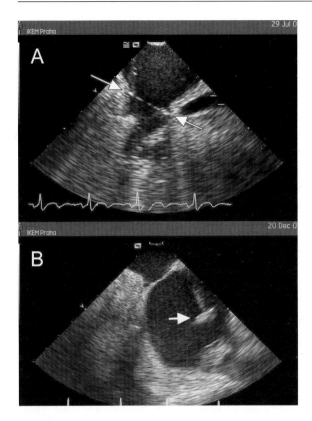

Fig. 3. Intracardiac echo-cardiograms that show: **a** precise positioning of the circular mapping catheter (Lasso) at the level of ostium of the right inferior PV (*arrows* mark ostial margins); **b** mobile thrombus attached to the tip of the trans-septal sheath in the left atrial cavity before introduction of the ablation catheter (*arrow*). The thrombus was safely removed by suction

Implications for Catheter Ablation

All the above data suggest that arrangement of the PV ostia is highly vari-able, and even results obtained by the same imaging technique may vary sig-nificantly. This underlines the need for pre-procedural 3D imaging (i.e. MRA or CTA), which is important for understanding the anatomy and provides a basis for subsequent evaluation of PV stenosis. To achieve maximum safety of catheter ablation, there appears to be a need for on-line visualisation of the PV ostia and the position of the ablation catheter by means of ICE. However, most centres use only electroanatomical mapping to support catheter ablation around the PV ostia. Although this provides a certain degree of 3D navigation for catheter ablation, one must not forget that it is virtual anatomy that is being displayed, and certainly this is not the ideal technique for description of the true anatomy of the PV ostia.

Following previous experience with segmental isolation and then with circumferential ablation, we started to employ pre-procedural MRA of the left atrium and PVs in every ablation case. In addition, we adopted the use of ICE in association with electroanatomical mapping system and the Lasso catheter. One of the reasons for this move was the observed variability in the PV ostial arrangement, which does not allow accurate location of the PV ostia by the electroanatomical mapping system. The other reason was to improve the efficacy and safety of ablation in the same way as reported by Marrouche et al. [24]. The strategy is to integrate data obtained by pre-procedural 3D MRA with the virtual anatomical map constructed during the procedure under ICE guidance (Fig. 4). ICE further enables precise placement of the Lasso catheter at the level of the venoatrial junction and deployment of ablation lesions proximal to it. In addition, it may help to create adequate radiofrequency lesions by monitoring the power delivery and the creation of microbubbles as a sign of tissue overheating. So far, we have performed 38 procedures in 37 patients without structural heart disease, and 23 of them have a minimum follow-up of 2 months. Nineteen (83%) are without AF, partial effect was observed in another subject, and three patients continue to have AF and symptoms. No case of PV stenosis or thromboembolism were observed. Although it is early to analyse the efficacy of the above approach, we believe that ICE provides significant help in catheter ablation of AF.

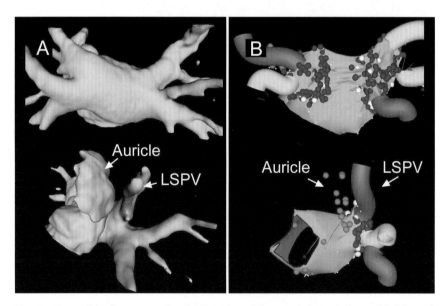

Fig. 4. a Examples of pre-procedural MRA viewed from posteroanterior and left lateral projections in a patient who subsequently underwent circumferential ablation around the PV ostia. **b** Corresponding projections as obtained by electroanatomical mapping and tagging PV ostia under intracardiac echocardiographic navigation. Left auricle is labelled as floating points. Note the good correlation between the two methods of reconstruction

Conclusions

Lessons learned from sophisticated imaging techniques such as MRA or CTA suggest that anatomy of the left atrium and PVs is very complex and highly variable. This agrees with clinical experience derived from catheter ablation of AF and leads to a paradigm shift from navigation of catheter ablation solely by mapping to the need for imaging of the PV ostia. It appears that detailed knowledge of the anatomy diminishes the risk of PV stenosis as the lesions are applied outside the tube-like portions of the PVs. Imaging techniques also allow postoperative detection of PV stenosis. Intraoperative use of ICE supports precise catheter positioning, and allows energy delivery to be monitored and/or complications to be reduced.

References

1. Haïssaguerre M, Shah DC, Jais P et al (2000) Electrophysiological breakthroughs from the left atrium to the pulmonary veins. Circulation 102:2463–2465
2. Haïssaguerre M, Shah DC, Jais P et al (2000) Mapping-guided ablation of pulmonary veins to cure atrial fibrillation. Am J Cardiol 86(Suppl 1):K9-K19
3. Pappone C, Rosanio S, Oreto G et al (2000) Circumferential radiofrequency ablation of pulmonary vein ostia: a new anatomic approach for curing atrial fibrillation. Circulation 102:2619–2628
4. Pappone C, Oreto G, Rosanio S et al (2001) Atrial electroanatomic remodeling after circumferential radiofrequency pulmonary vein ablation: efficacy of an anatomical approach in a large cohort of patients with atrial fibrillation. Circulation 104:2539–2544
5. Nademanee K, McKenzie J, Kosar E et al (2004) A new approach for catheter ablation of atrial fibrillation: mapping of the electrophysiologic substrate. J Am Coll Cardiol 43:2044–2053
6. Nathan H, Eliakin M (1966) The junction between the left atrium and the pulmonary veins. Circulation 34:412–422
7. Ho SY, Sanchez-Quintana D, Cabrera JA et al (1999) Anatomy of the left atrium: implications for radiofrequency ablation of atrial fibrillation. J Cardiovasc Electrophysiol 10:1525–1533
8. Ho SY, Cabrera JA, Tran VH et al (2001) Architecture of the pulmonary veins: relevance to radiofrequency ablation. Heart 86:265–270
9. Moubarak JB, Rozwadowski JV, Strzalka CT et al (2000) Pulmonary veins—left atrial junction: anatomic and histological study. Pacing Clin Electrophysiol 23:1836–1838
10. Lin WS, Prakash VS, Tai CT et al (2000) Pulmonary vein morphology in patients with paroxysmal atrial fibrillation initiated by ectopic beats originating from the pulmonary veins: implications for catheter ablation. Circulation 101:1274–1281
11. Wittkampf FHM, Vonken EJ, Derksen R et al (2003) Pulmonary vein ostium geometry: analysis by magnetic resonance angiography. Circulation 107:21–23
12. Vasamreddy CR, Jayam V, Lickfett L et al (2004) Technique and results of pulmonary vein angiography in patients undergoing catheter ablation of atrial fibrillation. J Cardiovasc Electrophysiol 15:21–26

13. Tsao HM, Yu WC, Cheng HC et al (2001) Pulmonary vein dilation in patients with atrial fibrillation: detection by magnetic resonance imaging. J Cardiovasc Electrophysiol 12:809–813

14. Dill T, Neumann T, Ekinci O et al (2003) Pulmonary vein diameter reduction after radiofrequency catheter ablation for paroxysmal atrial fibrillation evaluated by contrast-enhanced three-dimensional magnetic resonance imaging. Circulation 107:845–850

15. Kato R, Lickfett L, Meininger G et al (2003) Pulmonary vein anatomy in patients undergoing catheter ablation of atrial fibrillation: lessons learned by use of magnetic resonance imaging. Circulation 107:2004–2010

16. Takase B, Nagata M, Matsui T et al (2004) Pulmonary vein dimensions and variation of branching pattern in patients with paroxysmal atrial fibrillation using magnetic resonance angiography. Jpn Heart J 45:81–92

17. Mansour M, Holmvang G, Sosnovik D et al (2004) Assessment of pulmonary vein anatomic variability by magnetic resonance imaging: implications for catheter ablation techniques for atrial fibrillation. J Cardiovasc Electrophysiol 15:387–393

18. Mlcochová H, Cihák R, Tintera J et al (2004) Variability of pulmonary veins in patients undergoing ablation of AF. Europace 6(1):80

19. Scharf C, Sneider M, Case I et al (2003) Anatomy of the pulmonary veins in patients with atrial fibrillation and effects of segmental ostial ablation analyzed by computed tomography. J Cardiovasc Electrophysiol 14:150–155

20. Schwartzman D, Lacomis J, Wigginton WG (2003) Characterisation of left atrium and distal pulmonary vein morphology using multidimensional computed tomography. J Am Coll Cardiol 16:1349–1357

21. Marom EM, Herndon JE, Kim YH et al (2004) Variations in pulmonary venous drainage to the left atrium: implications for radiofrequency ablation. Radiology 230:824–829

22. Cooper JM, Epstein LM (2001) Use of intracardiac echocardiography to guide ablation of atrial fibrillation. Circulation 104:3010–3013

23. Kalman JM, Fitzpatrick AP, Olgin JE et al (1997) Biophysical characteristics of radiofrequency lesion formation in vivo: dynamics of catheter tip-tissue contact evaluated by intracardiac echocardiography. Am Heart J 133:8–18

24. Marrouche N, Martin D, Wayni O et al (2003) Phased-array intracardiac echocardiography monitoring during pulmonary vein isolation in patients with atrial fibrillation: impact on outcome and complications. Circulation 107:2710–2716

25. Ren JF, Marchlinski FE, Callans DJ (2004) Left atrial thrombus associated with ablation for atrial fibrillation: identification with intracardiac echocardiography. J Am Coll Cardiol 43:1861–1867

26. Saad EB, Rosillo A, Saad CP et al (2003) Pulmonary vein stenosis after radiofrequency ablation of atrial fibrillation: functional characterisation, evolution, and influence of the ablation strategy. Circulation 108:3102–3107

Atypical Atrial Flutter

A.S. MONTENERO

Background

With the use of endocardial activation mapping and stimulation studies, several investigators have shown that different types of macroreentrant atrial tachycardias are possible. The circuit is usually located in the right atrium and a critical component of slow conduction is frequently present, often located at the isthmus of atrial tissue which is between the tricuspid annulus, the inferior vena cava, and the coronary sinus with eustachian valve and ridge. Of the different types of atrial flutter, the typical common or type 1 atrial flutter is the most frequent. In this type of flutter right atrial activation rotates in a counterclockwise direction. Less common are reverse (clockwise) typical flutter. More recently, other types of isthmus-dependent and non-isthmus-dependent flutter patterns have been described, even including left atrial flutter [1–3].

Lower Loop Atrial Flutter

Lower loop reentry is defined as macroreentrant tachycardia maintained by circus movement of the activation wave front around the inferior vena cava instead of around the tricuspid annulus as in typical right atrial flutter. An earlier study from Cheng et al. [1] showed that early breakthrough over the tricuspid annulus occurred over the low lateral right atrium. Later on the same group extended these observations showing that one annular break or more could occur at the lateral or anterolateral regions of the annulus [2]. Lower loop reentry uses the same isthmus between the tricuspid annulus and inferior vena cava as in common atrial flutter and therefore is similarly

Department of Cardiology and Arrhythmia Centre, Policlinico MultiMedica, Sesto S. Giovanni (Milan), Italy amendable by ablation of the isthmus. Recently Zhang et al. [4] have investigated the exact reentry circuit in patients with atrial flutter that was associated with surface ECG flutter wave morphology and endocardial recordings that are characteristic of clockwise atrial flutter. The major finding of this study is that most of the isthmus between the tricuspid annulus and the inferior vena cava dependent-flutter with positive flutter wave in the inferior ECG leads involves a reentrant circuit around the inferior vena cava. It provided the first evidence that figure-of-eight double loop reentry may occur around the inferior vena cava and tricuspid annulus and mimic typical clockwise atrial flutter in patients without prior atriotomy. Because the tricuspid isthmus constitutes the common pathway between the two reentrant loops, this double loop reentry is also amendable by ablation that results in bidirectional conduction block.

SI Short Circuit

Earlier studies by Olgin et al. [5] and Nakagawa et al. [6] showed that breakthrough over the eustachian ridge posterior to the coronary sinus (CS) ostium may be observed in 25–50% of patients with typical forms of flutter. In these reports, there was almost simultaneous activation of the septum by wave fronts advancing both anterior and posterior to the CS. Later Yang et al. [2] showed another novel finding: demonstration of a circuit with early activation of the CS region. In this circuit, a typical counterclockwise wave front negotiated the lateral portion of the isthmus and skirted posterior to the CS ostium and the septum. One possible explanation is the presence of a pectinate muscle band from the crista effectively separating the isthmus into anterior and posterior compartments. The authors defined this type of flutter as 'partial isthmus-dependent' atrial flutter. Bidirectional isthmus block induced by a radiofrequency lesion would terminate the tachycardia.

Upper Loop Reentry Tachycardia

Upper loop reentry (ULR) is interpreted as the 'converse' of lower loop reentry (LLR), with a clockwise circuit and break over the lateral or anterolateral annulus with impulse collision in the isthmus. It should be emphasised that electroanatomic mapping studies were not available during ULR; hence, the precise confines of the circuit are not clear, although detailed entrainment mapping in some of these patients showed concealed entrainment at the posterior right atrial septal region between the fossa ovalis and either the superior or the inferior vena cava. In addition, work by Yang et al. [2] supports the finding of spontaneous conversion of either typical clockwise flutter or

LLR to ULR. In one patient with LLR and multiple breakthroughs, conduction block over the isthmus was associated with the start of an ULR loop.

Previous reports [7] have described an atypical flutter circuit similar to the ULR described by Yang et al. [2]. In addition, a very complete report by Shah et al. [8], who used electroanatomic mapping, revealed a variable pattern of activation of the superior right atrium in patients with typical counterclockwise flutter. They showed an apparent isthmus between the superior vena cava and the superior portion of the tricuspid annulus. They hypothesise that ULR might use the channel between these structures. The descriptions provided by Yang et al. [2] of hypothetical circuits were derived largely from deductive reasoning based on typical flutter circuits. They appreciated that precise delineation of the tachycardia circuit(s) was not possible without advanced imaging techniques.

Scar-Related Atrial Tachycardia

Patients with who have previously undergone atriotomy may suffer from a scar-related tachycardia that mimics a counterclockwise atrial flutter. This tachycardia arises from a large low-voltage area of the posterolateral right atrium and travels around the scar with more than one critical isthmus. The identification and ablation of these isthmi may represent a challenge.

Left Atrial Flutter

Few data are available about left atrial flutters. In a dog model, Schuessler et al. [9] demonstrated atrial flutters, usually rotating around anatomical and functional zones of block. However, in dogs with enlarged and/or hypertrophied left atria, most of the circuits were located in the right atrium. Pure left atrial circuits were rarely found, usually rotating around the pulmonary vein (four dogs in Schuessler's experience). Therefore, both human and animal data suggest that the right atrium is more frequently involved in flutters than the left. However, the exact incidence of left atrial flutters in humans is currently unknown.

The diagnosis of left atrial flutter can be established by comprehensive mapping, including a 3D electroanatomic system, and confirmed by the results of catheter ablation achieving sinus rhythm. Various circuits can be demonstrated. In most cases, the arrhythmia may rotate around the mitral annulus, a zone of block including the pulmonary veins, or a silent area. Lines of block and silent areas also act as lateral barriers, probably allowing stabilisation of the circuit and preventing short circuiting. In a few patients, the circuit is more complex, with two or three loops rotating concomitantly.

There is no marked area of slow conduction in these macroreentrant circuits, in contrast to the cases of small reentrant circuits, in which a zone of very slow conduction has been demonstrated, accounting for more than two-thirds of the cycle length. Slow-conduction areas have been frequently reported in animal models, usually being the centre of the circuit, either alone or in association with anatomical obstacles. In contrast, a silent area has not previously been reported clinically. It seems to be a distinctive and relatively common feature of human left atrial flutter, present in 50% of the patients in the series of Jaïs et al. [10]. This is probably related to severe atrial fibrosis (and atrial myocardial cell modification/disappearance), a common phenomenon in patients with structural heart disease. It may also be possible that in patients who have suffered from atrial arrhythmias for many years, histological changes have occurred as a result of atrial arrhythmia. Marrouche et al. [11] recently reported on patients with a novel macroreentrant left atrial arrhythmia: the so-called left septal atrial flutter. Most of the patients in this study developed left atrial flutter after initiation of anti-arrhythmic therapy for atrial fibrillation. Slowing of atrial conduction by anti-arrhythmic drugs may be a factor that allows left septal flutter. The zone of double potentials anterior to the right pulmonary veins, corresponding to the limbus of the fossa ovalis for the right atrium, and the mitral annulus represent functional and anatomical barriers for left septal atrial flutter, respectively. In addition, the results from the Marrouche series appeared to suggest that the anterior ablation approach is more likely to provide a long-term cure. Concealed entrainment has been used to identify a protected isthmus between barriers, which are critical for the maintenance of arrhytmia. Concealed entrainment documented by pacing between the zone of double potentials between the right pulmonary veins and the septum primum and between the septum primum and the mitral annulus. Thus, the left septal atrial flutter circuit appeared to revolve around the septum primum with the use of two protected isthmi. The zone of double potential seems to play a role similar to that of the crista terminalis during typical atrial flutter. The zone of double potentials recorded in patients corresponds to the limbus of the fossa ovalis on the right septum, which seems to complete the embryological separation of the two atria. The region between the septum primum and the mitral annulus defines another critical isthmus for the left septal atrial flutter circuit. A similar situation has been described by Nagakawa et al. [6] in the right atrium, where the tricuspid annulus forms a continuous anterior barrier in patients with typical flutter. Marrouche has also demonstrated a similar role of the septal part of the mitral annulus in forming an anterior anatomical barrier for the left septal flutter circuit. The left atrial septum possesses a unique muscular architecture that would allow the maintenance of left septal atrial flutter. Moreover, Jaïs et al. [10] also recognised the mitral annulus as a critical anatomical barrier in 36% of patients with left atrial flutter. Linear radiofrequency lesions between the membranous septum and the mitral annulus seem to be an effective and safe therapy for this arrhythmia.

Conclusions

The identification of the macroreentrant nature of atrial flutter and the ability to localise the circuit by endocardial activation mapping and pacing resulted in attempts to interrupt the circuit by ablative interventions. Nowadays, catheter ablation of atrial flutter has become a safe, curative, and highly successful procedure, particularly when the right atrial isthmus is incorporated in the flutter circuit. Demonstration of bidirectional isthmus block after ablation predicts a high long-term success rate. Scar-related and left atrial flutters present more complex patterns of activation, making the ablation more difficult and the 3D system often mandatory.

References

1. Cheng J, Cabeen WR, Scheinman MM (1999) Right atrial flutter due to lower loop reentry: mechanism and anatomic substrates. Circulation 99:1700–1705
2. Yang YF, Cheng J, Bochoeyer A et al (2001) Atypical right atrial flutter patterns. Circulation 103:3092–3098
3. Kalman JM, Olgin JE, Saxon LA et al (1996) Activation and entrainment mapping defines the tricuspid annulus as the anterior barrier in typical atrial flutter. Circulation 94:398–406
4. Zhang S, Younis G, Hariharan R et al (2004) Lower loop reentry as a mechanism of clockwise right atrial flutter. Circulation 109:1630–1635
5. Olgin JE, Kalman JM, Fitzpatrick AP et al (1995) Role of right atrial endocardial structures as barriers to conduction during human type I atrial flutter: activation and entrainment mapping guided by intracardiac echocardiography. Circulation 92:1839–1848
6. Nakagawa H, Lazzara R, Khastgir T et al (1996) Role of the tricuspid annulus and the eustachian valve/ridge on atrial flutter: relevance to catheter ablation of the septal isthmus and a new technique for rapid identification of ablation success. Circulation 94:407–424
7. Lai LP, Lin JL, Tseng CD et al (1999) Electrophysiologic study and radiofrequency catheter ablation of isthmus-independent atrial flutter. J Cardiovasc Electrophysiol 10:728–735
8. Shah DC, Jaïs P, Haïssaguerre M et al (1997) Three-dimensional mapping of the common atrial flutter circuit in the right atrium. Circulation 96:3904–3912
9. Schuessler RB, Boineau JP, Bromberg BI et al (1995) Normal and abnormal activation of the atrium. In: Zipes DP, Jalife J (eds) Cardiac electrophysiology from cell to bedside, 2nd edn. Saunders Philadelphia, pp 543–562

10. Jais P, Shah D, Haïssaguerre M et al (2000) Mapping and ablation of left atrial flutters. Circulation 101:2928–2934
11. Marrouche NF, Natale A, Wazni O et al (2004) Left septal atrial flutter: electrophysiology, anatomy, and results of ablation. Circulation 109:2440–2447

Advances in Surgical Treatment of Atrial Fibrillation

L. Patanè, A. Cavallaro

Epidemiology

Atrial fibrillation (AF) is the most common cardiac rhythm disturbance, affecting 2.2 million people within the United States and 5.5 million worldwide. The incidence of AF increases with age, with a prevalence of 0.5% of people in the fifth decade of life, rising to 10% of people in the eighth decade [1]. AF is associated with a number of predisposing cardiovascular disorders, including coronary artery disease, valvular heart disease, congestive heart failure, and hypertension, and occurs in as many as 50% of patients undergoing cardiac operations. However, in up to 31% of cases AF is not associated with an underlying cardiovascular disorder [2]. AF contributes significantly to cardiovascular morbidity and mortality (Framingham study) [3]. It is an independent risk factor for death, with a relative risk of approximately 1.5 for men and 1.9 for women even after adjustment for associated cardiovascular disorders [4]. Because of the loss of effective atrial contraction, stasis of blood in the atria predisposes affected patients to thromboembolism. Patients with AF have a five-fold increased risk for stroke compared to age-matched controls, and AF is responsible for as many as 15% of all strokes [4, 5].

Persistence of AF after cardiac surgery carries significant cardiovascular morbidity and mortality despite medical treatment. In mitral valve disease up to 80% of the patients remain in AF after surgical correction of the valvular cardiac disease [3, 6]. Therefore, the goal for patients with organic heart diseases and permanent AF is not only the cure of lesions but also return to permanent normal sinus rhythm, restoration of biatrial transport function, and preventing thromboembolism. Building upon the pioneering work of

Centro Cuore Morgagni, Pedara (Catania), Italy

Cox et al., recent reported series have demonstrated the feasibility of treating patients undergoing cardiac surgery for other structural heart disease with limited left-atrial ablation lesion sets using alternative energy sources. This review summarises recent advances in surgery for AF.

Classification of Atrial Fibrillation

According to the American College of Cardiology, American Heart Association, and European Society of Cardiology task force, classification of AF begins with the first detected episode of this arrhythmia [7]. If a patient has two or more episodes, AF is considered recurrent. Recurrent AF is designated as paroxysmal, persistent, or permanent. Paroxysmal AF lasts 7 or fewer days and terminates spontaneously. Persistent AF does not terminate spontaneously, but requires electrical or pharmacological cardioversion to restore normal sinus rhythm; if the first detected episode of AF does not terminate spontaneously, it is also designated persistent. Permanent AF is defined as a condition in which sinus rhythm cannot be sustained after cardioversion or the patient and physician have decided against further efforts to restore sinus rhythm.

Physiopathology

Using computer simulation, Moe et al. [8, 9] postulated that multiple wandering wavelets are present during AF. An important further advance in our understanding of AF has been the recognition that AF itself alters atrial electrophysiological and structural properties, a process called 'electrical remodelling', in such a way that maintenance of the arrhythmia is favoured [10, 11]. The approximately 10-fold increase in atrial rate associated with AF causes intracellular calcium loading. As a compensatory response, atrial myocytes down-regulate calcium channel activity, which shortens the action potential duration, reduces the refractory period, and promotes the induction and maintenance of AF by multiple-circuit re-entry [1]. Over the past several years, a number of observations have been made that challenge this conventional viewpoint, that is that all AF results from multiple circuit re-entry. Experimental mapping studies have suggested the importance of a primary local generator, such as a single small re-entry circuit or ectopic focus [12, 13]. This notion has been supported by the finding that left atrial sources of ectopic activity are of particular importance in a subset of patients. In patients with paroxysmal AF, Haïssaguerre et al. have shown that arrhythmias originate from ectopic foci in the pulmonary veins up to 94% of the time [14]. This probably relates to the anatomic transition from pulmonary vein endothelium to left atrial endocardium; at this juncture, local ionic differences may lead to shorter refractory periods in left atrial tissue, favouring re-entry [15]. Although this observation demonstrates the critical importance of pulmonary veins in patients with paroxysmal AF, it may not apply to persistent or permanent AF, where the posterior left atrium and possibly the pulmonary veins are implicated in their pathogenesis and maintenance. Harada et al. [16] performed intraoperative atrial activation mapping in 10 patients with persistent AF, demonstrating that for most patients the left atrium acted as the electrical driving chamber. However, such patients also tend to have pathological right atrial changes [17]. Collectively, these recent findings challenge the long-held view that all AF results from multiple-circuit re-entry and explains both why the left atrium and pulmonary veins are so important for the ablation to be successful and why more limited procedures aimed at the electrical isolation of discrete atrial regions.

Surgical Treatment of Atrial Fibrillation

The long-term medical treatment of AF with anti-arrhythmic drug therapy is associated with a failure rate of 50% at 1 year and up to 84% at 2 years [5, 18]. In addition, currently available anti-arrhythmic agents are not specific for atrial activity and therefore can have profound effects on ventricular electrophysiology. The medical treatment for AF has therefore largely focused on ventricular rate control and management of thromboembolic risk with oral anticoagulants. While warfarin therapy has been shown to have a decisive benefit in reducing thromboembolism in patients with chronic AF, this treatment is cumbersome and exposes patients to significant haemorrhagic risk [19]. Dissatisfaction with medical therapy has spurred efforts to develop a surgical treatment for AF.

Cox Maze III

The pioneering work of Cox et al. in 1991 culminated in the development of the Cox maze III procedure, which remains the gold standard for the surgical treatment of AF [20–23]. This procedure, by making a series of single-line incisions and cryolesions in both the right and left atria, reduces atrial critical mass and interrupts all possible multiple re-entrant circuits necessary for the propagation of AF (Fig. 1). The interrupting incisions allow sinus node impulses to be transmitted across the atria to the atrioventricular node. The treatment of the left atrium includes isolation of the pulmonary veins and excision of the left atrial appendages. These elements of the Cox maze III procedure were retained in the majority of subsequently developed operations aimed at the treatment of AF. The outstanding results of the Cox maze

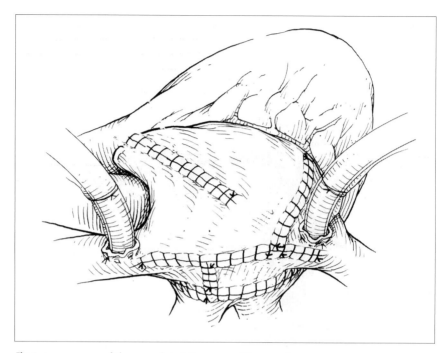

Fig. 1. Appearance of the completed Cox-maze III procedure

III procedure justify its status as the 'gold standard' surgical procedure for AF. Cox et al. report an overall success rate of 99% in curing patients with AF [24]. No instances of sinus node damage have been identified. Left and right atrial function have been documented in 93% and 98% of patients, respectively. High rates of freedom from AF have been reported by other investigators performing the Cox maze III procedure [25–27].

Despite this high degree of success, the procedure has not gained widespread clinical application due to its perceived complexity and invasiveness (requiring median sternotomy, long cardiopulmonary bypass, cardioplegic arrest, extensive cardiac dissection, and multiple atrial incisions) and its significant mortality and morbidity [28]. In an attempt to make the procedure simpler and less time-consuming, and potentially obviate the need for cardiopulmonary bypass, a number of investigators have developed the so-called partial maze procedures where the incisions are made only on the left atrium. Kress et al. have validated one such left atrial lesion set for the treatment of AF [29]. These procedures have generally focused on the left atrium, with the pulmonary veins being isolated by a series of lesions and the left atrial appendage being either excluded or excised. Alternative energy sources are typically used to reduce procedure time. The coronary sinus is typically not treated in partial maze procedures. Cox and Ad have previously emphasised the importance of ablating the coronary sinus during procedures for the treatment of AF in order to minimise the risk of atrial flutter [30, 31]. In patients undergoing a concomitant right atrial procedure and in those with a history of atrial flutter (in whom right-sided initiating foci are common), many surgeons also perform a limited right atrial ablation procedure.

Alternative Energy Sources

One of the obstacles to widespread clinical application of the Cox maze III procedure is the time required to cut and sew the left atrium to interrupt atrial re-entry circuits. The development of alternative energy sources that can ablate atrial tissue by topical application has been a necessary advance in the evolution toward faster, less invasive procedures for AF. The ideal energy source would be fast, reliable, yield a full-thickness lesion, would not damage surrounding tissues, and would be amenable to off-pump and minimally invasive application. Recently developed alternative energy sources now possess a number of these desirable characteristics.

Three alternative energy sources are used surgically to treat AF: radiofrequency, cryothermy, and microwave. Laser and ultrasound are not completely proven at this point. The goal of all five procedures is to develop controlled lesions of coagulative necrosis and ultimately scar tissue to block the abnormal electrical impulses from being conducted through the heart and promote the normal conduction of impulses through the proper pathway [32]. The lesion sets created with this alternative energy are similar, generally including pulmonary vein isolation. Cryothermy and microwave have also been used as part of Cox maze III.

Radiofrequency

Special probes uses radiofrequency energy, an alternating current from 350 kHz to 1 MHz, to heat tissue and create transmural epicardial and/or endocardial linear lesions that block atrial conduction similarly to the lesions of the maze procedure [33]. Experimental data demonstrate that heating tissue for approximately 1 min at 70–80 °C produces lesions 3–6 mm deep, usually sufficient to create a transmural line of conduction block [34]. With this energy source there has been a significant experience and a variety of surgical techniques [35–38], related to the different radiofrequency catheter systems available (unipolar, bipolar, dry or saline-cooled) [39–42], the amount of energy and variety of lesion sets (Melo pulmonary veins encircling, Alfieri set, and so on) (Fig. 2). Radiofrequency ablation by epicardial application holds promise for developing off-pump and minimally invasive procedures for AF.

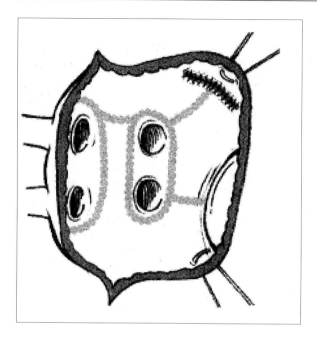

Fig. 2. Left-sided partial maze procedure. Complete radiofrequency endocardial lines ablation. ⬤⬤⬤⬤⬤⬤, ablative lines

The majority of radiofrequency ablation procedures to date have been performed with unipolar systems that have a number of limitations related, particularly with dry probes, to the unfocused nature of the energy that is delivered. Local temperatures can exceed 100 °C, leading to surface charring and potential thromboembolic complications. Heat is conducted to surrounding tissues, raising the risk of damage to surrounding structures. Oesophageal perforations have been reported with this technique [43, 44]. Recently developed saline-cooled bipolar radiofrequency clamps address these limitations and allow the creation of more precise and uniform transmural lesions. The early clinical experience with bipolar radiofrequency ablation has demonstrated consistent conduction block with epicardial and off-pump application [45]. Creation of left-sided lesion sets generally requires 10–20 min [34, 40–42, 46–53]. This amount of time contrasts with the 1 h required to perform the Cox maze III procedure [54, 55].

Cryothermy

Cryoablation is performed with a nitrous-oxide-cooled probe that when applied to atrial tissue at very cold temperature (–60 or –80 °C for 2 min) reliably produces transmural lesions that block atrial conduction. An advantage of this technique is that there is no tissue vaporisation or charring and the endocardial surface remains smooth following cryoablation. Cox et al. were the first to incorporate this modality into surgery for AF, to complete

[20–23] or replace ('cryo-maze' procedure) [20] the lesions of the Cox maze III operation. Sueda et al. have demonstrated the feasibility of left sided partial maze procedures using cryoablation [56–58]. This procedure is demanding and technically difficult. Ongoing development of minimally invasive procedures using cryoablation has been somewhat limited by currently available cryoprobe systems, which are rigid [33].

Microwave

Microwave ablation probes are commercially available and have been successfully used in partial maze operations to treat chronic AF [59, 60]. At present, 2-, 4-, and 10-cm probes are available for microwave-based AF ablation. A special wand-like catheter (the Flex-4 catheter) is used to direct microwave energy to create several lesions on the heart. Microwave ablation makes use of high-frequency electromagnetic radiation (microwaves), which upon application to atrial tissue causes oscillation of water molecules, converting electromagnetic energy into kinetic energy and producing heat. This heat causes thermal injury leading to conduction block. However, unlike radiofrequency heating, microwave heating does not cause endocardial surface charring, which may reduce the risk of thromboembolism [59]. Microwave ablation has greater tissue penetration than radiofrequency ablation, increasing the likelihood of a transmural lesion. These advantages, particularly before irrigated radiofrequency probes, have led to increasing interest in the use of microwave ablation in surgical procedures for AF. Oesophageal injury has been reported with radiofrequency surgery, but not with microwave.

Ultrasound

Ultrasound ablation is in very early development; the feasibility of this modality for the treatment of AF in humans has been demonstrated in early catheter-based approaches [61, 62]. Ultrasound wave propagation causes compression/refraction of the tissue, resulting in motions that produce heat (mechanical hyperthermia). Both focused (very short lesion times) and non-focused ablation are possible with ultrasound.

Laser

Light energy produces harmonic oscillation of water with the development of kinetic energy and subsequent heat that causes the lesions. Today, two devices have been used experimentally to produce linear myocardial lesions, the neodymium:yttrium–aluminium garnet (Nd:YAG) lasers and an infrared coagulator [63–66]. These methods produce well-demarcated transmural photocoagulation necrosis with relatively low peak tissue temperatures and without tissue vaporisation.

Postoperative Care

Medical Protocols

Whatever the technique used to create atrial lesions (e.g. incision, cryoabla-tion, radiofrequency energy), the time course of lesion maturation and scar formation results in delayed onset of complete electrical isolation. Thus, iso-lation procedures are associated with a high incidence of postoperative AF and/or flutter, ranging from 38% to 69% and 5% to 10% respectively [20, 35–42, 56–62]. These atrial arrhythmias are generally treated aggressively with pharmacological agents or external/internal electrical cardioversion or ablation procedures. The drug of choice is amiodarone, started immediately in the operating theatre with an intravenous loading dose, followed by a daily dose of 200 mg for up to 6 weeks or months postoperatively. If amiodarone is contraindicated, beta-blockers are administered. Several surgeons use DDD stimulation during the first 48 h. Using this protocol, most patients leave the hospital in sinus rhythm [67]. Anticoagulation treatment of patients remains controversial. Because of the high incidence of AF in the early perioperative period and the unpredictability of early atrial function in patients who remain in sinus rhythm, many surgeons recommend 3 or more months of anticoagulation treatment for all patients, regardless of the rhythm at hospi-tal discharge. Patients who are discharged in AF are maintained on oral anti-coagulants until sinus rhythm is documented at 3- to 6-month follow-up. These medical protocols are extremely variable [35–42, 67–69].

Diagnostic Protocols

The postoperative follow-up controls take place generally at hospital dis-charge, at the 1st, 3rd, 6th, and 12th month, and annually thereafter, by means of electrocardiogram, Holter monitoring, and echocardiogram. Echocardiogram examinations are used for sizing atrial dimension and assessing atrial contractility. The superoinferior diameter (D1), measured on B-mode in the four-chamber apical view, from the mitral valve plane towards the pulmonary veins, is usually considered as the left atrial diameter. The lat-eromedial (D2) and anteroposterior (D3) left atrial diameters are also mea-sured to enable calculation of the left atrial volume by the formula: (D1 x D2 x D3 x 0.53)/1000 [70]. Postoperative atrial contractility is assessed with pulsed Doppler, in four-chamber apical view, with effective restoration of atrial transport function considered present when the transvalvular peak A wave is equal to or greater than 10–30 cm/s. Other authors [69] aiming to assess biatrial contractility evaluate: (a) transmitral and trans-tricuspidal peak E wave and its velocity time integral (VTI_E); (b) transmitral and trans-tricuspidal peak A wave and its velocity time integral (VTI_A); (c) total transmitral or trans-tricuspidal velocity time integral (VTI$_{total}$); (d) E/A wave ratio. These data enable calculation of the atrial function fraction (AFF) by the formula: VTI$_A$/(VTI$_A$ + VTI$_E$). An AFF below 20% expresses severe left atrial impairment, between 20% and 29% mild to moderate impairment, and over 29% normal contractility. Results of biatrial contraction function can also be expressed in terms of the Santa Cruz Score [71, 72].

In order to assess the presence of tachy-brady arrhythmias and to calculate heart rate variability, Holter monitoring is performed generally at least 6 and 12 months postoperatively and annually thereafter in patients without AF [70]. If AF persists despite two or more electrical cardioversions, especially for more than 6 months postoperatively, electroanatomical computerised mapping (CARTO system) is indicated to reveal any discontinuities in the ablative line lesions [41]. If incomplete ablative lines are found, the patient is put forward for percutaneous partial radiofrequency catheter ablation. Electrical cardioversion, CARTO system, and percutaneous radiofrequency catheter ablation allow the restoration of sinus rhythm in about 100% of patients independently of the procedure and ablative set used.

Results of Surgery for Atrial Fibrillation

According to the protocol recently suggested by Gillinov [33], success or failure of surgical AF ablation is determined 6 months after surgery. Failure of surgery for AF is defined by the presence of AF 6 months or more after operation that is permanent or paroxysmal and unresponsive to anti-arrhythmic medications. If a patient can be maintained in sinus rhythm with anti-arrhythmic medications, AF surgery has not failed. Similarly, requirement for a pacemaker (range: 5–20%) does not constitute failure [24, 25]. If a patient requires an additional surgical or percutaneous procedure for AF or atrial flutter ablation, this is noted as failure of the initial procedure. However, subsequent interventions may restore sinus rhythm, representing ultimate success of combined therapy for AF. Based in the number of recurrences, other authors considered the surgical ablation procedure to have been ineffective when the discharged patients need more than three cardioversions for recurrences of AF/atrial flutter during the first 3 months after surgery. Cox et al. demonstrated both that temporary postoperative AF was common (38% of patients), due to a shortened atrial refractory period in the postoperative period [21], and that their 99% successful ablation of AF was unaffected by presence of mitral valve disease, left atrial size, and type of AF (paroxysmal versus persistent). Other centres have published results with the Cox maze III procedure [25, 73], but in general efficacy has been less than that reported by Cox et al. At the Cleveland Clinic and the Mayo Clinic, late freedom from AF is reported to be around 90% [25–27]. In other series, combining mitral valve surgery with the Cox maze III cured AF in only 75–82% of patients [53, 55, 74, 75].

The results in recently published series of patients undergoing left-sided partial maze procedures are summarised in Table 1 [43, 55, 56, 76-78]. These series in general share a number of limitations, which include relatively low numbers of patients, incomplete long-term follow-up, and non-standardised definitions of surgical success and failure. The vast majority of patients in these series had structural heart disease requiring additional procedures to be performed at the time of their partial maze, including mitral valve replacement and repair and coronary artery bypass.

Despite some limitations, the results of these early series have been an important incremental advance in the development of surgery for AF. These investigators have shown the feasibility of adding partial maze procedures to complex operations for structural heart disease. This has been accomplished with only a modest increase in procedure time and maintenance of low complication rates [39–47]. Mid- and long-term results have been encouraging, with success rates generally in the 70–80% range. Pasic et al. have reported success rates as high as 92% at 6-month follow-up [55]. While the results of partial maze procedures should be examined in the context of the outstanding experience Cox et al. have documented with the Cox maze III procedure, these studies have shown the potential for partial maze procedures to treat AF effectively with a simple, short, and less invasive procedure.

Although less frequently than in cases of underlying cardiopathy, surgical ablation has also been applied to treat lone AF. The reasons that have limited its use for this indication are probably the necessity of a sternotomy and underevaluation of AF consequences.

Table 1. Results of published series of patients undergoing left-sided partial maze procedures

Authors	Year	Patients (n)	Lesion type	Percentage in SR at mid-/long-term follow-up
Pasic et al. [55]	2001	48	RF	92
Mohr et al. [43]	2002	234	RF	81.1
Benussi et al. [76]	2002	132	Epicardial RF	77
Kress et al. [77]	2002	23	RF	86
Knaut et al. [78]	2002	105	Microwave	61
Kondo et al. [56]	2003	31	Cryoablation/RF	79.3

RF, radiofrequency; SR, sinus rhythm

Conclusions

Recent technological advances, focused on developing faster, simpler, and less invasive procedures with an efficacy similar to that achieved with the Cox maze, and demonstration that the pulmonary veins and posterior left atrium are the drivers of AF in most patients, justify a return of interest in direct surgical ablation of AF. A number of investigators have published results of left-sided partial maze procedures.

These procedures, performed in only 10–20 min using alternative energy sources to make ablative lesions, are safe and restore sinus rhythm in 70–80% of patients. These studies have demonstrated the feasibility of performing ablative procedures with limited lesion sets to effectively treat patients with medically refractory AF, and have established that the complete lesion set developed by Cox et al. is unnecessary to treat successfully all patients with AF. Preoperative identification of this subset of patients for whom left atrial sources of ectopic activity may be amenable to a simple left-sided partial maze would potentially improve the success rates of these procedures without further advancements in technique. On the other hand, a number of preoperative clinical criteria, such as enlarged left atrial size, prolonged duration of AF, electrocardiogram voltage criteria, advanced age, and associated coronary artery disease, have been associated with failure of the left-side partial maze procedure. This second subset could be treated by the classic Cox maze. Further advancements in our understanding of the pathophysiology of AF as well as improved electrophysiological screening of individual patients' ectopic foci, for instance with advanced mapping techniques, will lead to better patient selection and surgical cure rates [79–81].

The optimal lesion set has not yet been defined, although minor variations appear to produce little difference in outcome. Left atrial appendage exclusion or excision using surgical staplers [82] remains an important advantage of surgical approaches that should be included in all partial maze procedures. In fact, left atrial appendage excision/exclusion has been proposed as a stand-alone treatment for permanent or persistent AF, both because it removes the most important thromboembolic source for patients with chronic AF [83–85] and because anecdotal data suggest that the left atrial appendage contributes electrically to the initiation or propagation of AF. Minimally invasive off-pump ablation of AF is on the horizon, and in the near future it is likely that new probes, coupled with thoracoscopic stapling instruments, will facilitate off-pump epicardial ablation of AF performed through thoracoscopy. Emerging technologies that can be used for epicardial and beating heart application and ablation of atrial tissues, such as bipolar saline-cooled radiofrequency probes, show great promise as investigators work to develop minimally invasive approaches [86, 87]. As new procedures are developed that effectively treat AF, have low morbidity, and are minimally invasive, they will be increasingly utilised to restore sinus rhythm permanently, potentially in all patients affected by AF. Rigorous evaluation of developing procedures will be important in order to evaluate competing therapies, including medical, catheter-based, and surgical treatments. A standardised analysis and reporting system has been proposed to facilitate the fair comparison of emerging treatments for AF [33].

Many surgeons currently offer 'pulmonary vein isolation only' to patients who have had paroxysmal AF, and left atrial partial maze to patients who have had persistent or permanent AF for at least 6 months, or to those who have failed at least two cardioversion attempts. Most frequently this procedure is performed in patients undergoing mitral valve operations, but also it is applied in patients undergoing atrial sept defect (ADS) closure, aortic valve operations, and coronary artery bypass grafting. Because of the potential to completely discontinue anticoagulation by restoring sinus rhythm, ablation is performed more aggressively in patients undergoing valve repairs or tissue valve replacements. However, many others perform the procedure in patients receiving mechanical valves, since the elimination of AF may allow lower anticoagulation levels as well as improved cardiac function and avoidance of anti-arrhythmic medications. A left atrium diameter more than 60–65 mm is considered a contraindication for ablation procedure in many reports. Others also treat left atrium diameter more than 60-65 mm but associated atrial plasty.

Nowadays surgical ablation is the most effective procedure in the treatment of AF resistant to medical therapy. The Cox maze operation permits restoration of sinus rhythm in the great majority of patients, but is employed only by a few teams in selected cases (huge left atrium, long-standing AF, and so on). In the other cases, the left-sided partial maze (with new energy sources and lesion sets limited to the left atrium) is able to restore sinus rhythm in more than 70% of patients. The emerging technologies and the development of minimally invasive approaches will probably lead to an increase in the treatment of lone AF. Rigorous evaluation and standardised analysis of medium- and long-term results will permit tailoring of the best treatment for each subset of patients with AF.

References

1. Nattel S (2002) New ideas about atrial fibrillation 50 years on. Nature 415:219–226
2. Kannel WB, Abbott RD, Savage DD et al (1982) Epidemiologic features of chronic atrial fibrillation: the Framingham study. N Engl J Med 306:1018–1022
3. Benjamin EJ, Wolf PA, D'Agostino RB et al (1998) Impact of atrial fibrillation on the risk of death. The Framingham study. Circulation 98:946–952

4. Falk RH (2001) Atrial fibrillation. N Engl J Med 344:1067–1078
5. Ezekowitz MD, Netrebko PI (2003) Anticoagulation in management of atrial fibrillation. Curr Opin Cardiol 18:26–31
6. Obaida JF, El Farra M, Bastien OH et al (1997) Outcome of atrial fibrillation after mitral valve repair. J Thorac Cardiovasc Surg 114:179–185
7. Fuster V, Ryden LE, Asinger RW et al (2001) ACC/AHA/ESC guidelines for the management of patients with atrial fibrillation. A report of the American College of Cardiology/American Heart Association Task Force on Practice Guidelines and the European Society of Cardiology Committee for Practice Guidelines and Policy Conferences (Committee to develop guidelines for the management of patients with atrial fibrillation) developed in collaboration with the North American Society of Pacing and Electrophysiology. Eur Heart J 22:1852–1923
8. Moe GK, Rheinboldt WC, Abildskov JA (1964) A computer model of atrial fibrillation. Am Heart J 67:200–220
9. Moe GK (1962) On the multiple wavelet hypothesis of atrial fibrillation. Arch Int Pharmacodyn Ther 140:183–188
10. Wijffels MC, Kirchhof CJ, Dorland R et al (1995) Atrial fibrillation begets atrial fibrillation. A study in awake chronically instrumented goats. Circulation 92:1954–1968
11. Cox JL (2003) Atrial fibrillation I: a new classification system. J Thorac Cardiovasc Surg 126:1686–1692
12. Mandapati R, Skanes A, Chen J et al (2000) Stable microreentrant sources as a mechanism of atrial fibrillation in the isolated sheep heart. Circulation 101:194–199
13. Mansour M, Mandapati R, Berenfeld O et al (2001) Left-to-right gradient of atrial frequencies during acute atrial fibrillation in the isolated sheep heart. Circulation 103:2631–2636
14. Haïssaguerre M, Jaïs P, Shah DC et al (1998) Spontaneous initiation of atrial fibrillation by ectopic beats originating in the pulmonary veins. N Engl J Med 339:659–666
15. Li D, Zhang L, Kneller J et al (2001) Potential ionic mechanism for repolarization differences between canine right and left atrium. Circ Res 88:1168–1175
16. Harada A, Sasaki K, Fukushima T et al (1996) Atrial activation during chronic atrial fibrillation in patients with isolated mitral valve disease. Ann Thorac Surg 61:104–112
17. Nitta T, Imura H, Bessho R et al (1999) Wavelength and conduction inhomogeneity in each atrium in patients with isolated mitral valve disease and atrial fibrillation. J Cardiovasc Electrophysiol 10:521–528
18. Lundstrom T, Ryden L (1988) Chronic atrial fibrillation. Long-term results of direct current conversion. Acta Med Scand 223:53–59
19. Connolly SJ (2003) Preventing stroke in patients with atrial fibrillation: current treatments and new concepts. Am Heart J 145:418–423
20. Cox JL, Schuessler RB, Boineau JP (2000) The development of the Maze procedure for the treatment of atrial fibrillation. Semin Thorac Cardiovasc Surg 12:2–14
21. Cox JL, Boineau JP, Schuessler RB et al (1995) Electrophysiologic basis, surgical development, and clinical results of the maze procedure for atrial flutter and atrial fibrillation. Adv Card Surg 6:1–67
22. Cox JL, Jaquiss RD, Schuessler RB, Boineau JP (1995) Modification of the maze procedure for atrial flutter and atrial fibrillation. II. Surgical technique of the maze III procedure. J Thorac Cardiovasc Surg 110:485–495

23. Cox JL, Schuessler RB, D'Agostino HJ Jr et al (1991) The surgical treatment of atrial fibrillation. III. Development of a definitive surgical procedure. J Thorac Cardiovasc Surg 101:569–583

24. Cox JL, Ad N, Palazzo T et al (2000) Current status of the Maze procedure for the treatment of atrial fibrillation. Semin Thorac Cardiovasc Surg 12:15–19

25. McCarthy PM, Gillinov AM, Castle L et al (2000) The Cox-Maze procedure: the Cleveland Clinic experience. Semin Thorac Cardiovasc Surg 12:25–29

26. McCarthy PM, Castle LW, Maloney JD et al (1993) Initial experience with the maze procedure for atrial fibrillation. J Thorac Cardiovasc Surg 105:1077–1087

27. Schaff HV, Dearani JA, Daly RC et al (2000) Cox-Maze procedure for atrial fibrillation: Mayo Clinic experience. Semin Thorac Cardiovasc Surg 12:30–37

28. Kosakai Y, Kawaguci AT, Isobe F et al (1995) Modified maze procedure for patients with atrial fibrillation undergoing simultaneous open heart surgery. Circulation 92(9 Suppl):II359-364

29. Kress DC, Krum D, Chekanov V et al (2002) Validation of a left atrial lesion pattern for intraoperative ablation of atrial fibrillation. Ann Thorac Surg 73:1160–1168

30. Cox JL, Ad N (2000) New surgical and catheter-based modifications of the Maze procedure. Semin Thorac Cardiovasc Surg 12:68–73

31. Cox JL, Ad N (2000) The importance of cryoablation of the coronary sinus during the Maze procedure. Semin Thorac Cardiovasc Surg 12:20–24

32. Benussi S, Pappone C, Nascimbene S et al (2000) A simple way to treat chronic atrial fibrillation during mitral valve surgery: the epicardial radiofrequency approach. Eur J Cardiothorac Surg 17:524–529

33. Gillinov AM, Blackstone EH, McCarthy PM (2002) Atrial fibrillation: current surgical options and their assessment. Ann Thorac Surg 74:2210–2217

34. Williams MR, Stewart JR, Bolling SF et al (2001) Surgical treatment of atrial fibrillation using radiofrequency energy. Ann Thorac Surg 71:1939–1944

35. Haïssaguerre M, Jaïs P, Shah DC et al (1996) Right and left atrial radiofrequency catheter therapy of paroxysmal atrial fibrillation. J Cardiovasc Electrophysiol 7:1132–1144

36. Roithinger FX, Steiner PR, Goseki Y et al (1999) Electrophysiologic effects of selective right versus left atrial linear lesions in a canine model of chronic atrial fibrillation. J Cardiovasc Electrophysiol 10:1564–1574

37. Chen SA, Hsieh MH, Tai CT et al (1999) Initiation of atrial fibrillation by ectopic beats originating from the pulmonary veins: electrophysiological characteristics, pharmacological responses, and effects of radiofrequency ablation. Circulation 100:1879–1886

38. Gaita F, Riccardi R, Calo L et al (1998) Atrial mapping and radiofrequency catheter ablation in patients with idiopathic atrial fibrillation. Electrophysiological findings and ablation results. Circulation 97:2136–2145

39. Williams MR, Stewart JR, Bolling SF et al (2001) Surgical treatment of atrial fibrillation using radiofrequency energy. Ann Thorac Surg 71:1939–1944

40. Hindricks G, Mohr FW, Autschbach R, Kottkamp H (1999) Antiarrhythmic surgery for treatment of atrial fibrillation – new concepts. Thorac Cardiovasc Surg 47:365–369

41. Sie HT, Beukema WP, Misier AR et al (2001) Radiofrequency modified maze in patients with atrial fibrillation undergoing concomitant cardiac surgery. J Thorac Cardiovasc Surg 122:249–256

42. Sie HT, Beukema WP, Ramdat Misier AR et al (2001) The radiofrequency modified maze procedure. A less invasive surgical approach to atrial fibrillation during

open-heart surgery. Eur J Cardiothorac Surg 19:443–447

43. Mohr FW, Fabricius AM, Falk V et al (2002) Curative treatment of atrial fibrillation with intraoperative radiofrequency ablation: short-term and midterm results. J Thorac Cardiovasc Surg 123:919–927

44. Gillinov AM, Pettersson G et al (2001) Esophageal injury during radiofrequency ablation for atrial fibrillation. J Thorac Cardiovasc Surg 122:1239–1240

45. Gillinov AM, McCarthy PM (2002) Atricure bipolar radiofrequency clamp for intraoperative ablation of atrial fibrillation. Ann Thorac Surg 74:2165–2168

46. Benussi S, Pappone C, Nascimbene S et al (2000) A simple way to treat chronic atrial fibrillation during mitral valve surgery: the epicardial radiofrequency approach. Eur J Cardiothorac Surg 17:524–529

47. Patwardhan AM, Dave HH, Tamhane AA et al (1997) Intraoperative radiofrequency microbipolar coagulation to replace incisions of maze III procedure for correcting atrial fibrillation in patients with rheumatic valvular disease. Eur J Cardiothorac Surg 12:627–633

48. Melo J, Adragao PR, Neves j et al (1999) Electrosurgical treatment of atrial fibrillation with a new intraoperative radiofrequency ablation catheter. Thorac Cardiovasc Surg 47 (Suppl 3):370–372

49. Kottkamp H, Hindricks G, Hammel D et al (1999) Intraoperative radiofrequency ablation of chronic atrial fibrillation: a left atrial curative approach by elimination of anatomic 'anchor' reentrant circuits. J Cardiovasc Electrophysiol 10:772–780

50. Chen MC, Guo GB, Chang JP et al (1998) Radiofrequency and cryoablation of atrial fibrillation in patients undergoing valvular operation. Ann Thorac Surg 65:1666–1672

51. Hammer W, Botha C, Ickrath O et al (2001) Background and early results of a modified left atrial radiofrequency procedure concomitant with cardiac surgery. Cardiovasc J S Afr 12:19–28

52. Pasic M, Bergs P, Muller P et al (2001) Intraoperative radiofrequency maze ablation for atrial fibrillation: the Berlin modification. Ann Thorac Surg 72:1484–1491

53. Chen MC, Chang JP, Guo GB et al (2001) Atrial size reduction as a predictor of the success of radiofrequency maze procedure for chronic atrial fibrillation in patients undergoing concomitant valvular surgery. J Cardiovasc Electrophysiol 12:867–874

54. Handa N, Schaff HV, Morris JJ et al (1999) Outcome of valve repair and the Cox Maze procedure for mitral regurgitation and associated atrial fibrillation. J Thorac Cardiovasc Surg 118:628–635

55. Raanani E, Albage A, David TE et al (2001) The efficacy of Cox/maze procedure combined with mitral valve surgery: a matched control study. Eur J Cardiothorac Surg 19:438–442

56. Kondo N, Takahashi K, Minakawa M, Daitoku K (2003) Left atrial maze procedure: a useful addition to other corrective operations. Ann Thorac Surg 75:1490–1494

57. Sueda T, Nagata H, Shikata H et al (1996) Simple left atrial procedure for chronic atrial fibrillation associated with mitral valve disease. Ann Thorac Surg 62:1796–1800

58. Sueda T, Nagata H, Orihashi K et al (1997) Efficacy of a simple left atrial procedure for chronic atrial fibrillation in mitral valve operations. Ann Thorac Surg 63:1070–1075

59. Spitzer SG, Richter P, Knaut M et al (1999) Treatment of atrial fibrillation in open heart surgery – the potential role of microwave energy. Thorac Cardiovasc Surg 47:374–378

60. Knaut M, Spitzer SG, Karolyi L et al (1999) Intraoperative microwave ablation for

curative treatment of atrial fibrillation in open heart surgery – the MICRO-STAF and MICRO-PASS pilot trial. MICROwave Application in Surgical Treatment of Atrial Fibrillation. MICROwave Application for the Treatment of Atrial Fibrillation in Bypass Surgery. Thorac Cardiovasc Surg 47:379–384

61. Saliba W, Wilber D, Packer D et al (2002) Circumferential ultrasound ablation for pulmonary vein isolation: analysis of acute and chronic failures. J Cardiovasc Electrophysiol 13:957–961

62. Natale A, Pisano E, Shewchik J et al (2000) First human experience with pulmonary vein isolation using a through-the-balloon circumferential ultrasound ablation system for recurrent atrial fibrillation. Circulation 102:1879–1882

63. Fried NM, Lardo AC, Berger RD et al (2000) Linear lesions in myocardium created by Nd:YAG laser using diffusing optical fibers: in vitro and in vivo results. Lasers Surg Med 27:295–304

64. Keane D, Ruskin JN (1999) Linear atrial ablation with a diode laser and fiberoptic catheter. Circulation 100:59–60

65. Kubota H, Furuse A, Takeshita M et al (1998) Atrial ablation with an IRK–151 infrared coagulator. Ann Thorac Surg 66:95–100

66. Kubota H, Takamoto S, Takeshita M et al (2000) Atrial ablation using an IRK–151 infrared coagulator in canine model. J Cardiovasc Surg 41:835–847

67. Hornero F, Montero JA, Canovas S et al (2002) Biatrial radiofrequency ablation for atrial fibrillation: epicardial and endocardial surgical approach. Interactive Cardiovasc Thorac Surg 1:72–77

68. Gillinov AM, McCarthy PM, Blackstone EH et al (2003) Bipolar radiofrequency to ablate atrial fibrillation in patients undergoing mitral valve surgery. Heart Surg Forum 7:147–152

69. Nascimbene S, Benussi S, Calvi S et al (2004) Trattamento combinato della fibrillazione atriale in pazienti candidati ad intervento chirurgico a cuore aperto: risultati clinici e funzionali a distanza. Ital Heart J Suppl 5(3):199–204

70. Troise G, Cirillo M, Brunelli F et al (2004) Mid-term results of cardiac autotransplantation as method to treat permanent atrial fibrillation and mitral disease. Eur J Cardiothorac Surg 25:1025–1031

71. Melo J (2002) How to establish normal biatrial contraction and sinus rhythm without drug therapy. Heart Surg Forum Rev 1:5–6

72. Melo JQ, Neves J, Adragao P et al (1997) When and how to report results of surgery on atrial fibrillation. Eur J Cardiothorac Surg 12:739–744

73. Arcidi JM Jr, Doty DB, Millar RC et al (2000) The Maze procedure: the LDS Hospital experience. Semin Thorac Cardiovasc Surg 12:38–43

74. Kamata J, Kawazoe K, Izumoto H et al (1997) Predictors of sinus rhythm restoration after Cox maze procedure concomitant with other cardiac operations. Ann Thorac Surg 64:394–398

75. Izumoto H, Kawazoe K, Kitahara H et al (1998) Operative results after Cox/maze procedure combined with a mitral valve operation. Ann Thorac Surg 66:800–804

76. Benussi S, Nascimbene S, Agricola E et al (2002) Surgical ablation of atrial fibrillation using the epicardial radiofrequency approach: mid-term results and risk analysis. Ann Thorac Surg 74:1050–1057

77. Kress DC, Sra J, Krum D et al (2002) Radiofrequency ablation of atrial fibrillation during mitral valve surgery. Semin Thorac Cardiovasc Surg 14:210–218

78. Knaut M, Tugtekin SM, Spitzer S et al (2002) Combined atrial fibrillation and mitral valve surgery using microwave technology. Semin Thorac Cardiovasc Surg 14:226–231

79. Gepstein L, Hayam G, Shpun S et al (1999) Atrial linear ablations in pigs. Chronic effects on atrial electrophysiology and pathology. Circulation 100:419–426

80. Ernst S, Ouyang F, Lober F et al (2003) Catheter-induced linear lesions in the left atrium in patients with atrial fibrillation: an electroanatomic study. J Am Coll Cardiol 42:1271–1282

81. Patel VV, Ren JF, Marchlinski FE (2002) A comparison of left atrial size by two-dimensional transthoracic echocardiography and magnetic endocardial catheter mapping. Pacing Clin Electrophysiol 25:95–97

82. Landymore R, Kinley CE (1984) Staple closure of the left atrial appendage. Can J Surg 27:144–145

83. Blackshear JL, Odell JA (1996) Appendage obliteration to reduce stroke in cardiac surgical patients with atrial fibrillation. Ann Thorac Surg 61:755–759

84. Blackshear JL, Johnson WD, Odell JA et al (2003) Thoracoscopic extracardiac obliteration of the left atrial appendage for stroke risk reduction in atrial fibrillation. J Am Coll Cardiol 42:1249–1252

85. Odell JA, Blackshear JL, Davies E et al (1996) Thoracoscopic obliteration of the left atrial appendage: potential for stroke reduction? Ann Thorac Surg 61:565–569

86. Chevalier P, Obadia JF, Timour Q et al (1999) Thoracoscopic epicardial radiofrequency ablation for vagal atrial fibrillation in dogs. Pacing Clin Electrophysiol 22:880–886

87. Manasse E, Infante M, Ghiselli S et al (2002) A video-assisted thoracoscopic technique to encircle the four pulmonary veins: a new surgical intervention for atrial fibrillation ablation. Heart Surg Forum 5:337–339

CARDIAC RESYNCHRONISATION THERAPY: NEW THERAPEUTIC AND DIAGNOSTIC PERSPECTIVES IN HEART FAILURE MANAGEMENT

Guidelines for the Management of Patients with Heart Failure

G. Sinagra, G. Sabbadini, S. Rakar, A. Perkan, M. Zecchin, L. Salvatore, F. Longaro, A. Di Lenarda

Chronic congestive heart failure (HF) is a highly disabling, costly, and deadly syndrome which affects a hundred million people worldwide [1]. Large clinical trials have shown that drugs which antagonise the renin–angiotensin–aldosterone system [angiotensin converting enzyme (ACE) inhibitors, angiotensin II receptor blockers (ARBs), aldosterone receptor antagonists] and sympathetic nervous system (beta-blockers) are highly effective in reducing the rates of mortality and morbidity in patients with left ventricular (LV) chamber dilation/systolic dysfunction cardiomyopathies, whether of ischaemic or non-ischaemic aetiology (Tables 1–3) [2–5]. Although no survival benefit has been documented with diuretics and digoxin, the former remain a cornerstone in the treatment of HF patients as the most efficacious means of counteracting fluid retention [6], while the latter can be of value to achieve further improvements in symptoms and quality of life [7].

In addition, several randomised controlled trials have recently demonstrated the effectiveness of implantable cardioverter defibrillator (ICD) therapy for the primary and secondary prevention of unexpected cardiac sudden death (Table 4) [8–10].

Despite the availability of these useful therapies, HF patients continue to be affected by progressively worsening symptoms, the need for recurrent high-cost hospitalisations, poor quality of life, and shortened life expectancy [11]. It is indisputable that the persistence of high morbidity and mortality rates can be explained, at least in part, by the fact that treatments proven to be effective in randomised controlled trials have not been applied to all suitable patients encountered in the clinical arena [12]. Following from this, guidelines for the management of the syndrome have emerged in the last years as an helpful tool to translate scientific evidence into daily practice, providing indications for a more appropriate use of currently available therapeutic strategies [13, 14].

Department of Cardiology, Trieste Hospital and University, Trieste, Italy

Table 1. Randomised controlled trials with ACE inhibitors in HF

Trial drug tested	Patients (n)	HF aetiology	NYHA (I–IV)	LVEF (%)	Mean follow-up (months)	HF-related hospitalisations (RR, %)	All-cause mortality (RR, %)	HF-related mortality (RR, %)	Sudden mortality (RR, %)
CONSENSUS Enalapril	253	Mixed	IV	NA	6	NV	↓ 27 P = 0.003	↓ 50 P < 0.001	– P = NS
SOLVD-T Enalapril	2569	Mixed	II–III	≤ 35	41	↓ 26 P < 0.0001	↓ 16 P = 0.0036	↓ 22 P = 0.0045	↓ 10 P = NS
SOLVD-P Enalapril	4228	Mixed	I–II	≤ 35	37	↓ 44 P < 0.001	↓ 8 P = NS	↓ 21 P = NS	↗ 7 P = NS
SAVE Captopril	2231	Ischaemic[a]	I	≤ 40	42	↓ 22 P = 0.019	↓ 19 P = 0.019	↓ 36 P = 0.032	– P = NS
AIRE Ramipril	2006	Ischaemic[a]	II–III	NA	15	NE	↓ 27 P = 0.002	NE	NE
TRACE Trandolapril	1749	Ischaemic[a]	I–IV	≤ 35	24	NE	↓ 22 P = 0.001	↓ 25 P = NS	↓ 24 P = 0.03

ACE, angiotensin converting enzyme; HF, heart failure; LVEF, left ventricular ejection fraction; NA, not available; NE, not evaluated; NS, not significant; NV, New York Heart Association functional class; RR, relative risk; ↓, reduced; —, unchanged; [a] Recent acute myocardial infarction

Table 2. Randomised controlled trials with ARBs and aldosterone receptor blockers in HF

Trial drug tested	Patients (n)	HF aetiology	NYHA (I–IV)	LVEF (%)	Mean follow-up (months)	HF-related hospitalisations (RR, %)	All-cause mortality (RR, %)	HF-related mortality (RR, %)	Sudden mortality (RR, %)
ELITE-II Losartan[a]	3152	Mixed	II–IV	≤40	18	NE	– P = NS	NE	– P = NS
VAL-HeFT Valsartan	5010	Mixed	II	5010	Mixed	II–IV	≤40	23	↓27 P = 2
CHARM Candesartan	7601	Mixed	II–IV	≤40	38	↓23 P < 0.0001	↓13[c] P = 0.006	↓ P < 0.00001	↓ P < 0.00001
RALES Spironolactone	1663	Mixed	IIIb–IV	≤35	24	↓35 P < 0.001	↓30 P < 0.001	↓36 P < 0.001	↓29 P < 0.02
EPHESUS Eplerenone	6632	Ischaemic[b]	I–IV	↓ or —	16	NE	↓15 P = 0.008	NE	↓21 P = 0.03

ARBs, angiotensin receptor blockers; HF, heart failure; LVEF, left ventricular ejection fraction; NE, not evaluated; NS, not significant; NYHA, New York Heart Association functional class; RR, relative risk; ↓, reduced; —, unchanged; [a] Versus captopril; [b] Recent acute myocardial infarction; [c] For cardiovascular reasons

Table 3. Large randomised controlled trials with beta-blockers in HF

Trial drug tested	Patients (n)	HF aetiology	NYHA (I–IV)	LVEF (%)	Mean follow-up (months)	HF-related hospitalisations (RR, %)	All-cause mortality (RR, %)	HF-related mortality (RR, %)	Sudden mortality (RR, %)
US TRIAL Carvedilol	1094	Mixed	II–III	≤ 35	6	↓ 27[c] P = 0.036	↓ 65 P < 0.001	↓ P = NA	↓ P = NA
ANZ TRIAL Carvedilol	415	Ischaemic	I–III	≤ 45	19	↓ 23 P = 0.05	↓ 24 P = NS	– P = NS	– P = NS
CIBIS-II Bisoprolol	2647	Mixed	III	≤ 35	16	↓ 20 P = 0.0006	↓ 34 P < 0.0001	↓ 26 P = NS	↓ 44 P < 0.0001
MERIT-HF Metoprolol	3991	Mixed	II–III	≤ 40	12	NV	↓ 35 P < 0.0001	↓ 49 P < 0.0023	↓ 41 P < 0.0002
COPERNICUS Carvedilol	2289	Mixed	III–IV	< 25	21	↓ 24[d] P < 0.001	↓ 35 P < 0.00014	NV	NV
CAPRICORN Carvedilol	1959	Ischaemic[b]	I–II	≤ 40	16	↓ 14[e] P = NS	↓ 23 P = 0.031	↓ 40 P = NS	↓ 26 P = NS
COMET Carvedilol[a]	3029	Mixed	II–IV	≤ 35	58	↓ 3[e] P = NS	↓ 17 P = 0.0017	↓ 17 P = NS	↓ 19 P = 0.021

HF, heart failure; LVEF, left ventricular ejection fraction; NA, not available; NS, not significant; NYHA, New York Heart Association functional class; RR, relative risk; ↓, reduced; —, unchanged; [a] Versus metoprolol; [b] Recent acute myocardial infarction; [c] For cardiovascular reasons; [d] For HF; [e] Plus all-cause deaths

Table 4. Main primary and secondary prevention trials with ICD in asymptomatic/symptomatic left ventricular dysfunction

Trial (PP or SP)	Patients (n)	IHD (%)	NYHA	MI	LVEF	Arrhythmia profile	RCA	Control therapy	Mean follow-up (months)	All-cause mortality (HR, 95% CI)	Sudden mortality (HR, 95% CI)
	—	—		—	—		—				
MADIT (PP)	196	100	II–III (~65%)	100	26±7	ns-VT, ind-VT	0	Various anti-arrhythmic drugs	27	0.41 (0.24–0.69)	0.25 (0.07–0.83)
MUSTT (PP)	704	100	I–II (~75%)	95	30 (<40)	ns-VT, ind-VT	0	Placebo	39	0.49 (0.35–0.67)	0.29 (0.16–0.52)
MADIT II (PP)	1232	100	I–II (~70%)	100	23±6	No arrhythmias	0	Placebo	20	0.71 (0.56–0.92)	0.39 (0.24–0.61)
DEFINITE (PP)	458	0	I–II (~70%)	0	21 (7–35)	ns-VT, frequent PVC	0	Placebo	29	0.65 (0.40–1.06)[b]	0.20 (0.06–0.71)
COMPANION (PP)[a]	1520	55	III (~85%)	NA	21 (<35)	QRS > 120 ms	0	CRT alone, placebo	16	0.80 (0.68–0.95)[c-d]	NA
SCD-HeFT (PP)	2521	51	II–III (100%)	NA	25 (20–30)	No arrhythmias	0	Amiodarone, placebo	48	0.77 (0.62–0.96)[d]	NA
AVID (SP)	1016	82	I–II (~90%)	67	32±13	VF, s-VT	45	Amiodarone, sotalol	18	0.66 (0.51–0.85)	0.44 (0.28–0.70)
CASH (SP)	288	73	I–II (~80%)	51	45±17	VF, s-VT	100	Amiodarone, metoprolol, propafenone	57	0.82 (0.60–1.11)	0.39 (0.22–0.67)
CIDS (SP)	659	83	I–II (~90%)	77	34±14	VF, s-VT, ind-VT	48	Amiodarone	35	0.85 (0.67–1.10)	0.70 (0.45–1.09)

HF, heart failure; IHD, ischaemic heart disease; ind-VT, inducible sustained ventricular tachycardia; LVEF, mean left ventricular ejection fraction; MI, previous myocardial infarction; NA, not available; ns-VT, nonsustained ventricular tachycardia; NYHA, New York Heart Association functional class; HR, hazard ratio; PP, primary prevention of sudden death; PVC, premature ventricular complexes; RCA, resuscitated cardiac arrest; SP, secondary prevention of sudden death; s-VT, sustained ventricular tachycardia; VF, ventricular fibrillation; [a] Implantable cardioverter defibrillator plus cardiac resynchronisation therapy; [b] Statistically not significant; [c] Plus all-cause hospitalisation ; [d] Versus placebo

Conventional Pharmacological Therapies

All patients who are symptom-free [New York Heart Association (NYHA) class I] and have impaired LV pump function (ejection fraction, EF < 40–45%) should receive an ACE inhibitor; the addition of a beta-blocker can be recommended only in those who have asymptomatic LV systolic dysfunction following an acute myocardial infarction.

The established treatment for HF patients with NYHA class II–IV symptoms and reduced LVEF comprises an ACE inhibitor (or, if not tolerated, an ARB), a beta-blocker, one or more diuretics (including an aldosterone receptor antagonist), and possibly digoxin. The first step is to introduce an ACE inhibitor, which can be initiated before diuretic therapy in patients who show a low tendency to develop fluid retention; however, most patients exhibit congestive signs/symptoms, and thus these two forms of treatment are usually initiated at the same time. ACE inhibitor drugs must be started at low doses and slowly titrated up to those proven to be effective in the clinical trials (or, alternatively, to the maximum tolerated). ACE inhibitor treatment should not be initiated (or, if already started, it must be stopped) in patients with evidence of bilateral renal artery stenosis, angio-oedema, intractable dry cough, hypotension (systolic blood pressure < 80 mmHg), severe renal impairment (creatininaemia > 3.0 mg%) or electrolyte abnormalities (kalaemia > 5.5 mmol/l).

Some mildly symptomatic cases can be managed with a thiazide diuretic, but most patients require to be treated with a loop diuretic, perhaps given at high doses or in combination with metolazone in the presence of severe congestive signs/symptoms. During chronic diuretic therapy, it is necessary to check serum creatinine, electrolytes, uric acid, and glucose frequently.

In clinically stable patients on optimised treatment with an ACE inhibitor and diuretics, addition of a beta-blocker is indicated (only bisoprolol, long-acting metoprolol, and carvedilol can be recommended at present), unless they are intolerant or have any contraindication to this form of treatment (contraindications include bronchial asthma, severe bronchial disease, symptomatic bradycardia, advanced heart block, and symptomatic hypotension). Patients who undergo beta-blocker therapy should be closely followed during the up-titration phase and thereafter in order to ensure prompt recognition of the occurrence of major side effects (bradycardia, hypotension, fluid retention, worsening HF). Initial doses must be very low and must be increased slowly up to the optimal ones. If side effects occur, all attempts should be made to avoid discontinuation of the beta-blocker, by changing the ACE inhibitor and/or diuretic doses. If there is a need to reduce or stop the beta-blocker therapy, every effort should be made to reintroduce it when the patients become clinically stable.

Although ARBs have not been shown to be superior to ACE inhibitors, they are also effective on major clinical end points. Thus, if ACE inhibitors are contraindicated or not tolerated, ARBs represent the best alternative choice. Moreover, in patients receiving an ACE inhibitor and a beta-blocker, the addition of an ARB may provide further clinical benefits. Side effects are less frequent with ARBs than with ACE inhibitors.

The addition of spironolactone or eplerenone to an ACE inhibitor, a beta blocker, and possibly diuretics and digoxin is recommended in patients with severe HF and in those with symptomatic LV systolic dysfunction following an acute myocardial infarction. Renal function and serum electrolytes must be checked periodically. The administration of an aldosterone receptor antagonist should be avoided or stopped in patients with creatininaemia > 2.5 mg/dl, kalaemia > 5.0 mmol/l, or painful gynaecomastia.

Digoxin is indicated in HF in order to slow the ventricular rate when atrial fibrillation is present or to improve clinical status when symptoms persist despite optimal ACE inhibition and diuretic therapy; there is no clear evidence that the drug may be of value in patients on sinus rhythm receiving an ACE inhibitor, a beta-blocker, and diuretics. Digoxin therapy is contraindicated in the presence of bradycardia, advanced heart block, sick sinus syndrome, carotid sinus syndrome, Wolff-Parkinson-White syndrome, hypokalaemia, or hypercalcaemia. Serum creatinine and potassium should be assessed before initiating the treatment.

Adjunctive Pharmacological Therapies

Given the disappointing results that have emerged from large randomised controlled trials on pure vasodilating, positive inotropic, and anti-arrhythmic agents, there is no firm recommendation to use such classes of drug for the treatment of HF. However, nitrates remain an essential pharmacological tool to manage patients with concomitant angina or acute dyspnoea, and felodipine and amlodipine represent an additional option for patients with active ischaemic cardiomyopathy or arterial hypertension. Intravenous inotropic support may be unavoidable to counteract severe episodes of worsening HF or as a bridge to heart transplant in end-stage HF. The use of amiodarone may be indicated in association with a beta-blocker to treat some patients with atrial fibrillation/flutter or with non-sustained/sustained ventricular tachycardia.

In HF patients with prior myocardial infarction, either aspirin or oral anticoagulants are recommended as secondary prevention. Anticoagulation therapy is also firmly indicated in HF patients with atrial fibrillation, a history of previous thromboembolic events, or evidence of a mobile LV thrombus.

Nonpharmacological Therapies

The prevention of sudden death in patients with HF continues to represent a hard challenge since medical treatments have had only a limited impact on this mode of death. Recent clinical trials have shown that ICD therapy reduces the rate of mortality among patients resuscitated from a cardiac arrest or with a history of sustained ventricular tachycardia poorly tolerated and/or associated with low LVEF. There is also evidence that the use of ICD as the primary prevention strategy improves the survival rate of patients with NYHA class II–III symptoms and LVEF below 35%. Moreover, when associated with biventricular pacing to treat ventricular dyssynchrony (QRS width > 120 ms), the ICD has been shown to reduce all-cause deaths and/or hospitalisations in patients with LVEF below 35% and NYHA class III–IV symptoms. All these benefits observed with the ICD therapy are additive to optimal pharmacological treatment, regardless of the aetiology of the cardiac disease.

Given the high costs and the subsequent low availability of these devices, it is necessary to define better their short-term and long-term cost-effectiveness and also to refine the selection of patients who are likely to benefit most from an ICD.

Treatment of Diastolic Heart Failure

There is little evidence from randomised controlled trials to support firm recommendations for the treatment of patients with HF due to exclusive or prevalent LV diastolic dysfunction.

ACE inhibitors, ARBs, beta-blockers, and verapamil-type calcium antagonists are useful to treat underlying conditions (myocardial ischaemia, arterial hypertension) and have the ability to improve LV diastolic properties through a number of different mechanisms; thus, there is the potential for beneficial effects from the use of these drugs.

Digoxin may be indicated in patients with concomitant atrial fibrillation, alone or in combination with a beta-blocker or verapamil. The administration of diuretics and nitrates may be necessary when episodes of fluid overload or acute dyspnoea occur, but they should be given cautiously in order to avoid an excessive preload reduction, which in turn might lead to a critical fall in cardiac output.

References

1. Murdoch DR, McMurray JJV (2000) Epidemiological perspective on heart failure: common, costly, disabling, deadly. In: Sharpe N (ed) Heart failure management. London, Martin Dunitz, pp 1–14

2. Fletcher MD, Yusuf S, Kober L et al (2000) Long-term ACE-inhibitor therapy in patients with heart failure or left ventricular dysfunction: a systematic overview of data from individual patients. ACE-Inhibitor Myocardial Infarction Collaborative Group. Lancet 355:1575–1581

3. Lee VC, Rhew DC, Dylan M et al (2004) Meta-analysis: angiotensin receptor blockers in chronic heart failure and high-risk acute myocardial infarction. Ann Intern Med 141:693–704

4. Struthers AD (2004) Aldosterone blockade in heart failure. J Renin Angiotensin Aldosterone Syst 5(Suppl 1):S23-S27

5. Foody JAM, Farrell MH, Krumholz HM (2002) Beta-blocker therapy in heart failure. JAMA 287:883–889

6. Faris R, Flather M, Purcell H et al (2002) Current evidence supporting the role of diuretics in heart failure: a meta-analysis of randomized controlled trials. Int J Cardiol 82:149–158

7. Wood WB, Dans AL, Guyatt GJ et al (2004) Digitalis for treatment of congestive heart failure in patients in sinus rhythm: a systematic review and meta-analysis. J Card Fail 10:155–164

8. Ezekowitz JA, Armstrong PW, McAlister FA (2003) Implantable cardioverter defibrillator in primary and secondary prevention: a systematic review of randomized, controlled trials. Ann Intern Med 138:445–452

9. Nanthakumar K, Epstein AE, Kay GN et al (2004) Prophylactic implantable defibrillator therapy in patients with left ventricular systolic dysfunction. A pooled analysis of 10 primary prevention trials. J Am Coll Cardiol 44:2166–2172

10. Bradley DJ, Bradley EA, Baughman KL et al (2003) Cardiac resynchronisation and death from progressive heart failure: a meta-analysis of randomised controlled trials. JAMA 289:730–740

11. Stewart S (2003) Prognosis of patients with heart failure compared with common types of cancer. Heart Fail Monit 3:87–94

12. Rich MW (1999) Heart failure disease management: a critical review. J Card Fail 5:64–75

13. Hunt SA, Baker DW, Chin MH et al (2001) Report of ACC/AHA guidelines for the evaluation and management of chronic heart failure in the adult. Circulation 104:2996–3007

14. Task Force for the Diagnosis and Treatment of Chronic Heart Failure (2001) European Society of Cardiology: WJ Remme and K. Swedberg (Co-Chairmen). Guidelines for the diagnosis and treatment of chronic heart failure. Eur Heart J 22:1527–1560

How to Detect Dyssynchrony and How to Correct It

L. Ascione, M. Accadia, R. Iengo, S.E. Rumolo, C. Muto, M. Canciello, G. Carreras, B. Tuccillo

Introduction

Despite remarkable advances, pharmacological treatment of heart failure suffers from serious limitations and the prognosis of these patients remains poor in terms of both mortality and morbidity [1]. In this context, cardiac resynchronisation therapy (CRT) has recently been introduced to improve symptoms, functional capacity, and functional parameters of the left ventricle in patients with heart failure that is refractory to optimal medical therapy [2, 3].

Patients with left ventricular systolic dysfunction and dilatation frequently have ventricular conduction delays [4], usually manifested as left bundle branch block (LBBB). This type of conduction abnormality is generally associated with delayed depolarisation and contraction of the lateral left ventricular wall whereas the interventricular septum shows a normal (early) contraction resulting in a paradoxical septal motion.

The abnormal activation sequence induced by LBBB changes regional ventricular loadings, redistributes myocardial blood flow, and creates a regional, non-uniform myocardial metabolism [5, 6]. The effects of this electromechanical dyssynchrony may contribute to disease progression in patients, with left ventricular systolic dysfunction revealing itself as an independent predictor of an adverse outcome [4, 7].

CRT was classified in the American College of Cardiology/American Heart Association/North American Society of Pacing and Electrophysiology/ Heart Rhythm Society 2002 guideline update for implantation of pacemaker and antiarrhythmic devices with level of evidence II A for patients with idiopathic or ischaemic cardiomyopathy, severe heart failure NYHA functional class III or IV despite optimised medical therapy, left ventricular ejection

Division of Cardiology, S. Maria di Loreto Hospital, Naples, Italy

fraction < 35%, QRS duration > 130 ms and left ventricular end-diastolic diameter > 55 mm [8]. However, approximately 20% to 30% of patients do not respond to this form of therapy, underscoring the need for additional selection to identify potential responder [9].

Mechanical Dissynchrony

It has been recently shown that mechanical dyssynchrony is not necessarily related to electrical dyssynchrony [10, 11]; furthermore, the major predictor of response to CRT is the presence of mechanical dyssynchrony. These considerations suggest that surface ECG may not be the optimal tool to detect dyssynchrony, while new, non-invasive imaging techniques may provide additional information for the selection of potential responders to CRT. Radionuclide imaging has been shown to be useful in assessing interventricular dyssynchrony, though the spatial and temporal resolution are limited and a detailed evaluation of intraventricular dyssynchrony may not always be possible. Cardiac magnetic resonance is a relatively luxurious investigation that is potentially useful to quantify regional wall motion and strain rate when combined with a tagging technique, though further tests are needed to evaluate this role. Echocardiography with its newer applications such as Doppler tissue imaging, strain, and strain rate has partly solved most of the aforementioned limitations of other imaging techniques and seems to be the technique of choice to select candidates for CRT. Before discussing the various echocardiographic approaches to detect asynchrony, the various forms of dyssynchrony are listed below.

Types of Mechanical Dyssynchrony

Atrioventricular Dyssynchrony

An abnormal conduction of the AV node results in:
- A delay between atrial and ventricular contraction
- Mitral valve incompetence with occurrence of late diastolic regurgitation
- Shortened ventricular filling time, limiting net diastolic stroke volume
- Often, immediate occurrence of atrial systole with early passive filling, hence reducing left ventricular filling

Interventricular Dyssynchrony

Altered electrical activation in patients with LBBB results in a delayed left ventricular contraction and relaxation compared with the right ventricle. This asynchronous right–left ventricular contraction and relaxation may produce dynamic alterations in trans-septal pressure and volume that may cause abnormal septal motion, resulting in altered regional ejection fraction with a reduced interventricular septal contribution to global left ventricular performance [12].

Intraventricular Dyssynchrony

A disorganised left ventricular contraction generates regions of both early and delayed contraction, reducing left ventricular performance, since early contraction occurs when pressure is low and does not lead to ejection while the late contraction occurs at higher stress and results in paradoxical stretch of early-contracting segments [13].

Echocardiographic Assessment of Dyssynchrony

Atrioventricular Dyssynchrony

Left ventricular performance can be improved by adequate atrioventricular timing. It has been proposed that the optimal atrioventricular delay should provide the longest left ventricular filling time without premature truncation of the A-wave by mitral valve closure [14]. This approach is widely accepted as a simple method by which to optimise atrioventricular delay, even if it is not clear whether atrioventricular timing optimisation is needed or whether an atrioventricular delay of 100 or 120 ms would be appropriate for all patients.

Interventricular Dyssynchrony

The asynchronous right–left ventricular contraction can be evaluated (Fig. 1) by assessing the extent of interventricular mechanical delay, defined as the time difference between left and right ventricular pre-ejection intervals (IVMD). A value of IVMD of 40 ms or greater is considered indicative of interventricular dyssynchrony, and in the MIRACLE trial this index of inter-ventricular dyssynchrony was reduced by 19% after CRT [15, 16]. Tissue Doppler imaging was also used to demonstrate interventricular dyssyn-chrony; Yu et al. found a large mechanical delay between the free right ven-tricular wall and the lateral wall of the left ventricle, which was completely reversed after CRT [17].

Intraventricular Dyssynchrony

Among the various forms of mechanical dyssynchrony, intra-left-ventricular electromechanical asynchrony seems to be the most important since it reflects the mechanical dispersion of motion within the left ventricle; fur-

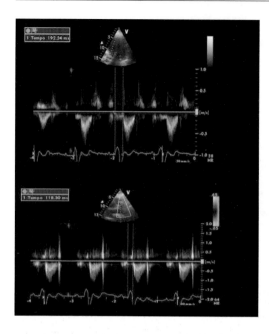

Fig. 1. Measurement of inter-ventricular mechanical delay by Doppler echocardiography. The right and left ventricular pre-ejection intervals are measured from the onset of QRS to the onset of aortic and pulmonary outflow

thermore, it has recently shown that it is an independent predictor of cardiac events in heart failure patients [18, 19].

Several echocardiographic methods have been proposed to assess intra-left-ventricular dyssynchrony, both with conventional echocardiography and with newer echocardiographic methods. Using an M-mode recording from the parasternal short axis view, Pitzalis et al. demonstrated that a value of 130 ms or greater of the septal-to-posterior wall motion delay is a marker of intraventricular dyssynchrony predicting reverse remodelling with high accuracy [20]. This method is simple but has only been employed in patients with very long QRS duration where the timing of isovolumic contraction of the anterior septum is compared to the contraction of the posterior wall during the ejection phase (Fig. 2); furthermore, this electromechanical delay frequently cannot be determined, either because the septum is akinetic after a large anterior infarction or because the maximal posterior motion is not well defined.

Tissue Doppler imaging (TDI) has proved an useful tool for non-invasive analysis of the left ventricular activation–contraction sequence on a regional basis, because of its high spatial (< 1 mm) and temporal (<100 Hz) resolution. Unfortunately, consensus on which TDI measurements should be used, and where to place the region of interest, has not yet been achieved; in fact, at least three different approaches for the assessment of intra-left-ventricular dyssynchrony have been proposed by the various groups that have evaluated TDI in the CRT context (Fig. 3). Some groups analyse the basal left ventricle in two orthogonal planes (anteroposterior and septal—lateral) and

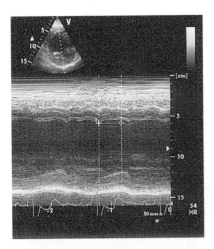

Fig. 2. Parasternal M-mode recording the left ventricular cavity in heart failure patient with left bundle branch block. A clear delay between peak systolic septal and posterior wall inward motion is observed

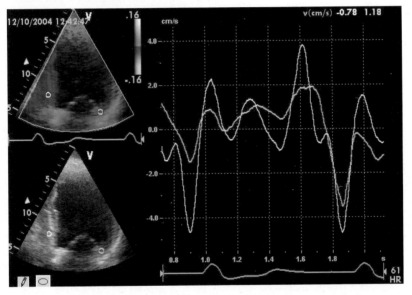

Fig. 3. Tissue Doppler curves taken from the basal septum and lateral wall in a patient with intra-left-ventricular dyssynchrony

focus on early systole, measuring the regional difference between the onset of the QRS complex and the onset of systolic movement [18, 21]; on the other hand, the method used by Søøgard et al. focuses on late or post-systolic longitudinal contraction at the base of left ventricle [22]; while Yu et al. evaluate the regional difference between the interval from QRS onset to peak systolic velocity of both basal and middle left ventricular segments in a 12-segment model [17]. Results may be completely different depending on which one of these approaches is used.

One of the most important limitations of TDI analysis with velocity imaging is its inability to determine whether the motion represents contraction or is merely passive. To overcome these limits, strain and strain rate, two new imaging modalities, have been recently introduced into clinical practice. Using digitally stored, colour-coded tissue Doppler images, it is possible to obtain, off line, information regarding regional myocardial deformation, a property of particular importance in identifying the ideal CRT responder. Strain analysis allows direct assessment of the degree of myocardial deformation during systole and is expressed as the percentage of segmental shortening or lengthening in relation to its original length (Fig. 4), while strain rate measures the rate of local deformation and is expressed in centimetres per second (Fig. 5). Compared with TDI, the main advantage of strain rate imaging resides in its better differentiation between active systolic contraction and passive displacement, which is of particular importance in ischaemic patients with scar tissue [23, 24]. However the clinical applicability of this imaging modality is still limited by the acoustic artefacts, angle dependency, and a poor signal-to-clutter ratio, which render the image acquisition and analysis process tedious and time-consuming, decreasing its reproducibility and widespread use.

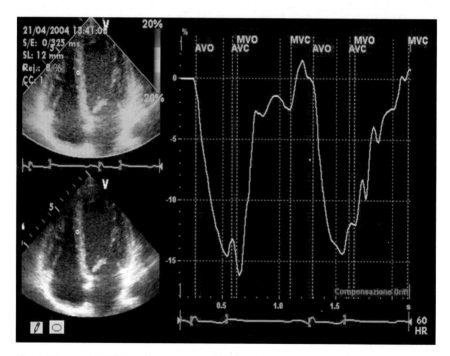

Fig. 4. Myocardial deformation as assessed by strain imaging

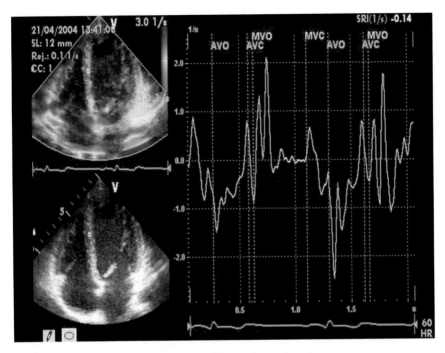

Fig. 5. Myocardial deformation as assessed by strain rate imaging

Echocardiography to Optimise Lead Positioning

The aim of CRT is early contraction of the most delayed left ventricular myocardial segments to improve left ventricular myocardial synchrony. In order to maximise the haemodynamic effect, it is of paramount importance to know the site of the latest mechanical activity. Ansalone et al. have shown that the most delayed wall is the lateral one (35%), followed by the anterior and posterior regions (26% and 23%), while the inferior wall and the septum infrequently show the latest mechanical activity; furthermore, these authors demonstrated that biventricular pacing provided additional benefit when applied at the most delayed site [25].

Conclusions

The response to CRT is largely determined by the baseline degree of inter- and intraventricular dyssynchrony, and echocardiography seems to be the ideal technique by which to identify responders to CRT. At present the definition of echocardiographic indices of ventricular dyssynchrony is undergoing intense research, and several indices have been proposed that may or may not prove useful in a prospective evaluation. It is time for a prospective trial to evaluate these different parameters with regard to their impact on the efficacy of CRT. These data will provide a better basis for the clinical decision as to which heart failure patients are likely to benefit from this new form of therapy.

References

1. Zannad F, Briancon S, Juillere Y et al (1999) Incidence, clinical and etiologic features and outcomes of advanced chronic heart failure: the epical study. J Am Coll Cardiol 33:734–742
2. Cazeau S, Leclerq M, Lavergne T et al (2001) Multisite Stimulation in Cardiomyopathies (MUSTIC) Study Investigators. Effect of multisite biventricular pacing in patients with heart failure and interventricular conduction delay. N Engl J Med 1344:873–880
3. St John Sutton M, Plappert T, Abraham WT et al (2003) Effect of cardiac resynchronization therapy on left ventricular size and function in chronic heart failure. Circulation 107:1985–1990
4. Baldasseroni S, Opasich C, Gorini M et al (2002) Left bundle-branch block is associated with increased 1-year sudden and total mortality rate in 5517 outpatients with congestive heart failure: a report from the Italian network on congestive heart failure. Am Heart J 143:398–405
5. Prinzen FW, Hunter WC, Wyman BT et al (1999) Mapping of regional myocardial strain and work during ventricular pacing: experimental study using magnetic resonance imaging tagging. J Am Coll Cardiol 33:1735–1742
6. Ukkonen H, Beankinds RSB, Burwash IG et al (2003) Effect of cardiac resynchronization on myocardial efficiency and regional oxidative metabolism. Circulation 107:28–31
7. Bader H, Garrigue S, Lafitte S et al (2004) Intra-left ventricular electromechanical asynchrony. A new independent predictor of severe cardiac events in heart failure patients. J Am Coll Cardiol 43:248–256
8. Gregoratos G, Abrams J, Epstein AE et al (2002) ACC/AHA/NASPE 2002 guidelines update for implantation of cardiac pacemakers and antiarrhythmia devices. J Am Coll Cardiol 40:1703–1719
9. Leclercq C, Kass DA (2002) Retiming the failing heart: principles and current clinical status of cardiac resynchronization. J Am Coll Cardiol 39:194–201
10. Yu CM, Lin H Zuang Q (2003) High prevalence of left ventricular systolic and diastolic asynchrony in patients with congestive heart failure and normal QRS duration. Heart 89:54–60
11. Auricchio A, Yu CM (2004) Beyond the measurements of QRS complex towards mechanical dyssynchrony: cardiac resynchronisation therapy in heart failure patients with a normal QRS duration. Heart 90:479–471
12. Grines CL, Bashore TM, Boudoulas H et al (1989) Functional abnormalities in isolated left bundle branch block: the effect of interventricular asynchrony. Circulation 79:845–853
13. Nelson GS, Curry CW Wyman BT et al (2000) Predictors of systolic augmentation from the left ventricular preexcitation in patients with dilated cardiomyopathy and intraventricular conduction delay. Circulation 101:2703–2709

14. Kindermann M, Frolhig G, Doerr T et al (1997) Optimizing the AV delay in DDD pacemaker with high degree AV block: mitral valve Doppler versus impedance cardiography. Pacing Clin Electrophysiol 20:2543–2562

15. Porciani MC, Puglisi A, Colella A et al (2000) Echocardiographic evaluation of the effect of biventricular pacing; the InSync Italian Registry. Eur Heart J Suppl 2 (Suppl J):J23–J30

16. St John Sutton MG, Plappert T Abraham WT et al (2003) Effect of cardiac resynchronization therapy on left ventricular size and function in chronic heart failure. Circulation 107:1985–1990

17. Yu CM, Chau E, Sanderson JE et al (2002) Tissue Doppler echocardiography evidence of reverse remodelling and improved synchronicity by simultaneously delaying regional contraction after biventricular pacing therapy in heart failure. Circulation 105:438–445

18. Bader H, Garrigue S, Lafitte S et al (2004) Intra-left ventricular electromechanical asynchrony. A new independent predictor of severe cardiac events in heart failure. J Am Coll Cardiol 43:248–256

19. Fauchier L, Marie O, Casset-Senon D et al (2002) Interventricular and intraventricular dyssynchrony in idiopathic dilated cardiomyopathy. A prognosis study with Fourier analysis of radionuclide angioscintigraphy. J Am Coll Cardiol 40:2002–2030

20. Pitzalis MV, Iacoviello M, Romito R et al (2002) Cardiac resynchronization therapy tailored by echocardiographic evaluation of ventricular asynchrony. J Am Coll Cardiol 40:1615–1622

21. Ghio S, Costantin C, Klersy C et al (2004) Interventricular and intraventricular dyssynchrony are common in heart failure patients, regardless of QRS duration. Eur Heart J 25: 571–578

22. Søøgard P, Egeblad H, Kim WY et al (2002) Tissue Doppler imaging predicts improved systolic performance and reversed left ventricular remodelling during long–term cardiac resynchronization therapy. J Am Coll Cardiol 40:723–730

23. Heimdal A, Stolen A, Torp H et al (1998) Real time strain-rate imaging of the left ventricle by ultrasound. J Am Soc Echocardiogr 11:1013–1019

24. D'Hooge J, Heimdal A, Jamal F et al (2000) Regional strain and strain rate measurements by cardiac ultrasound: principles, implementation and limitation. Eur J Echocardiogr 1:154–170

25. Ansalone G, Giannantoni P, Ricci R et al (2002) Doppler myocardial imaging to evaluate the effectiveness of pacing sites in patients receiving biventricular pacing. J Am Coll Cardiol 39:489–499

Advancements in 'Over-the-Wire' Versus Stylet-Guided Left Ventricular Leads

S. Boveda

Coronary Sinus and Target Vein Anatomy

It is now well known that cardiac resynchronisation therapy (CRT) achieved by biventricular pacing improves haemodynamics in advanced heart failure patients with interventricular and/or intraventricular dyssynchrony. The delivery of CRT is still challenging, as transvenous access to the left ventricle through the coronary sinus tributaries is required. When this technique was first introduced, stylet-delivered shaped leads were used for the left ventricular pacing, but the implantation success rate (around 90%) was very dependent on the coronary sinus anatomy, and on the access to and diameter of the lateral vein.

The usual anatomy of the coronary sinus consists of three groups of veins, designated according to their localisation along the left ventricle as posterior, lateral, and anterior. In fact, the coronary sinus configuration varies greatly from patient to patient. In some, there is no lateral vein. Sometimes, there is only a posterolateral or an anterolateral vein. Vessels may be large, medium-sized, or very small. In addition, left ventricular lead placement is performed by a retrograde approach, and the presence of venous valves or spasm phenomenon can make the progression very difficult.

For all these reasons, the left ventricular lead should be selected after a venogram has been performed, since the choice will depend on the size, tortuosity, and angulation of the target vein with the coronary sinus. To improve the implantation success rate, the industry proposes a range of stylet- and over-the-wire-guided leads to suit all venous anatomies [1]. Over-the-wire leads will be used in the case of small or medium-calibre tortuous

Cardiology Department, Clinique Pasteur, Toulouse, France

veins or when there is acute angulation with the coronary sinus. By contrast, stylet leads will be more appropriate for medium-sized and large straight veins and an open angle with the coronary sinus.

Angioplasty Technology: Over-the-Wire LV Leads

This great variability of the coronary sinus anatomy led to the development of a novel 'over-the-wire' approach, combining a standard pacing lead and angioplasty technology. The technique is based on shaped sheaths for coronary sinus catheterisation and angiography, and guide wires for the left ventricular lead [1]. The sheaths must be smooth and flexible, to avoid coronary sinus dissection. A special venography balloon catheter is inserted into the sheath to perform a coronary sinus angiogram that will help in identification of the target vein and thus in the selection of the most appropriate left ventricular lead. Then, using angioplasty techniques and tools, the left ventricular lead will be driven to the target vein using the inner stylet for a classical shaped lead, or a special guide wire for an over-the-wire left ventricular lead. After placement of the left ventricular lead, the sheath is removed by cutting (Medtronic, Biotronik), peeling (St. Jude Medical), or just dragging it away (Guidant, Ela Médical) all along the lead.

This logical approach to reaching the target vessel in the coronary sinus has interested many interventional cardiologists specialising in coronary angioplasty. They have adapted their skill, performing coronary vein balloon angioplasty and evolving new solutions for difficult cases.

Over-the-Wire/Stylet LV Leads

These over-the-wire systems have been improved more recently with new active fixation mechanisms and steroid-eluting leads to provide better pacing thresholds [2]. Among the recent advancements may be mentioned the distal tip silicone seal designed to reduce blood ingress into the lumen.

Some over-the-wire leads have no shape and a passive classical (Guidant Easytrak 1 and 2) [3] or active silicone screw (Ela Médical) fixation system on the distal tip. In many cases (Medtronic, Biotronik, St. Jude Medical, Guidant Easytrak 3) the leads have an angled lead body with two or more distal curves (Medtronic, St. Jude Medical) or a helix (Biotronik, Guidant Easytrak 3) for a better stability inside the vein.

Many over-the-wire leads can also be stylet-delivered (Medtronic, St. Jude Medical, Biotronik), depending on the configuration of the target vein. The Medtronic 4193 lead has a 4F flexible lead body for easier implantation in the small veins. One of the problems of these over-the-wire thin leads is the risk of phrenic nerve stimulation because of their placement in the distal part of the vein. In this situation, it is necessary to withdraw the lead until phrenic nerve stimulation stops.

Finally, all left ventricular leads have the standard IS-1 connection, except the Guidant Easytrak leads (original LV1 connection) [3].

Results

As has been demonstrated by Boriani et al. [4], it is obvious that CRT procedures require a learning curve, and the implant success rate increases dramatically from 52% in inexperienced hands to more than 90% in trained teams. There is also an improvement in the success rate when the implanter uses the complementarity of the left ventricular lead range: from 91.6% with over-the-wire leads only, up to 94.1% success when stylet and/or over-the-wire leads are used. This means that comprehensive knowledge of CRT tools and leads is necessary to achieve a success rate of 90% or more, which seems to be the goal at present. However, despite this, experience remains the most important factor of success.

Unfortunately, we know that in a small group of patients (around 5%) CRT is impossible to achieve. Peculiarities of anatomy are the main reasons for unsuccessful attempts, leading to inability to access the coronary sinus ostium or the coronary vein, or dislodgement or unstable positioning of the lead.

The electrical performances of over-the-wire left ventricular leads are similar to those observed for right ventricular leads, except for the pacing threshold, which is usually higher, around 1.5 V in our experience (Table 1). In addition, left ventricular pacing thresholds are not significantly different between over-the-wire- and stylet-delivered leads [5].

We compared the data of the MIRACLE [6] and InSync III [7] studies to assess whether there was an improvement in implantation success rates and complication rates with increased experience and the introduction of new left ventricular lead technologies. In each study, investigators were asked to first attempt the implant with a selected lead: the Attain 2187 (stylet-delivered) for the MIRACLE and the Attain 4193 (over-the-wire-guided) for the InSync III study. If unsuccessful, they could use other leads included in the protocols. Performance comparisons were made between the MIRACLE and the InSync III studies, both of which used CRT-only devices (Table 2). It is very interesting to observe that implantation success rate improved with experience. However, there was a highly significant decrease in implantation time and fluoroscopy time with the InSync III study which can be attributed to implanter experience and the addition of the over-the-wire lead (Fig. 1). Finally, perioperative complications decreased significantly with the addition

Table 1. Experience at the Clinique Pasteur, 2003-2004

	CRT implants 2003-2004
Enrollment period	January 2003 – December 2004
OTW vs stylet LV leads (%)	100% vs 0%
Implant attempts	128
Successful implants (% success rate)	122 (95%)
Number of patients needing 2 procedures	5 (4%)
Mean procedure time (min)	92 ± 53
Complications[a]	14 (11%)
Mean LV pacing thresholds (V)	1.53

[a] Complications: phrenic stimulation ($n = 5$), lead dislodgement ($n = 4$), > 5-V thresholds ($n = 3$), haematoma/infection ($n = 2$)

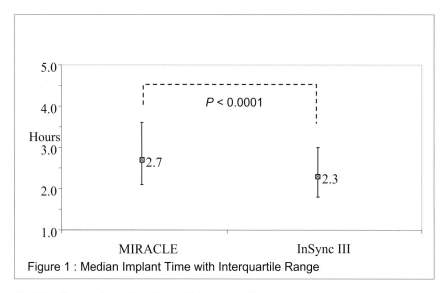

Figure 1 : Median Implant Time with Interquartile Range

Fig. 1. Median implantation time with interquartile range

of the Attain over-the-wire lead in InSync III (Table 3). These data suggest that an over-the-wire lead should be implanted primarily in order to significantly reduce procedure duration, fluoroscopy time, and the risk of perioperative complications.

It seems likely that implanter experience and coronary sinus anatomy have a strong impact on procedure times and outcomes.

Table 2. Over-the-wire or stylet guiding lead?

	MIRACLE	InSync III
Enrollment period	November 1998 December 2000	November 2000 June 2002
Primary Attain LV lead reference number (% used)	2187 (97.5%)	4193 (88.9%)
Generator model used	InSync 8040	8042
Implantation attempts	571	422
Successful implantations	528	397

P = n.s.

Table 3. Which lead is safer?

	MIRACLE	InSync III
Primary Attain LV lead reference number (% used)	2187 (97.5%)	4193 (88.9%)
Successful implants	528	397
Procedure-related deaths (%)	2 (0.4)	1 (0.2)
Patients with perioperative LV lead complications (%)	19 (3.3)*	5 (1.2)*
Patients with postoperative LV lead complications (%)	39 (7.4)*	16 (4.0)*
Patients with LV lead dislodgement (%)	26 (4.9)	15 (3.6)

* $P \leq 0.05$

Complications

Potential risks during the CRT procedure include complete heart block by traumatic right bundle branch block, induction of atrial or ventricular arrhythmias, and, especially, the risk of coronary sinus perforation or dissection with a pericardial effusion. During the perioperative period the most common complications are left ventricular lead dislodgement, phrenic nerve stimulation, and left ventricular high pacing thresholds.

In our experience, we reported an 11% rate of global complications (see Table 1). The global complication rate in the MIRACLE study was 16% and in the InSync III study it was 9% (Table 3). These data confirm that CRT remains a risky procedure.

Conclusions

Although the implantation success rate does not differ significantly between over-the-wire and stylet leads, procedure duration, fluoroscopy time, and perioperative complication decrease when an over-the-wire left ventricular lead is primarily implanted by experienced teams. This novel lead, sometimes combined with coronary vein angioplasty [8, 9], represents a decisive improvement of the technique, especially for pacing of the left ventricle in the optimal spot. Despite all these efforts, a 100% success rate will probably never be reached by the endovascular approach. A surgical approach via a minimally invasive thoracotomy should be considered for those 5% of patients in whom endovascular CRT device implantation has failed.

References

1. Lau CP, Barold S, Tse HF et al (2003) Advances in devices for cardiac resynchronization in heart failure. J Interv Card Electrophysiol 9:167–181
2. Achtelik M, Bocchiardo M, Trappe HJ et al (2000) Performance of a new steroid-eluting coronary sinus lead designed for left ventricular pacing. Pacing Clin Electrophysiol 23:741–743
3. Purerfellner H, Nesser HJ, Winter S et al (2000) Transvenous left ventricular lead implantation with the EASYTRAK lead system: the European experience. Am J Cardiol 86:157–164
4. Boriani G, Padeletti L, Bongiorni G et al (2002) Left ventricular pacing from the coronary sinus: implanters dependance of the success rate on learning curve (abstract). Cardiostim, Nice (abs)
5. Daoud EG, Kalbfleisch SJ, Hummel JD et al (2002) Implantation techniques and chronic lead parameters of biventricular pacing dual-chamber defibrillators. J Cardiovasc Electrophysiol 13:964–970
6. St John Sutton MG, Plappert T, Abraham WT et al (2003) Effect of cardiac resynchronisation therapy on left ventricular size and function in chronic heart failure. Circulation 107:1985–1990
7. Adamson PB, Smith AL, Abraham WT et al (2004) Continuous antonomic assessment in patients with symptomatic heart failure: prognostic value of heart rate variability measured by an implanted cardiac resynchronisation device. Circulation 110:2389–2394
8. Sandler DA, Feigenblum DY, Bernstein NE et al (2002) Cardiac vein angioplasty for biventricular pacing. Pacing Clin Electrophysiol 25:1788–1789
9. Hansky B, Lamp B, Minami K et al (2002) Coronary vein balloon angioplasty for left ventricular pacemaker lead implantation. J Am Coll Cardiol 40:2144–2149

Assessment of Diastolic Function in Heart Failure and Atrial Fibrillation

S. Carerj, S. Raffa, C. Zito

In the past three decades, Doppler echocardiography has emerged as a non-invasive alternative to cardiac catheterisation for evaluating haemodynamic variables [1]. A well-performed Doppler examination is able to provide as accurate data as conventional cardiac catheterisation does.

Diastolic function of the left ventricle (LV) plays a relevant role in producing the signs and symptoms of heart failure (HF) in cardiac diseases, the end result of which is the elevation of left ventricular pressure per unit volume of blood entering the LV [2-5]. This elevated filling pressure increases left atrial pressure, which is reflected back to the pulmonary circulation and causes symptoms of shortness of breath and signs of pulmonary congestion. Because of the complexity of the multiple interrelated events that comprise diastolic filling of the heart, assessment of LV diastolic function was in the past limited to the catheterisation laboratory, where complex measurements of pressure–volume relations and rates of decrease in pressure from high-fidelity pressure curves were used [6].

It has been speculated that Doppler echocardiography could be used to assess diastolic filling and function of the LV non-invasively [7, 8]. Kitabatake et al. [9] in 1982 described the different flow velocity curves that occur in different disease states from Doppler interrogation of transmitral flow. Multiple investigations in both animals and humans followed and provided insight into the interpretation of these flow velocity patterns [10, 11]. The mitral flow velocity curves can be viewed as determined by the relative driving pressure across the mitral valve from the left atrium to the LV. There is an initial rapid acceleration of flow as left ventricular pressure drops rapidly below left atrial pressure during ventricular relaxation (measured as the E wave velocity). As the LV fills in early diastole, there is a rise in pres-

Division of Cardiology, University of Messina, Italy

sure that exceeds the left atrial pressure, causing a deceleration of flow. The rate of deceleration of flow is measured as the mitral E wave deceleration time and is dependent mainly upon the effective operating compliance of the LV. During mid-diastole there is equilibration of left ventricular and left atrial pressures, with a low velocity of forward flow as a result of inertial forces. Finally, at atrial contraction there is a re-acceleration of transmitral flow as left atrial pressure rises above left ventricular pressure (measured as the A wave velocity). These flow velocity curves are dependent on multiple intrinsic factors that include the rate of left ventricular relaxation and elastic recoil (diastolic suction), left atrial and left ventricular compliance, and left atrial pressure, as well as varying patient conditions such as load, age, and heart rate [10, 11].

It has already been shown in experimental models of HF [12] that there is also a progression of abnormal diastolic patterns that occurs over time with cardiac diseases. In the early stage of dysfunction, impaired relaxation of the LV dominates, which decreases early diastolic filling although filling pressures remain normal in the rest state. This is reflected by a decrease in the initial E wave velocity, prolongation of E wave deceleration time, and increased proportion of filling due to atrial contraction. With disease progression, left atrial pressure rises, which increases the driving pressure across the mitral valve. This is accompanied by a gradual increase in E wave velocity and a decrease in effective operating compliance of the LV, which shortens the mitral E wave deceleration time. In advanced stages of disease, there will be even higher pressures, a higher E/A ratio, and a very abbreviated mitral deceleration time. This concept of a progression of the mitral flow velocity curves with worsening disease has a clinical application: the prognosis of patients with either dilated or infiltrative cardiomyopathy is indicated by a short mitral deceleration time, with values below 140 ms indicating a poor outcome, independently of the degree of systolic dysfunction [13, 14]. Furthermore, non-invasive assessment of left ventricular filling pressures in HF patients would be of great value in assessing their degree of left ventricular dysfunction and monitoring the effect of unloading therapies. Previous studies have shown that this can be estimated by combining various Doppler echocardiographic variables [10, 15–17]. Patients with atrial fibrillation (AF) have, however, been excluded from these studies, limiting the applicability of such estimates to patients in sinus rhythm.

It has been shown that in patients with HF and sinus rhythm elevated left atrial pressures can compensate for delayed left ventricular relaxation, thus increasing early diastolic mitral flow velocity and its deceleration and decreasing isovolumic relaxation time. High left atrial pressure before atrial contraction together with a stiff LV shortens and reduces mitral flow velocity wave at atrial contraction. This leads to the so-called pseudo-normal and restrictive patterns that in HF patients are reliable indexes of elevated left ventricular filling pressures. Pulmonary venous flow in sinus rhythm patients shows a triphasic pattern which is predominantly related to left atrial function and reflects the oscillations of left atrial pressures [18]. Thus, the systolic forward flow velocity is determined by the combined backward effect of the decrease in left atrial pressure, due to both left atrial relaxation and mitral annulus descent, and the forward propagation of systolic right ventricular pressure [19]. The diastolic forward flow velocity, which occurs when the mitral valve is open and the left atrium behaves as a passive conduit, slightly follows and is closely related to early diastolic mitral flow velocity. The reverse diastolic flow velocity wave is determined by atrial contraction and its duration depends mainly on left ventricular compliance. In patients with HF and sinus rhythm, when the left atrial pressure is high (and left atrial compliance is reduced) the systolic flow velocity is blunted; the diastolic forward flow velocity is high and its deceleration is rapid; the reverse flow is prolonged and its duration exceeds that of forward mitral flow at atrial contraction.

Unfortunately, approximately 20% of patients with chronic HF have AF [20, 21]. When AF is present, the loss of atrial contraction and of ventricular rate control affects both mitral and pulmonary venous flow and the relationship between Doppler variables and left ventricular filling pressure becomes more complicated. When AF occurs, the active atrial contraction is lost, so that the whole blood volume filling the LV is detected in a monophasic E wave. At the same time Doppler recording of pulmonary venous flow shows a loss of the late diastolic reverse flow. Loss of the active left atrial relaxation causes the disappearance of the first component of the systolic forward flow velocity. Besides these effects on left ventricular and atrial filling due to the loss of an active atrial contraction, irregular cardiac cycle lengths produce marked beat-to-beat variations in both mitral and pulmonary venous flow velocities.

Despite all these differences between Doppler echocardiographic findings in patients with sinus rhythm and AF, a relatively accurate estimation of pulmonary capillary wedge pressure (PCWP) can be achieved in HF patients who are in AF. In particular, in patients with AF, indexes of early left ventricular diastolic filling, i.e. isovolumic relaxation time, deceleration time, and deceleration rate, and the systolic fraction of pulmonary venous flow are almost as strongly correlated with PCWP as they are in patients with sinus rhythm [22, 23]. Temporelli et al. [24] have recently found that a value of 120 ms in E wave deceleration time seems to be the best cut-off point in predicting high values of PCWP in HF patients with AF, the sensitivity and specificity of a mitral E wave deceleration time below 120 ms in predicting PCWP above 20 mmHg being 100% and 96%, respectively.

AF is characterised by an irregular heart rate that produces beat-to-beat variations in contractility, preload, after-load, and mitral regurgitation, which leads to increased variability in Doppler measurements. To minimise this problem it would be preferable to investigate patients when they are receiving optimal medical therapy including medications that are able to reduce sufficiently (and synchronise as much as possible) their ventricular heart rate. Moreover, short cardiac cycles (< 600 ms) should not be analysed because they are often associated with fusion of pulmonary venous flow waves. The optimal number of beats to be analysed and averaged for Doppler measurements of diastolic function in AF should be approximately three times that necessary in sinus rhythm, i.e. from 5 to 10.

Problems related to variability of haemodynamic conditions in HF patients with AF may constitute a limit of flow Doppler; furthermore, to obtain meaningful data, a strict and time-consuming methodology must be followed, which may limit the everyday application of this parameters in a busy clinical practice.

In order to limit the load dependence of flow Doppler measurements on left ventricular diastolic function, new methods have recently been introduced. Nagueh et al. [25] found that peak acceleration of the E wave (PkAcc), isovolumic relaxation time, deceleration time of the E wave, and the ratio of E velocity to propagation velocity (E/Vp) were strongly related to left ventricular filling pressure. In particular, the velocity of propagation of the early inflow from the LV base to the apex (Vp), determined using colour M-mode, correlated well with the time constant of isovolumetric left ventricular relaxation (τ) [26]. In patients with abnormal left ventricular relaxation and elevated left ventricular end-diastolic pressure, filling flow propagation is rapidly attenuated in spite of the increased early transmitral velocity. Therefore, as the severity of HF increases, the E/Vp also increases and may be a more sensitive index than E velocity or Vp alone. Recently Oyama et al. [27] found that a cut-off value of E/Vp of 1.7 was able to predict with acceptable accuracy the presence of high PCWP (> 15 mmHg) in HF patients with AF.

Tissue Doppler imaging has recently become a common tool of modern ultrasound systems. This allows the recording of myocardial contraction and relaxation velocities. The early diastolic mitral annular velocity (Ea) has been shown to be a relatively load-independent measure of myocardial relaxation in patients with cardiac disease [28]. When tissue Doppler imaging is combined with pulsed Doppler transmitral flow in early diastole (E), the resultant E/Ea ratio has been correlated with left ventricular filling pressure measured invasively in patients with sinus rhythm [29]. E/Ea values above 15 have been shown to be highly predictive (sensitivity 92%, specificity 90%) of a PCWP greater than 15 mmHg in patients with depressed ejection fraction and sinus rhythm [30]. In conclusion, Doppler echocardiography is now well accepted as a reliable and reproducible method for assessing diastolic function in various cardiac diseases. Several studies have demonstrated that left ventricular pressure and mean PCWP can be estimated from variables of mitral and pulmonary venous flow. In particular, an excellent inverse correlation has been found between the deceleration time of transmitral E wave and PCWP in patients with severe left ventricular dysfunction and sinus rhythm. In the case of HF patients with AF, however, few data have been published so far. The presence of irregular rhythm associated with high variability of haemodynamic conditions and absence of atrial contraction constitute an obstacle to the accurate evaluation of left ventricular diastolic function by means of flow Doppler imaging. Tissue Doppler imaging could be of great utility in this particular clinical setting thanks to its relative load-independence. Further clinical studies are needed in order to assess the value of tissue Doppler variables in estimating left ventricular filling pressures and to compare them to flow Doppler parameters in HF patients with AF.

References

1. Nishimura RA, Tajik AJ (1994) Quantitative hemodynamics by Doppler echocardiography: a noninvasive alternative to cardiac catheterization. Prog Cardiovasc Dis 36:309–342
2. Grossman W, Barry WH (1980) Diastolic pressure-volume relations in the diseased heart. Fed Proc 39:148–155
3. Levine HJ, Gaasch WH (1978) Diastolic compliance of the left ventricle: chamber and muscle stiffness, the volume/mass ratio and clinical implications. Mod Concepts/Cardiovasc Dis 47:99–102
4. Gaasch WH, Levine HJ, Quinones MA et al (1976) Left ventricular compliance: mechanisms and clinical implications. Am J Cardiol 38:645–653
5. Grossman W, McLaurin LP (1976) Diastolic properties of the left ventricle. Ann Intern Med 84:316–326
6. Mirsky I (1984) Assessment of diastolic function: suggested methods and future considerations. Circulation 69:836–841
7. DeMaria AN, Wisenbaugh T (1987) Identification and treatment of diastolic dysfunction: role of transmitral Doppler recordings. J Am Coll Cardiol 9:1106–1107
8. Labovitz AJ, Pearson AC (1987) Evaluation of left ventricular diastolic function: clinical relevance and recent Doppler echocardiographic insights. Am Heart J 114:836–851
9. Kitabatake A, Inoue M, Asao M et al (1982) Transmitral blood flow reflecting diastolic behaviour of the left ventricle in health and disease – a study by pulsed Doppler technique. Jpn Circ J 46:92–102
10. Appleton CP, Hatle LK, Popp RL (1988) Relation of transmitral flow velocity patterns to left ventricular diastolic function: new insights from a combined hemodynamic and Doppler echocardiographic study. J Am Coll Cardiol 12:426–440
11. Appleton CP, Hatle LK, Popp RL (1988) Demonstration of restrictive ventricular

physiology by Doppler echocardiography. J Am Coll Cardiol 11:757–768

12. Ohno M, Cheng CP, Little WC (1994) Mechanism of altered filling patterns of left ventricular filling during the development of congestive heart failure. Circulation 89:2241–2250

13. Rihal CS, Nishimura RA, Hatle LK et al (1994) Systolic and diastolic dysfunction in patients with clinical diagnosis of dilated cardiomyopathy: relation to symptoms and prognosis. Circulation 90:2772–2779

14. Xie GY, Berk MR, Smith MD et al (1994) Prognostic value of Doppler transmitral flow patterns in patients with congestive heart failure. J Am Coll Cardiol 24:132–139

15. Pozzoli M, Capomolla S, Opasich C et al (1992) Left ventricular filling pattern and pulmonary wedge pressure are closely related in patients with recent anterior myocardial infarction and left ventricular dysfunction. Eur Heart J 13:1067–1073

16. Brunazzi MC, Chirillo F, Pasqualini M et al (1994) Estimation of left ventricular diastolic pressures from precordial pulsed-Doppler analysis of pulmonary venous and mitral flow. Am Heart J 128:293–300

17. Appleton CP, Galloway JM, Gonzales MS et al (1993) Estimation of left ventricular filling pressures using two-dimensional and Doppler echocardiography in adult patients with cardiac diseases. Additional value of analyzing left atrial size, left atrial ejection fraction, and the difference in duration of pulmonary venous and mitral flow velocity at atrial contraction. J Am Coll Cardiol 22:1972–1982

18. Keren G, Sherez J, Megidish R, Levitt B, Laniado S (1985) Pulmonary venous flow pattern: its relationship to cardiac dynamics. Circulation 71:1105–1112

19. Smiseth OA, Thompson CR, Lohavanichbutr K et al (1999) The pulmonary venous systolic flow pulse: its origin and relationship to left atrial pressure. J Am Coll Cardiol 34:802–809

20. Kopecky SI, Gersh BJ, McGoon MD et al (1987) The natural history of lone atrial fibrillation: a population-based study over three decades. New Engl J Med 317:669–674

21. Kannel WB, Abbott RD, Savane DD et al (1982) Epidemiologic features of chronic atrial fibrillation. N Engl J Med 306:1018–1022

22. Traversi E, Corbelli F, Pozzoli M (2001) Doppler echocardiography reliably predicts pulmonary artery wedge pressure in patients with chronic heart failure even when atrial fibrillation is present. Eur J Heart Fail 3:173–181

23. Pozzoli M, Capomolla S, Pinna G et al (1996) Doppler echocardiography reliably predicts pulmonary artery wedge pressure in patients with chronic heart failure with and without mitral regurgitation. J Am Coll Cardiol 27:883–893

24. Temporelli PL, Scapellato F, Corrà U et al (1999) Estimation of pulmonary wedge pressure by transmitral Doppler in patients with chronic heart failure and atrial fibrillation. Am J Cardiol 83:724–727

25. Nagueh SF, Kopelen HA, Quinones MA (1996) Assessment of left ventricular filling pressure by Doppler in the presence of atrial fibrillation. Circulation 94:2138–2145

26. Brun P, Tribouilloy C, Duval AM et al (1992) Left ventricular flow propagation during early filling is related to wall relaxation: a color M-mode Doppler analysis. J Am Coll Cardiol 20:420–432

27. Oyama R, Murata K, Tanaka N et al (2004) Is the ratio of transmitral peak E-wave velocity to color flow propagation velocity useful for evaluating the severity of heart failure in atrial fibrillation? Circ J 68:1132–1138

28. Nagueh SF, Middleton KJ, Kopelen HA et al (1997) Doppler tissue imaging: a noninvasive technique for evaluation of left ventricular relaxation and estimation

of filling pressures. J Am Coll Cardiol 30:1527–1533

29. Ommen S, Nishimura RA, Appleton CP et al (2000) Clinical utility of Doppler echo-cardiography and tissue Doppler imaging in the estimation of left ventricular filling pressures: a comparative simultaneous Doppler-catheterization study. Circulation 102:1788–1794

30. Dokainish H, Zoghbi WA, Lakkis NM et al (2004) Optimal noninvasive assessment of left ventricular filling pressures: a comparison of tissue Doppler echocardiography and B-type natriuretic peptide in patients with pulmonary artery catheters. Circulation 109:2432–2439

Is CRT Useful in Patients with Atrial Fibrillation?

L. Paperini, M. Carluccio, E. Pardini

The Scale of the Problem

Despite improvements in the medical therapy of chronic heart failure (CHF) some patients remain refractory to full medical treatment, with limited therapeutic options and poor prognosis. Cardiac resynchronisation therapy (CRT) by biventricular pacing has recently been demonstrated to represent a valuable therapeutic strategy in improving the clinical course of patients with advanced heart failure and intraventricular conduction delay [1–5].

Atrial fibrillation (AF) is common in patients with CHF and its incidence increases with the severity progression of the syndrome. In all CHF patients, the prevalence of permanent AF is relatively high (approximately 20%) [6], but it may reach 40% in patients with advanced heart failure [7]. From an epidemiological point of view, AF in CHF is a relevant clinical problem. In fact the incidence of both CHF and AF markedly increases in the elderly, so that in the light of the ageing population these two diseases have been called 'the new epidemics' of cardiovascular disease. However, the prognostic significance of AF in the CHF population remains the subject of controversy. While Middelkauf et al. [7] in 1991 reported an increased mortality associated with AF in CHF patients, more recent data [8, 9] did not support the concept that the presence and/or development of AF correlates independently with an adverse outcome during long-term follow-up. The usually observed higher mortality in AF patients seems to be related to factors other than, but related to, AF (i.e. age, left ventricular ejection fraction, NYHA class, and serum urea) and closely linked to haemodynamic control of the syndrome. Therefore the improvement in heart failure therapy might significantly reduce the prognostic impact of this pathological rhythm on CHF patients.

U.O. Cardiologia ed UTIC, Azienda USL 6, Livorno, Italy

Multivariate models may possibly underestimate the true effect of the arrhythmic disturbance. AF, per se, may lead to haemodynamic and pathological changes interacting with heart failure prognosis: loss of atrial contribution, irregular ventricular filling, and inappropriately high ventricular rates (particularly during exercise) [8]. As a consequence, left ventricular ejection fraction (EF), exercise capacity, and peripheral perfusion decrease, worsening signs and symptoms of heart failure and NYHA functional class.

CRT has been shown to improve left ventricular contractile function and symptoms in CHF patients by reversing intraventricular dyssynchrony, optimising ventricular filling, and reducing mitral regurgitation [10]. Most published studies testing biventricular pacing excluded patients with chronic AF, so that few data exist for this subset of patients [1–5]. As approximately 40% of potential candidates for biventricular pacing were in AF, controlled data validating the efficacy of CRT in such patients are required in order to avoid excluding a large part of the CHF population from the benefits of this therapy.

Candidates for CRT Among AF Patients: Open Questions

We will discuss data from the literature in relation to three main subsets of patients with AF and potential indication for CRT:

1. Patients with CHF and primary indication for permanent ventricular pacing owing to spontaneous slow ventricular rate or for atrioventricular (AV) nodal ablation for control of heart rate. In this group, haemodynamic and observational [11–14] studies suggest an additional benefit of biventricular (or left ventricular) over right ventricular pacing.
2. Patients with advanced heart failure, AF, and chronic right ventricular apical pacing. In these patients, upgrading the pacing system to a biventricular one provides cardiac resynchronisation and improves ventricular performance, quality of life, and symptoms of heart failure in the same manner described in patients with sinus rhythm and interventricular conduction delay who undergo biventricular pacing [15].
3. Patients with advanced heart failure and AF candidates for CRT as supplemental non-pharmacological therapy in refractory heart failure. Data in this field are sparse and probably non-conclusive as few randomised studies have been conducted [16–22].

Haemodynamic Studies

Haemodynamic studies investigate the short-term changes in left ventricle (LV) mechanics during different stimulation modalities under controlled conditions. Patients with AF provide an optimal model for examining the isolated effect of biventricular pacing on ventricular performance independently of any AV timing considerations. By eliminating the confounding factor of AV conduction on LV haemodynamics during pacing one may attribute any change during different pacing modes to a 'pure' effect of stimulation on LV function [23].

In a small series, Etienne et al. [11] assessed the acute haemodynamic effect of biventricular pacing in patients with severe heart failure and AF. Patients with congestive heart failure and sinus rhythm served as control group. The 11 patients with AF, compared with 17 patients in sinus rhythm, exhibited comparable acute haemodynamic effects of biventricular pacing in terms of capillary wedge pressure reduction, V wave amplitude reduction, and rise in systolic blood pressure (Fig. 1). These data support the hypothesis that biventricular pacing may be beneficial in patients with severe cardiac failure and intraventricular conduction disease, regardless of whether the patients are in sinus rhythm or in AF.

Similar results were recently reported by Hay et al. [12] in nine patients with heart failure, low EF, chronic AF, and AV nodal block (six patients with AV node ablation). This acute haemodynamic study compared biventricular-based to right univentricular pacing (apex or outflow tracts) at 80 and 120 bpm. Biventricular pacing significantly improved both systolic (dP/dt_{max} 983 ± 102 vs 810 ± 83 mmHg/s, $P < 0.05$) and diastolic ventricular function

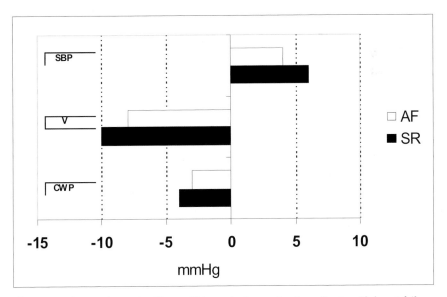

Fig. 1. Acute haemodynamic effects of biventricular pacing in patients with heart failure and atrial fibrillation or sinus rhythm. SBP, systolic blood pressure; V, V wave amplitude; CWP, capillary wedge pressure. (Data from [11])

(isovolumetric relaxation). Similar results were obtained for both methods of heart rate pacing and were not influenced by a right ventricular pacing site.

Another recent acute haemodynamic evaluation was conducted by Simantirakis et al. [13] in 12 patients who had undergone 'ablate and pace' therapy with biventricular pacemaker implantation [24] for drug-refractory AF. With a conductance catheter left ventricular pressure–volume loops were analysed to evaluate LV mechanics during apical right ventricular versus left ventricular pacing (left free wall or biventricular). The results confirm the superiority of left ventricular-based pacing in terms of contractile function and left ventricular filling.

Puggioni et al. [14] tested the hypothesis that left ventricular pacing was superior to right ventricular apical pacing after AV junction ablation. An acute intrapatient echocardiographic evaluation of LV performance parameters (EF and mitral regurgitation) and QRS width demonstrated in 44 patients the superiority of left ventricular pacing compared with right ventricular pacing in improving EF (EF% 43 ± 14.2 vs 40 ± 14.9, $P < 0.002$) and decreasing mitral regurgitation (MR score 1.5 ± 0.7 vs 1.8 ± 0.9, $P < 0.001$) and QRS width (178 ± 36 vs 187 ± 39 ms, $P < 0.04$). A significant finding of this study was that AV ablation appeared acutely to improve EF with both pacing modalities, although left ventricular-based pacing would give an additive favourable haemodynamic effect.

In summary, published data support the hypothesis of an acute superiority of biventricular versus right apical pacing in terms of LV mechanics. Acute haemodynamic data represent the basis for verifying a possible beneficial clinical effect of such therapy in heart failure patients with chronic AF.

Clinical Data

Few data support the hypothesis that re-synchronising a left ventricle dyssynchronised by right pacing may produce a clinical benefit on heart failure patients with AF. Leon et al. [15] evaluated 20 patients with severe heart failure, permanent AF, prior AV nodal ablation, and at least 6 months of right ventricular apical pacing. All patients underwent upgrading of the pacing system from right ventricular only to biventricular. Evaluated after a mean follow-up of 17 months, patients showed a significant reduction of NYHA functional class and number of hospitalisations and a significant improvement of Minnesota Quality of Life scores (Table 1). These results provide evidence that upgrading to biventricular pacing of patients with CHF, AF, and right ventricular apical pacing reverses asynchrony and improves ventricular performance and quality of life.

Although a robust series of haemodynamic preliminary data support a beneficial effect of biventricular pacing on left ventricular performance, few

Table 1. Effect of upgrading to biventricular pacing in patients with heart failure, atrial fibrillation, prior junctional ablation, and right ventricular pacing [15]

	Baseline	Follow-up	*P*
NYHA functional class	3.4 ± 0.5	2.4 ± 0.6	< 0.001
Hospitalisations (number)	1.9 ± 0.8	0.4 ± 0.6	< 0.001
Quality of life (Minnesota score)	78 ± 24	52 ± 23	< 0.01

data are available about the long-term effect of permanent biventricular stimulation in patients with advanced heart failure, AF, and no primary indication for pacing. Moreover, all the haemodynamic data were obtained in patients without severe heart dysfunction.

In a preliminary report by Leclercq et al. [16] chronic biventricular pacing significantly improved exercise tolerance and NYHA functional class after a mean follow-up of 14 ± 9.4 months in 15 patients with advanced CHF and AF. The results in this subset of patients closely resembled those obtained in patients with normal sinus rhythm.

The only randomised trial which tried to assess the clinical efficacy and safety of CRT in patients with chronic AF was the MUSTIC study [17], a single-blind, randomised, controlled, cross-over study enrolling 59 NYHA class III patients with left ventricular systolic dysfunction, chronic AF, slow ventricular rate requiring permanent ventricular pacing (63% after AV nodal ablation), and wide QRS complex (paced width > 200 ms). The primary end-point was the 6-min walked distance, while secondary end-points were peak oxygen uptake, quality of life, hospitalisations, and patients' preferred study period in relation to the different stimulation modes. The intention-to-treat analysis showed no statistically significant difference as to either primary or secondary end-points between conventional right ventricular and biventricular pacing. The statistical power of the study was, however, greatly limited by a high drop-out rate, so that only 37 patients completed the cross-over phases. An important reason for this – probably underestimated when the study was being designed – was the potential deleterious haemodynamic effect of right univentricular pacing during the (6- to 12-week) observation period. In the analysis of the 37 patients in whom therapy was effectively delivered (a pacing percentage > 75% at 24-h Holter ECG recording), a significant improvement of both 6-min walked distance and peak VO$_2$ uptake was revealed during biventricular pacing. The authors therefore concluded that, with all the methodological limitations imposed by the study design, 'effective' biventricular pacing seems to improve exercise tolerance in this group of patients. Long-term analysis of biventricular pacing results in AF MUSTIC patients confirmed positive and stable effects over 12 months of follow-up in terms of quality of life [18] and echocardiographic measurements of left ventricular reverse remodelling [19].

A not yet published study, PAVE, a controlled, randomised study, evaluates biventricular pacing after AV nodal ablation in patients with AF whatever their left ventricular systolic function or NYHA functional class [20]. The primary end-point is exercise capacity as measured by the distance walked during the 6-min walk test. Secondary end-points are functional capacity as measured by peak VO_2 during cardiopulmonary exercise testing and health-related quality of life as measured by SF-36 score. One hundred and two left ventricular and 82 right ventricular randomised paced patients were evaluated for 6 months. In patients with chronic AF treated with AV nodal ablation, biventricular pacing produces a statistically significant improvement in functional capacity over right ventricular pacing as measured by the 6-min walk test, peak VO_2 (Fig. 2) and exercise duration. Most of the benefit results from a progressive improvement of functional capacity in the biventricular group as compared to the right ventricular group. Therefore, the results of the PAVE study suggest that biventricular pacing should be the preferred mode of pacing in patients undergoing AV nodal ablation for control of chronic AF.

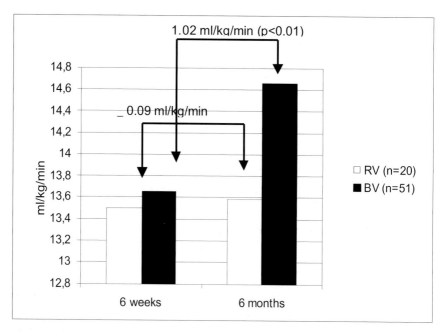

Fig. 2. Data from the PAVE study [20]. There is a significant improvement in peak VO_2 between 6 weeks and 6 months only in patients with a biventricular pacing system

Finally, two recent series reported data about long-term survival of patients with advanced heart failure and AF. The first one [21], in non-ablated patients who underwent biventricular pacing, demonstrated a significantly lower mortality in sinus rhythm patients than in those with AF (33.3% in AF vs 13.4% in SR, follow-up 36 months, $P < 0.05$). By contrast, when studying patients with AF all subjected to AV nodal ablation and biventricular pacing, Gasparini et al. [22] found a reduction of major events in 71 AF patients as compared with the sinus rhythm group (219 patients) after a mean follow-up of 27 ± 13 months (cardiac mortality 5.5%/year in sinus rhythm vs 3.4%/year in AF patients, $P = $ n.s.).

Conclusions

It may be said that CRT has a role in improving functional capacity over conventional right ventricular pacing in patients with left ventricular failure who require permanent ventricular stimulation and/or in those with an indication for AV nodal ablation. As for the great majority of patients with advanced heart failure and AF without conventional indications for permanent cardiac pacing – a wide and progressively expanding population in the 'border zone' of current indications for CRT – no definite data are available. Some promising results from ablated patients show a favourable trend in major cardiac event reduction after CRT. More controlled clinical data are required to achieve definite conclusions about the indications for CRT in heart failure patients with AF.

References

1. Gras D, Mabo P, Tang T et al (1998) Multisite pacing as a supplemental treatment of congestive heart failure: preliminary results of the Medtronic Inc. InSync Study. Pacing Clin Electrophysiol 21:2249–2255
2. Cazeau S, Leclercq C, Lavergne T et al (2001) Effects of multisite biventricular pacing in patients with heart failure and intraventricular conduction delay. N Engl J Med 344:873–880
3. Auricchio A, Stellbrink C, Block M et al (1999) Effect of pacing chamber and atrioventricular delay on acute systolic function of paced patients with congestive heart failure. Circulation 99:2993–3001
4. Abraham WT, Fisher WG, Smith AC et al (2002) Cardiac resynchronization in chronic heart failure. N Engl J Med 346:1845–1853
5. Bristow MR, Saxon LA, Borhmen J (2004) Cardiac resynchronization therapy with or without an implantable defibrillator in advanced heart failure. N Engl J Med 350:2140–2150
6. CIBIS II Investigators and Committees (1999) The Cardiac Insufficiency Bisoprolol Study II (CIBIS II): a randomized trial. Lancet 353:9–13

7. Middelkauf HR, Stevenson WG, Stevenson LW (1991) Prognostic significance of atrial fibrillation in advanced heart failure. A study of 390 patients. Circulation 84:40–48

8. Stevenson WG, Stevenson LW, Middelkauf HR et al (1996) Improving survival for patients with atrial fibrillation and advanced heart failure. J Am Coll Cardiol 28:1458–1463

9. Crijns HJGM, Tjeerdsma G, De Kam PJ et al (2000) Prognostic value of the presence and development of atrial fibrillation in patients with advanced chronic heart failure. Eur Heart J 21:1238–1245

10. Kerwin WF, Botnivick EH, O'Connell JW et al (2000) Ventricular contraction abnormalities in dilated cardiomyopathy: effect of biventricular pacing to correct interventricular dyssynchrony. J Am Coll Cardiol 35:1221–1227

11. Etienne Y, Mansourati J, Gilard M et al (1999) Evaluation of left ventricular based pacing in patients with congestive heart failure and atrial fibrillation. Am J Cardiol 83:1138–1140

12. Hay I, Melenovsky V, Barry J et al (2004) Short term effects of right-left sequential cardiac resynchronization in patients with heart failure, chronic atrial fibrillation and atrioventricular nodal block. Circulation 110:3404–3410

13. Simantirakis EN, Vardakis KE, Kochiadakis GE et al (2004) Left ventricular mechanics during right ventricular apical or left ventricular based pacing in patients with chronic atrial fibrillation after atrioventricular junction ablation. J Am Coll Cardiol 43:1013–1018

14. Puggioni E, Brignole M, Gammage M et al (2004) Acute comparative effect of right and left ventricular pacing in patients with permanent atrial fibrillation. Circulation 43:234–238

15. Leon AR, Greenberg JM, Kanuru N (2002) Cardiac resynchronization in patients with congestive heart failure and chronic atrial fibrillation. J Am Coll Cardiol 39:1258–1263

16. Leclercq C, Victor F, Alonso C et al (2000) Comparative effects of permanent biventricular pacing for refractory heart failure in patients with stable sinus rhythm or chronic atrial fibrillation. Am J Cardiol 85:1154–1156

17. Leclercq C, Walker S, Linde C et al (2002) Comparative effects of permanent biventricular and right univentricular pacing in heart failure patients with chronic atrial fibrillation. Eur Heart J 23:1780–1787

18. Linde C, Braunschweig F, Gadler F et al (2003) Long term improvements in quality of life by biventricular pacing in patients with chronic heart failure: results from the Multisite Stimulation In Cardiomyopathy study (MUSTIC). Am J Cardiol 91:1090–1095

19. Linde C, Leclercq C, Cazeau S et al (2002) Reverse mechanical remodeling by biventricular pacing in congestive heart failure: one-year results from patients in atrial fibrillation in the MUSTIC (Multisite Stimulation In Cardiomyopathy) Study. J Am Coll Cardiol 39:A95–A96

20. Doshi R for PAVE study group (2004) The Left Ventricular-Based Cardiac Stimulation Post AV Nodal Ablation Evaluation Study. Late breaking clinical trials, ACC 8 March, New Orleans, LA

21. Kawabata M, Regoli F, Fantoni C et al (2004) Outcome in patients with advanced heart failure and cardiac resynchronization therapy: a comparison between sinus rhythm and atrial fibrillation. Heart Rhythm 1:S59

22. Gasparini M, Galimberti P, Simonini S et al (2004) Long term results of cardiac resynchronization therapy in patients with permanent atrial fibrillation. Heart Rhythm 1:S59

23. Nishimura RA, Hayes DL, Holmes DR et al (1995) Mechanism of haemodynamic improvement by dual-chamber pacing for severe left ventricular dysfunction: an acute Doppler and catheterization haemodynamic study. J Am Coll Cardiol 25:281–288

24. Brignole M, Menozzi C, Gianfranchi L et al (1998) Assessment of atrio-ventricular junction ablation and VVIR pacemaker versus pharmacological treatment in patients with heart failure and chronic atrial fibrillation: a randomized, controlled study. Circulation 98:953–960

Future New Indications for CRT: Which Patients Might Benefit?

B. Pezzulich, P. Greco Lucchina

Cardiac resynchronisation therapy (CRT) is a non-pharmacological treatment for patients with severe congestive heart failure (CHF) due to systolic dysfunction who also present an intraventricular conduction abnormality and a QRS duration greater than 120 ms [1]. CRT has been shown to improve functional status, quality of life, and exercise tolerance and to decrease hospitalisation frequency in these patients: recent results of the MUSTIC [2] and MIRACLE [3] trials are consistent in showing an improvement in NYHA class, quality of life scores, and distance covered during a 6-min walking test. A decrease in dynamic mitral regurgitation, increase in left ventricular ejection fraction, and reverse remodelling effect on the left ventricle has also been noted. The COMPANION study has recently demonstrated that CRT provides significantly better results regarding a combined endpoint of mortality and heart failure hospitalisation [4].

Consequently, CRT has been included in the current American Heart Association/American College of Cardiology/North American Society of Pacing and Electrophysiology guidelines for the implantation of permanent pacemakers as a therapeutic option for patients with systolic heart failure, NYHA class $\geq$ 3, QRS duration $\geq$ 130 ms, left ventricular end-diastolic diameter $\geq$ 55 mm and ejection fraction < 35% [5]. According to these criteria, between 13% and 35% of patients with heart failure would be eligible for CRT [6, 7]. However, a growing body of evidence seems to suggest that a larger proportion of heart failure patients could benefit of CRT. Some of the 'new' indications for CRT are discussed in this paper.

Cardiology Department San Luigi Gonzaga Hospital, Turin, Italy

CRT in Patients with a Narrow QRS (≤ 130 ms)

Most of the work done in these years in the field of CRT has focused on the deleterious effects of a wide QRS, especially with LBBB morphology, and narrowing of the QRS complex was considered a major target. This approach has several pitfalls, namely it remains unclear whether a classical LBBB morphology is required or not, and what is the 'right' duration of QRS, which in different studies has ranged from 120 to more than 150 ms [2–4]. Moreover it became clear that atrio-left-ventricular pacing, often associated with a widening of QRS duration, can yield comparably positive clinical results. In recent years it has been appreciated that mechanical cardiac dyssynchrony has to be the target of CRT [8], and that the electrical phenomenon of QRS widening is just a marker of this condition [9]. To define ventricular dyssynchrony by the threshold QRS > 150 ms is easy but, while it is true that the larger the QRS, the more likely the dyssynchrony, many patients with mechanical dyssynchrony and narrow QRS can be misdiagnosed and not scheduled for CRT. In a study based on tissue Doppler analysis of regional longitudinal left ventricular function in normal subjects as opposed to patients with CHF and QRS > 140 ms, Faber et al. found that two-thirds of the CHF patients had intra-left-ventricular dyssynchrony with the lateral wall moving last, while in the other one-third the opposite was found. Of note, 12% of these patients had no detectable dyssynchrony, despite a large QRS [10]. Yu et al. found left ventricular systolic mechanical dyssynchrony to be common in patients with a narrow QRS complex, ranging from 51% to 69% [11]. These findings suggest that left ventricular dyssynchrony does not parallel the degree of conduction disturbance, and that different types of mechanical dyssynchrony may have similar ECG patterns.

A more recent study has suggested that, while patients with QRS > 150 ms have an almost immediate benefit, patients with QRS between 120 and 150 ms also showed an improvement in functional class and in exercise performance after 6 months.

Considering the limitations of conventional EKG, echocardiographic parameters are investigated in the ongoing CARE-HF study in which ventricular dyssynchrony is assessed in patients with QRS < 150 ms by considering (1) a prolonged aortic pre-ejection delay (> 140 ms), (2) an increased mechanical interventricular delay (> 40 ms), and (3) a left ventricular segmental post-systolic contraction [12].

It must be remembered that at present it is unclear which of these parameters [involving Tissue Doppler Imaging (TDI), strain, strain rate] provides optimal information on prospective identification of responders to CRT. Furthermore, it is becoming clear that various forms of dyssynchrony can be present, and it is unclear which form contributes most to heart failure.

Moreover, the underlying aetiology of heart failure can be important, as frequently scar tissue shows the latest activity, and it is unknown whether pacing of non-viable tissue results in clinical improvement.

CRT in Right Bundle Branch Block

The most frequent intraventricular conduction delay in heart failure patients is left bundle branch block; little is known about right bundle branch block. In 12 patients studied by Garrigue et al. with NYHA class II–III disease, ejection fraction 24%, and right bundle branch block (QRS average 189 ms) biventricular pacing resulted in a sustained increase in aortic time velocity integral, a significant decrease in mitral regurgitation, and a significant decrease in left ventricular end-diastolic diameter after 1 year [13]. In our experience five patients with dilated cardiomyopathy, NYHA class III, right bundle branch block, mean QRS duration 160 ms, showed sustained and significant improvement in functional class and in exercise capacity in cardiopulmonary testing. All of them at baseline showed significant ventricular dyssynchrony at TDI.

It may be speculated that biventricular pacing may be useful in patients with heart failure, right bundle branch block, and ventricular dyssynchrony, but this issue remains unproven.

CRT in Conventional Pacemaker Therapy

Right ventricular apical pacing may result in significant haemodynamic deterioration. An adverse effect of long-term ventricular pacing has been documented in patients with normal systolic and diastolic left ventricular function before pacemaker implantation [14]. In the Mode Selection Trial, which studied 1339 patients, percentages for normal ejection fraction, NYHA class I or II disease, baseline QRS duration < 120 ms, and hospitalisation for heart failure paralleled the percentage of right ventricular pacing. Patients paced in DDD less than 10% of the time had a 2% incidence of hospitalisation for heart failure, while patients paced for more than 90% of the time had a 12% incidence of hospitalisation. For patients paced with VVIR mode, hospitalisations for heart failure increased from 7% (for < 10% pacing) to 16% (for > 90% pacing) [15].

In the DAVID ICD trial, pacing in DDD-R mode with lower rate 70 bpm increased the relative risk of death or heart failure hospitalisation by 1.6 [16]. In terms of quality of life and exercise capacity, the PAVE study has recently shown biventricular pacing to be superior to conventional pacing after atrioventricular nodal ablation for atrial fibrillation.

Thus, for patients requiring conventional pacing, it may be speculated that right septal pacing or biventricular pacing may result in a lower incidence of heart failure during long-term follow-up. The BIOPACE study is addressing this issue in a randomised multicentre study [17].

It must be remembered that all trials were performed using lower rate 40 bpm or VDD mode, and whether atrial-biventricular pacing is equally effective remains unproven.

Prophylactic Effect of CRT in LBBB

Intraventricular conduction delay has been identified as a major negative prognostic indicator in patients with heart failure. In more than 5500 patients from the Italian Network of Congestive Heart Failure, mortality and hospitalisation due to heart failure after 1 year in patients with LBBB was 1.5-fold that in patients with a narrow QRS complex [18].

Acting through several mechanisms, including redistribution of regional ventricular loading, reduction or abolition of mitral regurgitation, reduction of sympathetic activity, increase of parasympathetic activity, and others, CRT also induces reverse remodelling of the failing left ventricle. Hence, the left ventricle gets smaller and contractility is improved after a period of CRT. Moreover, functional mitral regurgitation is reduced acutely and chronically during CRT. The effects of CRT on reverse ventricular remodelling have been consistently demonstrated in all randomised prospective controlled studies and in smaller mechanistic studies [19].

Recent data from Multicenter InSync Randomised Clinical Evaluation (MIRACLE) study have shown that reverse remodelling during CRT can also take place in patients not receiving beta-blocking agents. This effect of reverse remodelling, which has been demonstrated in all major cohorts, may be partly due to a decrease in mitral regurgitation and improved myocardial energetics as shown in acute and in chronically paced patients [20].

Moreover, recent data from the COMPANION study showed that patients assigned to optimal medical therapy had progressive reduction of systolic blood pressure, consistent with progression of the underlying disease, whereas patients assigned to CRT did not [21].

Reversing the natural course of the disease is an exciting promise, but a word of caution is necessary. Inadequate patient selection, lead selection, or device programming may impair survival or quality of life. Long follow-up periods are required to prove the hypothesis that early CRT influences disease progression and improves long-term survival.

References

1. Hlatky MA, Massie BM (2004) Cardiac resynchronization for heart failure. Ann Intern Med 141:409–410
2. Linde C, Leclercq C, Rex S et al (2002) Long-term benefits of biventricular pacing in congestive heart failure: results from the Multisite STimulation In Cardiomyopathy (MUSTIC) Study. J Am Coll Cardiol 40:111–118
3. Abraham WT, Fisher WG, Smith AL et al (2002). Cardiac resynchronization in chronic heart failure. N Engl J Med 346:1845–1853
4. Bristow MR, Saxon LA, Boehmer J et al (2004) Cardiac resynchronization therapy with or without an implantable defibrillator in advanced chronic heart failure. N Engl J Med 350:2140–2150
5. A Report of the American College of Cardiology/American Heart Association Task Force on Practice Guidelines (ACC/AHA/NASPE Committee on Pacemaker Implantation). ACC/AHA/NASPE 2002 guideline update for implantation of cardiac pacemakers and antiarrhythmia devices. American College of Cardiology website. Accessed October 12, 2002
6. Vardas PE, Simantirakis EN (2003) Resynchronization Therapy: Implications for Pacemaker Implantation in Europe. CEPR 7:27–29
7. Achilli A, Sassara M, Ficili S (2003) Long-term effectiveness of cardiac resynchronization therapy in patients with refractory heart failure and "narrow" QRS. J Am Coll Cardiol 42:2117–2124
8. Ghio S, Constantin C, Klersy C et al (2004) Interventricular and intraventricular dyssynchrony are common in heart failure patients, regardless of QRS duration. Eur Heart J 25:571–578
9. Yu CM, Lin H, Zhang Q et al (2003) High prevalence of left ventricular systolic and diastolic asynchrony in patients with congestive heart failure and normal QRS duration. Heart 89:54–60
10. Lamp B, Vogt J, Faber L et al (2004) Extended indications for cardiac resynchronization therapy? Eur Heart J 6(Suppl D): D128- D131
11. Yu CM, Lin H, Zhang Q et al (2003) High prevalence of left ventricular systolic and diastolic asynchrony in patients with congestive heart failure and normal QRS duration. Heart 89:54–60
12. Cleland JGF, Daubert JC, Erdmann E et al (2001) The CARE-HF study (CArdiac REsynchronisation in Heart Failure study): rationale, design and end-points. Eur J Heart Fail 3:481–489
13. Garrigue S, Reuter S, Labeque JN et al (2001) Usefulness of biventricular pacing in patients with congestive heart failure and right bundle branch block. Am J Cardiol 88:1436–1441
14. Askenazi J, Alexander JH, Koenigsberg DI et al (1984) Alteration of left ventricular performance by left bundle block simulated with atrioventricular sequential pacing. Am J Cardiol 53:99–104
15. Sweeney MO, Hellkamp AS, Ellenbogen KA et al (2003) Adverse effect of ventricular pacing on heart failure and atrial fibrillation among patients with normal QRS duration in a clinical trial of pacemaker therapy for sinus node dysfunction. Circulation 107:2932–2937
16. The DAVID trial investigators (2002) Dual chamber pacing or ventricular backup pacing in patient with an implantable defibrillator. The Dual Chamber and VVI Implantable Defibrillator (DAVID) trial. JAMA 288:3115-23

17. Funck RC, Mueller HH, Schade-Brittinger C et al (2003) Rationale, design and end points of a clinical study on biventricular pacing for atrioventricular block in left ventricular dysfunction to prevent cardiac desynchronization—the BIOPACE study. Europace, Suppl B, P-167 (B106)

18. Baldessaroni S, De Biase L, Fresco C et al (2002) Cumulative effect of complete left bundle-branch block and chronic atrial fibrillation on 1-year mortality and hospitalization in patients with congestive heart failure. A report from the Italian network on congestive heart failure. Eur Heart J 23:1692–1698

19. Nelson GS, Berger RD, Fetics BJ et al (2000) Left ventricular or biventricular pacing improves cardiac function at diminished energy cost in patients with dilated cardiomyopathy and left bundle branch block. Circulation 102:3053–3059

20. Young B, Abraham WT (2003) Cardiac resynchronization limits disease progression in patients with mild heart failure and an indication for ICD—results of a randomized study. Circulation 108:IV-629

21. Bristow MR, Feldman AM, Saxon LA et al (2003) Cardiac resynchronization therapy (CRT) reduces hospitalizations, and CRT with implantable defibrillator (CRT-D) reduces mortality in chronic heart failure: the COMPANION trial. Available at http://www.uchsc.edu/cvi/HFSA%20V3%20Late%20Breakerpresented%209.24.03.pdf. Accessed January 10

Economic Benefits of Cardiac Resynchronisation Therapy

K. Seidl

Introduction

Heart failure is a common condition with an estimated overall prevalence of 1–2%. Prevalence increases by age, with a marked rise above the age of 60 years [1, 2]. The progress in the pharmacological treatment of heart failure has been substantial [3, 4], but 1-year mortality is still around 10–14% [5, 6]. Healthcare expenditures for heart failure are significant, accounting for nearly 2% of the healthcare budget, 65–75% of which relates to hospital care [7, 8].

Patients with severe heart failure refractory to drug treatment can be offered heart transplantation or a cardiac assist device as a bridge to transplantation. Such treatment, however, is available for only a limited number of patients, so there is a clear need for additional treatment options.

It is estimated that 30% of patients with severe heart failure have intraventricular conduction disturbances characterised by wide QRS complexes and an uncoordinated ventricular contraction pattern [9, 10]. The delay in ventricular electrical activation may be overcome by biventricular pacing. A large number of uncontrolled and controlled randomised studies dealing with cardiac resynchronisation therapy (CRT) demonstrate improvements in central haemodynamics, exercise tolerance, and quality of life in patients with severe heart failure and wide QRS complexes [11–13].

The aim of the present study was to assess (1) the clinical effectiveness of a conventional individual optimised drug therapy for heart failure in comparison to the combination of drug treatment plus biventricular pacing, and (2) to evaluate its cost-effectiveness in respect of hospitalisations and outpatient visits.

Herzzentrum Ludwigshafen, Ludwigshafen, Germany

Methods

Between January 1995 and December 2002, 1118 consecutive patients with heart failure were included in a left ventricular dysfunction registry. The inclusion criterion was an ejection fraction below 45%. Mean age was 65 ± 11 years, 78% of patients were male, and the mean ejection fraction was 29 ± 8%. The aetiology of left ventricular dysfunction was coronary artery disease in 65%, non-ischaemic cardiomyopathy in 31%, and hypertensive heart disease in 4%. In this study population of 1118 patients, 97 patients received a CRT device because of severe heart failure which was refractory to optimised drug treatment (Table 1).

Table 1. Clinical data of patients included in the left ventricular dysfunction registry

	LVD patients ($n = 1021$)	CRT patients ($n = 97$)
Age (mean ± SD, years)	65 ± 9	65 ± 8
Male gender (%)	78	87
Coronary artery disease (%)	66	39
Non-ischaemic cardiomyopathy (%)	29	61
Diabetes mellitus (%)	28	22
Arterial hypertension (%)	59	43

LVD, left ventricular dysfunction; CRT, cardiac resynchronisation therapy

Within this study population we performed a matched controlled study for inter-individual comparison between similar patient groups in respect of clinical and economic data. Patients were matched for age, ejection fraction, NYHA functional class, and follow-up duration of 18 months. Overall 42 patients were enrolled in this comparison study: 14 patients in the control group versus 14 patients in the CRT pacemaker versus 14 patients in the CRT implantable cardioverter–defibrillator (ICD) arm. In this inter-individual comparison, cost-effectiveness was evaluated on the basis of the following data: symptoms, number of hospital stays, number of hospital days, and number of outpatient visits during a 12-month follow-up.

In addition, an intra-individual comparison was performed. For this purpose the clinical and economic data regarding these patients were collected for the entire year preceding the implantation and the year after implantation of a CRT device.

Results

Data for the patients of these three groups are shown in Tables 2 and 3. There was no significant difference in regard to age, gender, structural heart disease, diabetes, hypertension, ejection fraction, and NYHA functional class. However, there was a significant difference in QRS duration. Patients in the control arm had a mean QRS duration of about 107 ± 20 ms, patients in the CRT pacemaker arm had a mean QRS duration of 160 ± 23 ms, and patients in the CRT ICD arm had a mean QRS duration of 153 ± 40 ms.

During the 12-month period 71% of the patients in the control arm were in NYHA functional class III, 7% in NYHA class IV, and only 21% in NYHA class II. In contrast, during the same follow-up period 71% of the patients with the pacemaker were in NYHA class II, 21% remained in NYHA class III, and only 7% were in NYHA class IV. Similar results were obtained in the patients with the ICD: 79% of these patients were in NYHA class II, 14% in NYHA class III, and 7% in NYHA class IV (Fig. 1) during follow-up.

Table 2. Clinical data of patients in the inter-individual and intra-individual comparison groups

	Control (n = 14)	CRT pacemaker (n = 14)	CRT ICD (n = 14)	P value
Age (mean ± SD, years)	66 ± 7	67 ± 5	67 ± 5	0.61
Male gender (n)	14	14	14	1
Coronary artery disease (n)	8	6	6	0.68
Non-ischaemic CMP (n)	6	8	8	0.28
Diabetes mellitus (n)	1	2	1	0.76
Arterial hypertension (n)	4	5	6	0.73
Ejection fraction (%)	24 ± 6	25 ± 6	24 ± 6	0.89
QRS duration (mean ± SD, ms)	107 ± 22	160 ± 23	153 ± 40	0.009
NYHA class II (n, %)	4, 29	1, 7	2, 14	0.63
NYHA class III (n, %)	9, 64	11, 79	10, 71	
NYHA class IV (n, %)	1, 7	2, 14	1, 14	

Table 3. Drug treatments in the inter-individual and intra-individual comparison groups

	Control (%)	CRT pacemaker (%)	CRT ICD (%)	P value
Beta-blocker	67	67	71	0.67
ACE inhibitor	86	86	93	0.45
Diuretic	83	100	93	0.32
Digitalis	79	86	86	0.84

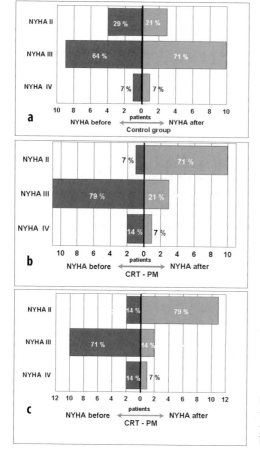

Fig. 1a–c. NYHA functional class in the control group (**a**) and in the pacemaker (**b**) and ICD groups (**c**) before and after implantation

Inter-individual Comparison

During a follow-up of 12 months patients in the control group had 2.3 ± 1.8 hospital stays, versus 1.5 ± 1.9 hospital stays in the patient population with the ICD device and only 0.6 ± 0.9 hospital stays in the patient population with the pacemaker. These differences were significant (Fig. 2). In respect of the mean number of hospital days during the 12-month follow-up, patients in the control group had 24 ± 22 days in hospital; patients in the CRT/ICD arm had 16 ± 22 days in hospital versus only 12 ± 19 days for the patients in the CRT pacemaker arm (Fig. 3).

No differences were noted in the number of outpatients visits (Fig. 4).

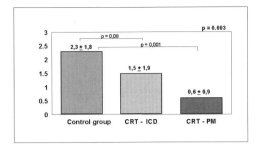

Fig. 2. Mean number (± SD) of hospital stays per patient in the three groups during 12-month follow-up

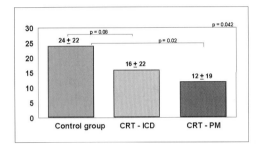

Fig. 3. Mean number (± SD) of days in hospital per patient in the three groups during 12-month follow-up

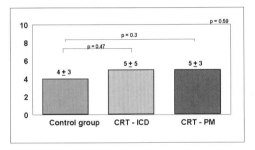

Fig. 4. Mean number (± SD) of outpatients visits per patient in the three groups during 12-month follow-up

Intra-individual Comparison

The mean number of hospital stays in CRT pacemaker patients was reduced from 2.4 ± 1.7 stays before pacemaker implantation to 0.6 ± 0.9 hospital stays after implantation (Fig. 5). Similar results were obtained in patients with the ICD (Fig. 6): during the year before implantation the mean number of hospital stays was 2.9 ± 1.1, after CRT implantation 1.5 ± 1.9.

The mean number of hospital days was reduced in the year after CRT device implantation in comparison to the year preceding the implantation: in the pacemaker group from 23 ± 18 to 12 ± 19 days, in the ICD group from 42 ± 22 to 16 ± 22 days (Figs. 7, 8).

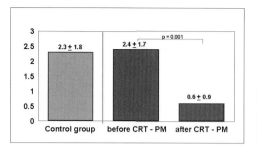

Fig. 5. Mean number (± SD) of hospital stays per patient in the control group and in the pacemaker group before and after implantation

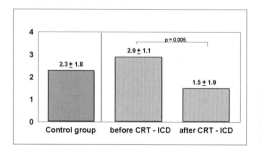

Fig. 6. Mean number (± SD) of hospital stays per patient in the control group and in the ICD group before and after implantation

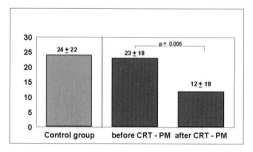

Fig. 7. Mean number (± SD) of days in hospital per patient in the control group and in the pacemaker group before and after implantation

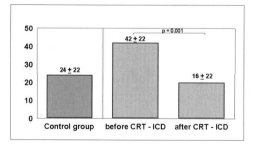

Fig. 8. Mean number (± SD) of days in hospital per patient in the control group and in the ICD group before and after implantation

The mean number of hospital stays and the mean number of hospital days during the year before CRT device implantation were similar and were in the same range as in the control group (2.3 ± 1.8 stays) (Figs. 5–8).

No differences were observed regarding outpatient visits in this study population (Figs. 9, 10). The important change after CRT implantation was the highly significant reduction in hospital stays and hospital days, which explained the cost reduction after CRT device implantation in this study.

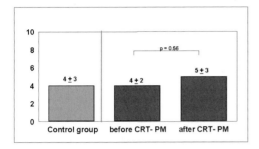

Fig. 9. Mean number (± SD) of outpatients visits per patient in the control group and in the pacemaker group before and after implantation

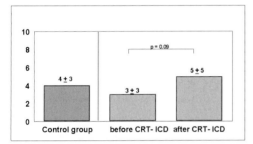

Fig. 10. Mean number (± SD) of outpatients visits per patient in the control group and in the ICD group before and after implantation

Discussion

This study demonstrates a reduction in the need for hospitalisation and hospital days in parallel to clinical improvements by CRT in selected patients with severe heart failure. Similar findings were obtained by Braunschweig et al., which showed that the need for hospital care decreased significantly after biventricular pacing [14]. The total number of hospital days for all patients was 253 days in the year before versus 45 days in the year after biventricular pacing. For heart-failure-related hospital days the respective figures were 183 and 39 days. Biventricular pacing led to improvement in 13 of 16 patients with severe heart failure and wide QRS complexes in this open study. The improvement resulted in reduced need for hospital care.

In 2004, Dixon et al. demonstrated that CRT results in a significant improvement in clinical parameters and considerable reductions in hospital admissions and costs in patients with chronic heart failure [15].

In heart failure management it is essential to bring down the costs relating to hospital care. Recent studies indicate that a comprehensive heart failure care programme can reduce the need for hospital care [16]. In the present study all patients were recruited from a left ventricular dysfunction registry with continued follow-up who still required a substantial amount of hospital care. We therefore believe that biventricular pacing rather than frequent follow-up was a reason for the improvement observed. Pacemaker therapy is not an inexpensive treatment and incurs costs for equipment, implantation procedure, and follow-up. The small number of patients does not justify more extensive cost–benefit analysis.

It is important to remember that it is hard to prove the cost-effectiveness of a novel treatment before it has been properly developed. For this reason, the pacemaker-related costs in the study were justifiable in view of the ongoing development and assessment of this treatment. In the future, the costs of biventricular pacing may be reduced as left ventricular lead technology is simplified and the patient selection improves. Nevertheless, these findings do indicate that CRT might reduce the costs for hospital care in selected patients with severe heart failure, at least over the first year. This treatment can therefore serve as a bridge to heart transplantation in those eligible, and improve the well-being and reduce the hospital care costs of these severely incapacitated patients [16].

The interpretation of our results is limited by the fact that the study was uncontrolled and enrolled only a small number of patients. Larger controlled studies are underway and will add valuable information to the issues discussed above.

In this uncontrolled study, biventricular device therapy improved NYHA functional class and the clinical improvement was accompanied by a significantly reduced need for hospital care.

References

1. Kannel WB, Ho K, Thom T (1994) Changing epidemiological features of cardiac failure. Br Heart J 72 (Suppl 2):S3–S9
2. Eriksson H, Svardsudd K, Larsson B et al (1989) Risk factors for heart failure in the general population: the study of men born in 1913. Eur Heart J 10:647–656
3. The SOLVD Investigators (1991) Effect of enalapril on survival in patients with reduced left ventricular ejection fractions and congestive heart failure. N Engl J Med 325:293–302
4. CONSENSUS trial study group (1987) Effects of enalapril on mortality in severe congestive heart failure. Results of the Cooperative North Scandinavian Enalapril Survival Study. N Engl J Med 316:1429–1434
5. MERIT-HF study group (1999) Effect of metoprolol CR/XL in chronic heart failure: Metoprolol CR/XL randomized intervention trial in congestive heart failure

(MERIT-HF). Lancet 353:2001–2007

6. Packer M, Carver JR, Rodeheffer RJ et al (1991) Effect of oral milrinone on mortality in severe chronic heart failure. The PROMISE Study Research Group. N Engl J Med 325:1468–1475

7. Rydén-Bergsten T, Andersson F (1999) The health care costs of heart failure in Sweden. J Intern Med 246:275–284

8. McMurray JHW, Rhodes G (1993) An evaluation of the cost of heart failure to the National Health Service in the UK. Br J Med Econ 6:99–100

9. Goldman S, Johnson G, Cohn JN et al (1993) Mechanism of death in heart failure. The Vasodilator-Heart Failure Trials. The V-HeFT VA Cooperative Studies Group. Circulation 87(Suppl 6):I24–I31

10. Xiao HB, Roy C, Gibson DG (1994) Nature of ventricular activation in patients with dilated cardiomyopathy: evidence for bilateral bundle branch block. Br Heart J 72:167–174

11. Cazeau S, Leclercq C, Lavergne T et al (2001) Effects of multisite biventricular pacing in patients with heart failure and intraventricular conduction delay. N Engl J Med 344:873–880

12. Abraham WT, Fisher WG, Smith AL et al for the Miracle Study Group (2002) Cardiac resynchronisation in chronic heart failure. N Engl J Med 346:1845–1853

13. Bristow MR, Saxon LA, Boehmer J et al (2004) Cardiac resynchronisation therapy with or without an implantable defibrillator in advanced chronic heart failure. N Engl J Med 350:2140–2150

14. Braunschweig F, Linde C, Gadler F et al (2000) Reduction of hospital days by biventricular pacing. Eur J Heart Fail 2:399–406

15. Dixon LJ, Murtagh GJ, Rechardson SG et al (2004) Reduction in hospitalisation rates following cardiac resynchronisation therapy in cardiac failure: experience from a single center. Europace 6:586–589

16. Cline CM, Israelsson BY, Willenheimer RB et al (1998) Cost effective management programme for heart failure reduces hospitalization. Heart 80:442–446

Cost-Effectiveness of Cardiac Resynchronisation Therapy in Heart Failure Patients

G. Mascioli, A. Curnis, L. Bontempi, T. Bordonali, L. Dei Cas

The rapidly growing incidence of heart failure (HF) is going to have an extremely large impact on costs for the management of decompensated patients. It has been calculated [1] that within the next 20 years, the prevalence of HF in Western countries will double, rising from 5.3 millions of persons suffering from this syndrome to 10.6 millions. Data furnished by the Italian Ministry of Health for the year 2000 showed that DRG 127 (cardiac failure and shock) already account for 13.5% of the total number of hospital admissions, with a mean of 9.6 hospital days: this means that – in Italy – 2.5% of the total number of hospital stays are due to HF [2]. If we consider that the course of HF is worse than that of lung cancer [3] in terms of frequent hospital re-admissions, and that hospitalisation represents the major component of the total expenditure on management of HF, it is easy to see that the economics of caring for these patients is set to grow exponentially.

What is cost-effectiveness? When a new therapy is introduced into treatment, four things can happen
- The new therapy is more effective than previous treatment, but at a major cost, or
- It is less effective and more expensive, or
- It is less effective but also less expensive, or, finally (and this is what we call cost-effective)
- It is more effective and less expensive

Many trials have now demonstrated that CRT is an effective tool for treating patients with episodes of acute HF refractory to optimised medical therapy. The results derived from PATH-CHF, MUSTIC, MIRACLE, and COMPANION [4–7] are all concordant and demonstrate not only that CRT can

Department and Chair of Cardiology, Spedali Civili and University of Brescia, Italy improve quality of life, but also that it affects instrumental and objective parameters, such as distance walked in the 6-min walking test, peak oxygen consumption during the effort test, ejection fraction as measured by echocardiography, etc. (Tables 1, 2).

Not only 'soft' end-points are improved: CRT also demonstrated a significant impact in relation to survival. In the COMPANION trial [7] the reduction in mortality almost reached statistical significance in the CRT-only group and was statistically significant in the CRT-D group (D=defibrillator). Even if the study was not designed to demonstrate this particular end-point, nevertheless the key message that can be obtained from the study is extremely important.

Table 1. Effect of CRT on quality of life (QoL) and functional capacity

Study	QoL Score	NYHA Class
French Pilot [8] ($n = 50$)		+
InSync Europe [9] ($n = 103$)	+	+
InSync ICD [10] ($n = 84$)	+	+
MIRACLE [6] ($n = 453$)	+	+
MIRACLE ICD [11] ($n = 247$)	+	+
MUSTIC [5] ($n = 67$)	+	+
PATH-CHF [4] ($n = 41$)	+	+
CONTAK CD [12] ($n = 203$)	+	+

+, improved; NYHA, New York Heart Association

Table 2. Effects of CRT on heart efficiency and disease progression

Study	LVEF	MR	LVEDV/LVESV	LV Filling time
Queen Mary Hospital [13]	+	-	-	+
MIRACLE [6]	+	-	-	+
MUSTIC [5]		-		+
MIRACLE ICD [11]	=	=	-	+

LVEF, left ventricular ejection fraction; MR, mitral regurgitation; LVEDV, left ventricular end-diastolic volume; LVESV, left ventricular end-systolic volume; +, increased; –, decreased; =, unchanged

The CARE-HF [14] study will address this issue, investigating whether CRT-P (without defibrillation back-up) could reduce mortality in patients with severe HF in comparison with optimised medical therapy.

In terms of the economical point of view, only two studies have specifically addressed this topic, but other trials have investigated reduction in hospital care after implantation of CRT devices (Table 3). This latter effect of CRT can be considered as a surrogate end-point of cost-effectiveness, considering – as has already been mentioned – that hospital care constitutes the main component of expenditure in HF management.

In the study by Braunschweig et al. [15], 16 patients in whom a biventricular device was implanted showed, in the 40 days after CRT, a significant reduction (82%) in HF-related hospitalisation and a 79% reduction in hospitalisation for all causes. Similar results were obtained in our study [16], in which 30 patients with a biventricular device implanted were followed in the year before and the year after implantation. At the end of follow-up, there was a 93% reduction in total hospital admissions and a 28% increase in outpatient visits: this translated into a 76% reduction of total hospital care. In the year before implantation, the expenditure was €12 784 per patient, compared with € 9663 per patient (device cost included) in the year after device implantation, so that economical breakeven was obtained only 1 year after implantation.

In the subanalysis of the MUSTIC study [11] there was a seven-fold decrease in monthly hospitalisations (0.14/month during the pacemaker-off period vs. 0.02/month in the pacemaker-on period). In the MIRACLE study [6], the reduction of event-free survival rate in the CRT group was 50% (absolute increase –11%), even if there was a 8.8% rate of device-related hospitalisations. In the same study, there was a 77% reduction in the number of total days of hospitalisation for worsening HF and a 59% reduction in days of hospitalisation due to all causes.

Table 3. Effects of CRT on hospitalisations

Study	Admissions	Stay	Hospital days due to HF
Karolinska Hospital, Sweden [15] ($n = 16$)	–	–	–79%
Belfast, Northern Ireland [18] ($n = 22$)	–	–	–96%
BRESCIA, Italy [16] ($n = 30$)	–	–	–93% (all causes)
MIRACLE [6] ($n = 453$)	–	–	–77%
MUSTIC [5] ($n = 67$)	–	–	–86%
PATH-CHF [4] ($n = 41$)	–	–	–77%

–, decreased

A preliminary analysis of 40 patients with at least 3 years of follow-up who underwent implantation in our centre seems to demonstrate that the positive cost-efficacy ratio is also maintained over the long term.

In conclusion, physicians who deal daily with HF patients now have a new 'more-than-promising' weapon in the struggle against this epidemic.

CRT seems to induce – at least in carefully selected patients – reverse remodelling [12] of the dilated heart, regardless the aetiology of dilation. It is extremely hard to calculate 'costs' in a health service like the Italian one, due to the fact that our system is funded and not reimbursed, so that speaking of DRG values is not directly related to costs. Nevertheless, many studies, and our study too (derived from an Italian experience), have demonstrated that a significant reduction in hospital care can be derived from biventricular pacing, and, however costs are calculated, a reduction in hospitalisations *does* equate to a reduction of costs.

It will be difficult to calculate the cost per year of life saved, but there is already a great deal of evidence that CRT can be considered a cost-effective procedure.

References

1. New Medicine Reports. 1999 Heart and Stroke Statistical Update. AHA
2. Ministero della Salute. Rapporto sulle schede di dimissione ospedaliera (SDO) 2000. Ministry of Health, Rome, Italy. www.ministerodellasalute.it
3. Stewart S, MacIntyre K, Hole DJ et al (2001) More 'malignant' than cancer? Five-year survival following a first admission for heart failure. Eur J Heart Fail 3:315–322
4. Auricchio A, Stellbrink C, Sack S et al (2002) Long-term clinical effects of haemodynamically optimised cardiac resynchronisation therapy in patients with heart failure and ventricular conduction delay. J Am Coll Cardiol 39:2026–2033
5. Cazeau S, Leclercq C, Lavergne T et al (2001) Effects of multisite biventricular pacing in patients with heart failure and intraventricular conduction delay. N Engl J Med 344:873–880
6. Abraham WT, Fisher WG, Smith AL et al (2002) Cardiac resynchronization therapy in chronic heart failure. N Engl J Med 346:1845–1853
7. Bristow MR, Saxon LA, Boehmer J et al (2004) Cardiac-resynchronization therapy with or without an implantable defibrillator in advanced chronic heart failure. N Engl J Med 350 :2140–2150
8. Leclercq C, Cazeau S, Ritter P et al (2000) A pilot experience with permanent biventricular pacing to treat advanced heart failure. Am Heart J 140:862–870
9. Gras D, Leclercq C, Teng AS et al (2002) Cardiac resynchronization therapy in advanced heart failure: the multicentre InSync clinical study. Eur J Heart Fail 4:311–320
10. Kuhlkamp V (2002) Initial experience with an implantable cardioverter–defibrillator incorporating cardiac resynchronization therapy. J Am Coll Cardiol 39:790–797
11. Abraham WT, Young JB, Leon AR et al (2004) Effects of cardiac resynchronization

therapy on disease progression in patients with left ventricular systolic dysfunction, an indication for an implantable cardioverter-defibrillator, on mildly symptomatic chronic heart failure. Circulation 110:2864–2868

12. Thackray S, Colette A, Jones P et al (2001) Clinical trials update: highlights of the Scientific Sessions of Heart Failure, a meeting of the Working Group on Heart Failure of the European Society of Cardiology. CONTAK-CD, CHRISTMAS, OPTI-ME-CHF. Eur J Heart Fail 3:491–494

13. Yu CM, Chau E, Sanderson JE et al (2002) Tissue Doppler echocardiographic evidence of reverse remodeling and improved synchronicity by simultaneously delaying regional contraction after biventricular pacing therapy in heart failure. Circulation 105:438–445

14. Cleland JG, Daubert JC, Erdmann E et al (2001) The CARE-HF study (CArdiac REsynchronization in Heart Failure study): rationale, design and end-points. Eur J Heart Fail 3:481–489

15. Braunschweig F, Linde C, Gadler F et al (2000) Reduction of hospital days by biventricular pacing. Eur J Heart Fail 2:399–406

16. Curnis A, Caprari F, Mascioli G et al (2003) Economic evaluation of cardiac resynchronization in patients with moderate-to-severe heart failure. PharmacoEconomics-Italian Research Articles 5:1–22

17. Linde C, Leclerq C, Rex S et al (2002) Long-term benefits of biventricular pacing in congestive heart failure: results from the MUltisite STimulation In Cardiomyopathy (MUSTIC) Study. J Am Coll Cardiol 40:111–118

18. Dixon LJ, Thompson G, Harbinson M et al (2002) Cardiac resynchronization therapy – a cost effective treatment for cardiac failure. Eur Heart J 23 (Suppl. August): abstract 3

MANAGING SUDDEN DEATH:
THE SELECTION OF PATIENTS, DRUGS AND DEVICES

Guidelines for the Prevention of Sudden Cardiac Death: Filling the Gap

A. Baranchuk, C. Morillo

Introduction

Sudden cardiac death (SCD) remains a major public health challenge in both North America and Europe. Identifying high-risk patients is of paramount importance in order to correctly select the population that derives the greatest benefit from ICD implantation. Unfortunately, risk markers developed to date are not universally applied and have low sensitivity and predictive values, limiting their use. Financial restraints on health care systems vary widely among different countries, adding complexity to global recommendations.

Cardiovascular disease is responsible for 40 000 deaths annually in Canada, and SCD related to ventricular tachyarrhythmias causes 50% of this mortality [1]. In the United States the annual figures for SCD range between 300 000 and 450 000 [2]. In addition, around 5 000 000 people live with chronic heart failure, with 550 000 new cases added every year. Almost 10% will die annually of either progressive pump failure or SCD [3]. The global incidence of SCD is difficult to estimate in Europe, but the Maastricht study showed an annual incidence of out-of-hospital SCD of 1 in 1000 inhabitants, which is similar to that reported in North America [4].

Several guidelines and recommendations have been published by most of the leading cardiovascular societies [5]. However, it is important to recognise that SCD is a moving target, and in the past 3 years important clinical trials not included in current guidelines have been reported. A thorough review of SCD guidelines is out of the scope of this review. This chapter will focus on the most recently published and presented trials and will place this new information in the framework of current SCD guidelines.

Department of Medicine, Arrhythmia Service, McMaster University, Hamilton Health Sciences Corporation, Hamilton, Ontario, Canada

Indications for ICD for Primary Prevention

Several studies have assessed the effectiveness of implantable cardioverter–defibrillators (ICDs) for the prevention of SCD in high-risk populations. These studies may be classified according to the underlying anatomical substrate:

1. Coronary artery disease + left ventricular ejection fraction (LVEF) < 30–35%: MADIT I, MADIT II, MUSTT, DINAMIT [6–9]
2. Non-ischaemic dilated cardiomyopathy + depressed LVEF: CAT, AMIOVIRT, DEFINITE [10–12]
3. LVEF ≤ 35% + NYHA class II/III regardless of the aetiology of the cardiomyopathy SCD-HeFT [13, 14]

Overall a 39% relative risk reduction in all-cause mortality [31% in non ischaemic dilated cordiomyopathy (NICM)] is achieved in the setting of primary prevention of SCD [15, 16] Current guidelines should be updated as follows:

1. *Class I:* Ischaemic heart disease with or without mild to moderate heart failure symptoms and LVEF ≤ 30%, measured at least 1 month after myocardial infarction and 3 months after coronary revascularisation procedure [percutaneous coronary interventions (PCI) and/or coronary artery bypass graft (CABG)] (level of evidence: A)
2. *Class IIa:*
   a) Patients with ischaemic heart disease and LV dysfunction (LVEF = 31–35%), measured at least 6 weeks after myocardial infarction and 3 months after coronary revascularisation procedure (PCI and/or CABG) with inducible ventricular fibrillation (VF)/sustained ventricular tachycardia (VT) at electrophysiology study (level of evidence: B)
   b) Patients with non-ischaemic cardiomyopathy ≥ 9 months, LVEF ≤ 30%, and NYHA functional class II–III heart failure (level of evidence: B)
   c) Patients with familial or inherited conditions such as but not limited to long QT syndrome, hypertrophic cardiomyopathy, Brugada syndrome, or arrhythmogenic right ventricular dysplasia (ARVD) and at a high risk for life-threatening ventricular tachyarrhythmias (level of evidence: B)
3. *Class IIb:*
   a) Patients with ischaemic heart disease, prior myocardial infarction, LV dysfunction (LVEF = 31–35%), with either no inducible VF/sustained VT at electrophysiology study, or without an electrophysiology study (level of evidence: C)
   b) Patients with non-ischaemic cardiomyopathy present for at least 9 months, LV dysfunction (LVEF = 31–35%) and NYHA functional class II–III heart failure (level of evidence: C)

ICD Indications after an Acute Myocardial Infarction

The first 6–12 months after an acute myocardial infarction (AMI) are a period of high risk for SCD. However, the benefit of ICDs in this setting has not been fully studied. The DINAMIT study was a randomised, open-label study that compared ICD therapy to no ICD therapy in 674 patients during the immediate period after an AMI (6–40 days). Inclusion criteria were: LVEF ≤ 35%, heart rate variability standard deviation of normal RR intervals (SDNN) ≤ 70 ms or a mean RR interval ≤ 750 ms (heart rate ≥ 80 bpm) by 24-h Holter monitoring. The primary outcome was total mortality. There was no difference in overall mortality between the two groups (95% CI, 0.76 to 1.55; P = 0.66; follow-up 30 ± 13 months). However, there was a reduction in arrhythmic deaths that was manifested by an increase in non-arrhythmic deaths in the ICD group [9].

Based on the DINAMIT study findings, the decision to implant an ICD should be delayed for at least 6 weeks and possibly more in patients with a recent myocardial infarction and reduced LV function. Reassessment of LV function is required in order to define the need for an ICD.

Indications for ICD for Secondary Prevention

There is conclusive evidence supporting the superiority of ICDs over drugs for the secondary prevention of SCD [17–19]. A meta-analysis of secondary prevention trials reported a 28% relative risk reduction in all-cause mortality. This reduction was almost entirely due to a 50% relative risk reduction in arrhythmic deaths. Greater benefit is derived in patients with an LVEF < 35% [20]. Current guidelines support the use of ICDs in patients surviving a cardiac arrest or having presented with symptomatic sustained VT with reduced LV function regardless of aetiology.

ICD Indications for Infrequent Clinical Conditions

The less common cardiac disorders such as hypertrophic cardiomyopathy, Brugada syndrome, long QT, and arrhythmogenic right ventricular dysplasia are difficult to include in general guidelines due to their low incidence. However, sudden death is relatively frequent and is a devastating clinical presentation that could affect young people, and ICDs are sometimes the only available alternative [21, 22] (Table 1). Risk stratification of diseases with low prevalence is challenging. However, some useful recommendations based on small non-randomised studies and expert opinions may be proposed.

The diagnosis of Brugada syndrome [23] is based on typical 12-lead ECG

Table 1. ICD recommendation for infrequent cardiac disorders

Disease	Primary prevention	Secondary prevention
Long QT	–	Class I
ARVD	Class IIa	Class I
HCM	Class IIa	Class I
Brugada	Class I[a]	Class I
CPVT	–	Class I

ARVD, arrhythmogenic right ventricular dysplasia; HCM, hypertrophic cardiomyopathy; CPVT, catecholaminergic polymorphic VT
[a] Patients with syncope and no documented VT

findings (ST segment elevation in leads V1–V3) in subjects with either a family history of unexplained SCD or syncope or presenting with symptoms. The role of an electrophysiology study in determining the risk of death remains uncertain; however, ICD implantation is recommended in patients who survive an episode of VT/VF [24]. The evidence is in favour of including as high-risk patients those with a previous history of syncope and a familial history of SCD.

SCD may frequently be the primary manifestation of the long QT syndrome. There are clinical indicators such as history of syncope, ECG characteristics, cardiac arrest and torsades de pointes, and genetic markers that may help identify subjects at higher risk. ICD is recommended for secondary prevention while primary prevention is based mostly in the treatment with beta-blockers and life-style changes [25].

Arrhythmogenic right ventricular dysplasia may be a cause of SCD in the younger groups. Evidence identifying high-risk subgroups is sparse. Nonetheless, ICD is indicated in patients with VT/VF that are refractory to anti-arrhythmic agents. Patients with LV involvement or severe compromise of the right ventricle are at higher risk [26].

There is sparse evidence to provide definitive recommendations regarding the role of ICD in patients with catecholaminergic polymorphic VT. Nonetheless, it is reasonable to recommend an ICD for secondary prevention or after beta-blockers have failed [27].

The level of evidence for all of these disorders is C, and larger studies assessing the role of primary prevention and better means for risk stratification are certainly needed. Careful assessment of family history, searching for early unexplained deaths, 'seizures', and recurrent syncope, may aid individualising the decision to implant an ICD in a young subject.

ICD or ICD and Cardiac Resynchronisation Therapy

A number of cardiac resynchronisation therapy (CRT) studies have demonstrated an improvement in quality of life, exercise tolerance, and NYHA class in patients with heart failure and prolonged QRS. However, the benefits in relation to mortality have not been clearly established. The COMPANION study was designed to evaluate the role of the addition of ICD therapy to CRT. The primary outcome was a composite of total mortality and hospitalisations related to heart failure. COMPANION showed a significant reduction in the primary outcome for both CRT and CRT-ICD. However, mortality was significantly reduced only in the CRT-ICD arm, a 40% relative risk reduction [28, 29, 31]. This effect was significant regardless of the aetiology of heart failure.

It still remains unclear whether the effect of CRT-ICD is due to a synergistic effect between the different therapies or if it is only caused by a reduction in arrhythmic deaths due to the presence of an ICD in high-risk patients. Ongoing studies are currently addressing this issue. Current evidence supports the use of CRT-ICD in patients who fulfill both criteria. This is a class IIa indication with level of evidence A.

Health-Economic Considerations

The economic implications of ICD implantation are unquestionable [31, 32]. The issue is rather how to scientifically and economically judiciously use the limited resources available. Further refining of risk-stratifying markers such as T wave alternans may aid in this decision. However, a prospective trial using a 'risk score' may need to be developed. Compared to other medical therapies, ICDs may be economically sound. Figure 1 shows the calculated number needed to treat to save one life in the different ICD-CRT clinical trials. These should provide a general perspective on the potential economic justification of ICD therapy. It is important to recognise that clinical trials are limited by the fact that they do not take into account the relentless progression of the disease in patients with impaired LV function. Nevertheless, the benefit is clear, and physicians and health authorities should team up to create responsible policies that should be adapted to each country's resources.

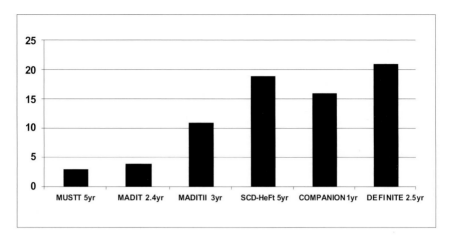

Fig. 1. Number needed to treat to prevent one death (all cause mortality/arrhythmic mortality)

Conclusions

Evidence-based large clinical trials have undoubtedly demonstrated the benefits of ICD in specific populations. Guidelines are intended only as a tool to aid in the decision whether to implant an ICD or CRT device. The responsibility of physicians is primarily towards their patients, but judicious use of health care resources is critical to be able to provide a fair share to all the patients in need of these devices.

References

1. Tang AS, Ross H, Simpson C et al (2005) Canadian Cardiovascular Society/Canadian Heart Rhythm Society. Position paper on implantable cardioverter defibrillator (ICD) use in Canada. Can J Cardiol (in press)
2. Josephson M, Wellens HJJ (2004) Implantable defibrillators and sudden cardiac death. Circulation 109:2685–2691
3. American Heart Association (2001) 2002 Heart and stroke statistical update. American Heart Association, Dallas, Texas
4. Vreede-Swagemakers JJM, Gorgels APM, Dubois-Arbouw WI et al (1997) Out-of-hospital cardiac arrest in the 1900s: a population-based study in the Maastricht area on incidence, characteristics and survival. J Am Coll Cardiol 30:1500–1505
5. Gregoratos G, Abrams J, Epstein AE et al (2002) ACC/AHA/NASPE 2002 guideline update for implantation of cardiac pacemakers and antiarrhythmia devices: summary article. Circulation 106:2145–2161
6. Moss AJ, Hall WJ, Cannom DS et al (1996) Multicenter Automatic Defibrillator Implantation Trial Investigators. Improved survival with an implanted defibrillator in patients with coronary disease at high risk for ventricular arrhythmia. N Engl J Med 335:1933–1940

7. Moss AJ, Zareba W, Hall WJ et al (2002) Prophylactic implantation of a defibrillator in patients with myocardial infarction and reduced ejection fraction. N Engl J Med 346:877–883

8. Buxton AE, Lee KL, Fisher JD et al (1999) Multicenter Unsustained Tachycardia Trial Investigators. A randomized study of the prevention of sudden death in patients with coronary artery disease. N Engl J Med 341:1882–1890

9. Hohnloser SH, Kuck KH, Dorian P et al (2004) Prophylactic use of an implantable cardioverter-defibrillator after acute myocardial infarction. DINAMIT investigators. N Engl J Med 351:2481–2488

10. Bansch D, Antz M, Boczor S et al (2002) Primary prevention of sudden cardiac death in idiopathic dilated cardiomyopathy: the cardiomyopathy trial (CAT). Circulation 105:1453–1458

11. Strickberger SA, Hummel JD, Bartlett TG et al (2003) Amiodarone versus implantable cardioverter-defibrillator: randomized trial in patients with nonischemic dilated cardiomyopathy and asymptomatic nonsustained ventricular tachycardia – AMIOVIRT. J Am Coll Cardiol 41:1707–1712

12. Kadish A, Dyer A, Daubert JP et al (2004) Prophylactic defibrillator implantation in patients with nonischemic dilated cardiomyopathy. N Engl J Med 350:2151–2158

13. The sudden cardiac death in heart failure trial (SCD-HeFT): http://www.sicr.org/scdheft

14. Klein H, Auricchio A, Reek S et al (1999) New primary prevention trials of sudden cardiac death in patients with left ventricular dysfunction: SCD-HeFT and MADIT-II. Am J Cardiol 83:91D–97D

15. Englestein ED (2003) Prevention and management of chronic heart failure with electrical therapy. AJC 91:62F–73F

16. Desai AS, Fang JC, Maisel WH et al (2004) Implantable defibrillators for the prevention of mortality in patients with nonischemic cadiomyopathy: a meta-analysis of randomized controlled trial. J Am Med Assoc 292:2873–2879

17. Connolly SJ, Gent M, Robert RS et al (2000) Canadian Implantable Defibrillator Study (CIDS): a randomized trial of the implantable cardioverter defibrillator against amiodarone. Circulation 101:1297–1302

18. Kuck KH, Cappato R, Siebels J et al (2000) Randomized comparison of antiarrhythmic drug therapy with implantable defibrillators in patients resuscitated from cardiac arrest: the Cardiac Arrest Study Hamburg (CASH). Circulation 102:748–754

19. Anderson JL, Hallstrom AP, Epstein AE et al, for the AVID Investigators (1999) Design and results of the Antiarrhythmic Vs. Implantable Defibrillators (AVID) registry. Circulation 99:1692–1699

20. Connolly SJ, Hallstrom AP, Cappato R et al (2000) Meta-analysis of the implantable cardioverter defibrillator secondary prevention trials. AVID, CASH and CIDS studies. Antiarrhythmic vs. implantable defibrillator study. Eur Heart J 21:2071–2078

21. Priori SG, Aliot E, Blomstrom-Lundqvist C et al (2002) Task force on sudden death, European Society of Cardiology. Summary of recommendations. Europace 4:3–18

22. Priori SG, Aliot E, Blomstrom-Lundqvist C et al (2003) Update of the guidelines on sudden cardiac death of the European Society of Cardiology. Eur Heart J 24:13–15

23. Brugada J, Brugada R, Brugada P (1998) Right bundle-branch block and ST-segment elevation in leads V1 through V3: a marker for sudden death in patients without demonstrable structural heart disease. Circulation 97:457–460

24. Priori SG, Napolitano C, Gasparini M et al (2000) Clinical and genetic heterogeneity of right bundle branch block and ST-segment elevation syndrome: a prospec-

tive evaluation of 52 families. Circulation 102:2509–2515

25. Priori SG, Napolitano C, Bloise R et al (2003) Risk stratification in the long-QT syndrome. N Engl J Med 348:1866–1874

26. Link MS, Wang PJ, Haugh CJ et al (1997) Arrhythmogenic right ventricular dysplasia: clinical results with implantable cardioverter defibrillators. J Interv Card Electrophysiol 1:41–48

27. Leenhardt A, Lucet V, Denjoy I et al (1995) Catecholaminergic polymorphic ventricular tachycardia in children. A 7-year follow-up of 21 patients. Circulation 91:1512–1519

28. Bristow MR, Saxon LA, Boehmer J et al (2004) Cardiac-resynchronisation therapy with or without an implantable defibrillator in advanced chronic heart failure. N Engl J Med 350:2140–2150

29. Morillo CA (2004) A prophylactic cardioverter-defibrillator prevented sudden death from arrhythmia in nonischemic cardiomyopathy. ACP J Club 141(3):61

30. Morillo CA (2004) Cardiac resynchronization therapy reduced all-cause death and hospitalization in chronic heart failure. ACP J Club 141(3):60

31. Priori SG, Klein W (2003) Medical practice guidelines. Separating science from economics. Eur Heart J 24:1962–1964

32. Chen L, Hay JW (2004) Cost-effectiveness of primary implanted cardioverter defibrillator for sudden death prevention in congestive heart failure. Cardiovasc Drug Ther 18:161–170

Management of Cardiac Arrhythmias in Post-PCI Patients

B. Gorenek

Introduction

Percutaneous coronary interventions (PCI) have been the fastest growing major invasive procedure in the past decade. Accompanying the obvious benefit, there are certain risks, including cardiac arrhythmias. A variety of arrhythmias and conduction disturbances can occur during PCI. In general, lethal ventricular arrhythmias, including serious ventricular tachycardia (VT) and ventricular fibrillation (VF), have been reported to occur in 1.5–4.4% of the patients undergoing coronary angioplasty. The frequency of these arrhythmias after primary PCI was analysed in data on 3065 patients from Primary Angioplastic in Myocardial Infarction (PAMI) trials [1]. Ventricular arrhythmias occurred in 133 patients (4.3%). Smoking, lack of preprocedural beta-blockers, shorter time from symptom onset to arrival in emergency room initial thrombolysis in myocardial infarction (TIMI) flow grade 0, and right coronary artery-related infarct were variables independently associated with a risk of serious ventricular arrhythmias. These patients had higher rates of complications including cardiopulmonary resuscitation and intubation in the catheterisation laboratory, but had similar frequencies of major adverse cardiac events in hospital and at 1 year.

These arrhythmias may be the result of excessive catheter manipulation, intracoronary dye injection, new ischaemic events, or reperfusion injury.

Role of Dye Injection and Intracoronary Solutions

Various contrast media have been developed for use in coronary angiography and PCI. These contrast media may be divided into ionic contrast media

Cardiology Department, Osmangazi University, Eskisehir,Turkey

of high osmolarity, those of low osmolarity, and non-ionic contrast materials. The risk of ventricular arrhythmia from intracoronary dye is greatest with the injection of ionic contrast agents into the right coronary artery, particularly in the setting of prolonged injection or a damped pressure tracing. VF may occur if dye is allowed to remain static in the coronary tree. The incidence of VF during PCI can be significantly decreased by using low-osmolarity non-ionic contrast media lacking calcium-binding additives. However, in some reports, contrary to the current belief in the overall safety of low-osmolarity ionic contrast agents compared with other agents in diagnostic coronary angiography procedures, such agents are associated with an increased risk of sustained ventricular arrhythmias [2].

VF is a serious complication during induction of hypothermia for surgical purposes [3]. In a study published 2 years ago, six patients were found to have VF during intracoronary saline, heparin, contrast medium, or nitrate delivery [4]. These medications did not warm up to body temperature. Immediate intracoronary flush would result in local hypothermia. Thus, to decrease the risk of VF, warmed-up fluid and warmed-up iso-osmolar non-ionic contrast agents must be preferred, especially in patients undergoing PCI on the right coronary artery.

Management of Ventricular Premature Beats

The first period of ventricular premature beats, which usually heralds malignant arrhythmias during acute coronary occlusion, develops after a quiescent period of 1.5–2.5 min and reaches a peak at 5 min. Both re-entrant and non-re-entrant mechanisms contribute to the development of premature beats and malignant ventricular arrhythmias during the early phase of myocardial ischaemia. Complex premature ventricular contractions and occasional non-sustained ventricular tachycardia are seen after 2–3% of apparently uncomplicated angioplasty procedures. These arrhythmias usually abate over 12–36 h and do not, in general, require treatment. However, hypokalaemia and hypomagnesaemia should be ruled out because potassium and magnesium may be depleted by diuretic-induced diuresis and may need to be replaced [5].

Arrhythmias Related to Ischaemia

Acute myocardial ischaemia often results in malignant arrhythmias owing to both the direct effects of ischaemia and the resultant haemodynamic compromise during PCI. Some of the most refractory ventricular ectopy is seen in the setting of profound transmural ischaemia or early myocardial infarction. Venticular fibrillation due to acute ischaemia is a not infrequent complication of PCI. As in diagnostic coronary angiography, it is readily treated by defibrillation and death rarely results. There appears to be no relation to the severity of coronary artery disease, and the cause is partially related to the use of contrast agents or post-PCI complications.

Arrhythmic Complications and Patient Characteristics

Vessel calibre is one of the important factors in the genesis of arrhythmias in PCI. Huang et al. observed that a small calibre of the right coronary artery and associated ST segment changes played important roles in the patients who experienced VF during the PCI. They suggested that the cause of acute ischaemia might be the size of the guiding catheter. Most of the catheters they used in patients with VF were 7F, except in two cases where a 6F catheter was used. So, small-size catheters should be preferred especially in high-risk patients [4].

The risk of cardiac arrhythmias in PCI is more pronounced in patients with heart failure. Three years ago, DeGeare et al. investigated the predictive value of Killip classification in patients undergoing primary PCI for acute myocardial infarction. Killip classification predicted the incidence of arrhythmias in those patients. This classification was a predictor of mortality in their study. Killip classification on hospital admission was a simple and useful independent predictor of in-hospital and 6-month mortality in patients with acute myocardial infarction who were undergoing primary PCI [6].

Importance of QT Dispersion and Heart Rate Variability

QT dispersion may serve as a measure of variability in ventricular recovery time and may be a means of identifying patients at risk of lethal ventricular arrhythmias and sudden death with coronary artery disease. Ashikaga et al. showed that increased QTc dispersion may predict the risk of lethal ventricular arrhythmias during angioplasty. The fact that successful angioplasty decreased QTc dispersion indicates that part of increased QTc dispersion is related to myocardial ischaemia in patients with coronary artery disease [7]. Thus, in patients with QTc dispersion we should be alert for serious ventricular arrhythmias. Nicorandil may precondition the myocardium and may prevent the occurrence of ventricular arrhythmias after coronary angioplasty by suppressing the increase in QT dispersion [8].

Abrupt coronary occlusion may cause a wide range of autonomic reactions as evidenced by changes in heart rate, blood pressure, and heart rate variability (HRV). Coronary occlusion-induced increase in HRV seems to have a protective effect against the occurrence of complex ventricular arrhythmias during the early stage of abrupt coronary occlusion, suggesting that vagal activation may modify the outcome of acute coronary events with coronary artery disease [9].

Reperfusion Arrhythmias

Reperfusion arrhythmias may be one of the manifestations of reperfusion injury. These arrhythmias are common in patients undergoing PCI, which include accelerated idioventricular rhythms, VT, and VF. Reperfusion arrhythmias, in addition to their importance as a marker of successful reperfusion, need special attention because haemodynamics may rapidly deteriorate during VT or VF.

Intracellular calcium overload is believed to play a critical role in the development of reperfusion arrhythmias. Accumulation of calcium in the cell causes damage to the respiratory chain and decreases ATP production, leading to depletion of mitochondrial energy [10]. The oxygen paradox is closely linked to the calcium overload or calcium paradox, since oxygen mediates the uptake of calcium by mitochondria [11]. Oxygen also leads to cell damage during reperfusion through the formation of oxygen radicals [12]. The role of free radicals in the genesis of reperfusion arrhythmias is uncertain. Free-radical-induced damage occurs in the 10 min after reperfusion [13]. Reduced levels of free radical scavengers have been observed within 3 h of angioplasty in patients with acute myocardial infarction [14].

Some strategies may be helpful for the prevention and treatment of reperfusion arrhythmias, but their beneficial affects are limited. Today we know a little about the effectiveness of antioxidant therapy. The results have largely been mixed and the investigation remains focused at the animal level. Magnesium can be a choice, but there are conflicting data on its benefit. Numerous studies have examined the efficacy of vasodilators as cardioprotective agents in ischaemic reperfusion injury. Intracoronary adenosine and papaverine may be effective as cardioprotective agents. Human studies with papaverine have also demonstrated success in improving angiographically documented TIMI flow grades in epicardial arteries [15]. Calcium channel blockers may block intracellular calcium overload and have positive effects on vascular flow. The effects have been demonstrated during the administration of nifedine and verapamil [16]. Two years ago Yoshida et al. showed that administration of dipyridamole can prevent and terminate reperfusion arrhythmias such as accelerated idioventricular rhythms and VT. They concluded that cAMP-mediated triggered activity may, at least in part, be responsible for reperfusion arrhythmias [17].

Role of Inhibition of the Renin–Angiotensin–Aldosterone System

In the normal heart, locally derived angiotensin II may modulate coronary blood flow, inotropy, and chronotropy [18–21], whereas under pathological conditions the renin–angiotensin–aldosterone system (RAS) may influence ventricular growth and myocardial metabolism, induce ventricular arrhythmias during ischaemia and reperfusion injury, and contribute to post-infarction ventricular remodelling [22]. We also know that bradykinin accumulation is a potent cardioprotective mechanism underlying RAS inhibition in ischaemia and reperfusion injury. A role for RAS in reperfusion arrhythmias was suggested by studies in angiotensin II type 1a receptor knockout mice which, compared to wild-type mice, showed less reperfusion arrhythmia despite a similar infarct size. In addition, administration of a selective angiotensin II type 1 receptor before ischaemia blocked reperfusion arrhythmias [23]. An experimental study showed us that losartan attenuates myocardial ischaemia-induced ventricular arrhythmias and reperfusion injury in hypertension, and may be useful in the treatment of ventricular arrhythmias induced by acute myocardial infarction and attenuation of reperfusion injury [24]. Intracoronary enalaprilat infusion in the infarct-related artery is feasible in the setting of primary angioplasty and is safe and well tolerated [25]. Effective cardiac RAS inhibition can be achieved by low-dose intracoronary enalaprilat, which primarily causes a potentiation of bradykinin [25].

Preconditioning and Arrhythmias

The incidence of serious ventricular arrhythmias in the presence of intracoronary thrombus was high in a report [26]. Sudden obstruction of the coronary artery without pre-existing coronary artery narrowing was associated with a higher incidence of VF than was obstruction occurring in association with pre-existing stenoses [26]. The profibrillatory effect of thrombus was not detectable in another report. Experimental studies have suggested that the phenomenon of ischaemic preconditioning may increase the VF threshold [27] and reduce the incidence of ischaemic and reperfusion arrhythmias [28]. The mitochondrial KATP channel seems to be important in prevention of myocardium by preconditioning. A study in dogs suggests that preconditioning may exert an antiarrhythmic effect during ischaemia by modifying cardiac autonomic receptor mechanisms, which results in an improved parasympathetic balance. A preceding short vessel occlusion-reperfusion cycle increases the electrical stability of ischaemic myocardium, so the repeated coronary artery occlusions during PCI protect against ischaemia-induced ventricular arrhythmias [29].

Benefits of Intra-aortic Balloon Counterpulsation

Intra-aortic balloon counterpulsation (IABC) has been used following primary PCI in high risk patients in an attempt to improve outcomes by increasing coronary blood flow reserve, decreasing preload and afterload, and augmenting systemic pressure [30]. In high risk patients prophylactic use of IABC may decrease the incidence of VF, especially in patients with cardiogenic shock [30]. Intra-aortic balloon counterpulsation used before primary PCI provides benefit to patients with cardiogenic shock by reducing the incidence of catheterisation laboratory events, including VT. So, we recommend the use of IABC in patients with cardiogenic shock who are undergoing primary PCI.

Supraventricular Arrhythmias and Atrial Fibrillation

Supraventricular arrhythmias including atrial fibrillation (AF) may be induced by PCI, but they are not as frequent as ventricular arrhythmias. However, AF especially has prognostic significance in patients treated with PCI. Because the patency of infarct-related artery is better, primary PCI is superior to thrombolytic therapy in restoring sinus rhythm in patients with acute myocardial infarction who have developed AF [31].

Kinjo et al. investigated the prognostic significance of AF and atrial flutter in patients with acute myocardial infarction treated with PCI. In their study, the patients with AF were older, were in higher Killip classes, had higher rates of previous myocardial infarction and previous cerebrovascular accident, had systolic blood pressure of less than 100 mmHg and heart rates of 100 beats/min or more, were less likely to smoke, and had a higher prevalence of multivessel disease and poorer reperfusion of infarct-related artery than those without AF. Atrial fibrillation was a common complication in patients with acute myocardial infarction who are treated with PCI and independently influenced 1-year mortality, they said [32].

Atrial fibrillation during PCI tends to revert spontaneously over a period of minutes to hours, but may require additional therapy if it produces ischaemia or haemodynamic instability. Intravenous beta-blockers (e.g.

esmolol, metoprolol), calcium channel blockers (e.g. verapamil), or digoxin may be given and up-titrated until adequate control of ventricular response is achieved. Electrical cardioversion is rarely required.

Conduction Defects and Heart Blocks

New conduction defects occur in about 0.9% of the patients undergoing coronary angioplasty [33]. Of these, right bundle branch block was the most common, followed by first-degree atrioventricular block. These defects almost always disappeared without treatment before the time of hospital discharge, but occasionally required the elimination of drugs depressing cardiac activity [5].

When complete heart block develops, atropine is rarely helpful in the setting of inadequate escape and deterioration, but should be given anyway. Coughing may help support the circulation and maintain consciousness while a temporary pacing catheter is inserted.

Conclusions

Either ventricular or atrial arrhythmias or conduction disturbances can be observed during PCI. Some of them occur as a complication of the procedure, but many of the arrhythmias are related to reperfusion injury. The patient's characteristics, the type of the procedure, the features of the target vessel and the type of the lesion play an important role in the occurrence of arrhythmias. The majority of the arrhythmias tend to revert spontaneously, but when necessary, special treatment must be given promptly.

References

1. Mehta RH, Harjai KJ, Grines L et al (2004) Sustained ventricular tachycardia or fibrillation in the cardiac catheterisation laboratory among patients receiving primary percutaneous coronary intervention: incidence, predictors, and outcomes. J Am Coll Cardiol 43:1765–1772
2. Hajj-Ali R, Ezzeddine R, Jadonath R et al (2001) Use of low-osmolar ionic contrast agents increases the risk of sustained ventricular arrhythmias during diagnostic coronary angiography. Am J Cardiol 88 (5A): TCT298 Suppl.
3. Kearns JB, Murnaghan MF (1969) Ventricular fibrillation during hypothermia. J Physiol Lond, 203(1):51P-53P
4. Huang JL, Ting CT, Chen YT, Chen SA (2002) Mechanisms of ventricular fibrillation during coronary angioplasty: increased incidence for the small orifice caliber of the right coronary artery. Int J Cardiol 82:221–228

5. Ellis SG (1994) Elective coronary angioplasty: technique and complications. In: Topol EJ (ed) Textbook of interventional cardiology. Saunders, Philadelphia, pp 186–206
6. DeGeare WS, Boura JA, Grines LL et al (2001) Predictive value of the Killip classification in patients undergoing primary percutaneous coronary intervention for acute myocardial infarction. Am J Cardiol 87:1035–1038
7. Ashikaga T, Nishizaki M, Arita M et al (1998) Increased QTc dispersion predicts lethal venticular arrhythmias complicating coronary angioplasty. Am J Cardiol 82:814–816
8. Kato T, Kamiyama T, Maruyama M et al (2001) Nicorandil, a potent cardioprotective agent, reduces QT dispersion during coronary angioplasty. Am Heart J 141:940–943
9. Airaksinen KE, Ylitalo A, Nimela MJ et al (1999) Heart rate variability and occurrence of ventricular arrhythmias during balloon occlusion of a major coronary artery. Am J Cardiol 83:1000–1005
10. Matsuma K, Jeremy RW, Schaper J et al (1998) Progression of myocardial necrosis during reperfusion of ischemic myocardium. Circulation 97:795–804
11. Opie LH, Coetzee WA (1988) Role of calcium ions in reperfusion arrhythmias: Relevance to pharmacologic intervention. Cardiovasc Drugs Ther 2:623–636
12. Hearse DJ, Tosak A (1988) Free radicals and calcium. Simultaneous interacting triggers as determinants of vulnerability to reperfusion-induced arrhythmias in the rat heart. J Mol Cell Cardiol 20:213–223
13. Ambrosio G, Weisfeldt ML, Jacobus WE et al (1987) Evidence for a reversible oxygen mediated component of reperfusion injury: reduction by recombinant human superoxide dismutase administered at the time of reflow. Circulation 75:282–291
14. Lafont A, Marwick TH, Chisolm GM et al (1996) Decreased free radical scavengers with reperfusion after coronary angioplasty in patients with acute myocardial infarction. Am Heart J 1996 131:219–23
15. Ishihara M, Sato H, Tateishi H et al (1996) Attenuation of the no-reflow phenomenon after coronary angioplasty for acute myocardial infarction with intracoronary papaverine. Am Heart J 132:959–963
16. Tillmanns H, Neumann FJ, Parekh et al (1990) Pharmacologic effects on coronary microvessels during myocardial ischemia. Eur Heart J 11:B10–B15
17. Yoshida Y, Hirai M, Yamada T et al (2000) Arrhythmic efficacy of dipyridamole in treatment of reperfusion arrhythmias. Circulation 101:624–630
18. Saito K, Gutkind JS, Saaverda JM (1987) Angiotensin II binding sites in the conduction system of rat hearts. Am J Physiol 253:1618–1622
19. Xiang JZ, Scholkens BA, Ganten D, Unger T (1984) Effects of sympathetic nerve stimulation is attenuated by the converting enzyme inhibitor Hoe 498 in isolated rabbit hearts. Clin Exp Hypertens 6:1853–1857
20. Xiang JZ, Linz W, Becker H et al (1985) Effects of converting enzyme inhibitors: ramipril and enalapril on peptide action and sympathetic neurotransmission in the isolated heart. Eur J Pharmacol 113:215–223
21. Rogers TB, Gaa ST, Allen IS (1986) Identification and characterization of functional angiotensin II receptors on cultured heart myocytes. J Pharmacol Exp Ther 236:438–444
22. Dostal DE, Baker KM (1993) Evidence for a role of an intracardiac renin-angiotensin system in normal and failing hearts. Trends Cardiovasc Med 3:67–74
23. Harada K, Komuro I, Hayashi D et al (1998) Angiotensin II type 1a receptor is involved in the occurrence of reperfusion arrhythmias. Circulation 97:315–317

24. Lee YM, Peng YY, Ding YA et al (1997) Losartan attenuates myocardial ischemia-induced ventricular arrhythmias and reperfusion injury in spontaneously hypertensive rats. Am J Hypertens 10:852–858

25. Kurz T, Schafer U, Dendorfer A et al (2001) Effects of intracoronary low dose enalaprilat as an adjunct to primary percutaneous transluminal coronary angiography in acute myocardial infarction. Am J Cardiol 88:1351–1357

26. Coronel R, Wilms-Schopman FJ, Janse MJ (1997) Profibrillatory effects of intracoronary thrombus in acute regional ischemia of the in situ porcine heart. Circulation 96:3985–3991

27. Gulker H, Kramer B, Stephan K et al (1977) Changes in ventricular fibrillation threshold during regional short-term coronary occlusion and release. Basic Res Cardiol 72:547–562

28. Lawson CS, Hearse DJ (1996) Anti-arrhythmic protection by ischemic preconditioning in anesthetised dogs and rats. Cardiovasc Res 31:655–662

29. Airaksinen KEJ, Huikuri HV (1997) Antiarrhythmic effect of repeated coronary occlusion during balloon angioplasty. J Am Coll Cardiol 29:1035–1038

30. Brodie BR, Stuckey TD, Hansen C et al (1999) Intra-aortic balloon counterpulsation before primary percutaneous transluminal coronary angioplasty reduces catheterization laboratory events in high-risk patients with acute myocardial infarction. Am J Cardiol 84:18–23

31. Gorenek B, Birdane A, Unalir A et al (2000) Restoring sinus rhythm in patients with atrial fibrillation complicating acute myocardial infarction: comparison of outcomes of primary angioplasty and thrombolytic therapy (abstract). Eur J Heart Fail, Suppl 1:32

32. Kinjo K, Sato H, Sato H et al (2003) Prognostic significance of atrial fibrillation/atrial flutter in patients with acute myocardial infarction treated with percutaneous coronary intervention. Am J Cardiol 92:1150–1154

33. Bredlau CE, Roubin GS, Leimgruber PP et al 81985) In-hospital mortality in patients undergoing elective coronary angioplasty. Circulation 72:1044–1052

Anti-tachycardia Pacing for Termination of Rapid Ventricular Tachycardia in Patients with Implantable Cardioverter-Defibrillators. The PITAGORA ICD Trial

M. GULIZIA[1], S. MANGIAMELI[2], F. MASCIA[3], V.A. CICONTE[4], R.M. POLIMENI[5], A. CAPUCCI[6], V. CALOGERO[7], C. PUNTRELLO[8], S. SAMMARTANO[9], M. SCHERILLO[10], O. PENSABENE[11], M.C. SCIANARO[12] ON BEHALF OF PITAGORA ICD STUDY INVESTIGATORS

Introduction

In patients with an implantable cardioverter–defibrillator (ICD) many episodes of rapid monomorphic ventricular tachycardia (VT) may be labelled ventricular fibrillation (VF) by the ICD and treated by painful shocks [1, 2]. Several observational studies have shown that ventricular anti-tachycardia pacing (ATP) is effective in VT termination [1–5].

The PainFREE Rx trial [6] has enrolled 220 patients with coronary artery disease and standard ICD indications, programmed a standardised ventricular detection and therapy algorithm (two burst sequences, eight pulses, 88%) for arrhythmias faster than 188 bpm (320 ms) and showed that:

- 43% of arrhythmias were detected in the traditional VF zone of < 320 ms
- 93% of arrhythmias detected in the VF zone were detected as fast VT (FVT)
- Empirical ATP therapy terminates 85% of FVT episodes with cycle length (CL) from 240 to 320 ms (250–190 bpm) at the first attempt
- The number of shocks saved by enabling ATP for FVT was 396 out of 446 detected episodes
- The low observed incidence of syncopes and FVT acceleration was no greater than that reported in other studies of ICD patients

[1]Cardiology Department, San Luigi, S. Currò Hospital, Catania; [2]Cardiology Department, Garibaldi Hospital, Catania; [3]Cardiology Department, S Sebastiano Hospital, Caserta; [4]Cardiology Department, Pugliese Ciaccio Hospital, Catanzaro; [5]Cardiology Department, S. Maria degli Ungheresi Hospital, Polistena; [6]Cardiology Department, Civile Hospital, Piacenza; [7]Cardiology Department, Umberto I Hospital, Enna; [8]Cardiology Department, S. Antonio Abate, Trapani; [9]Cardiology Department, Civico e Benfratelli Hospital, Palermo; [10]Cardiology Department, Rummo Hospital, Benevento; [11]Cardiology Department, Villa Sofia Hospital, Palermo; [12]Cardiology Department, Perrino Hospital, Brindisi, Italy

The PainFREE trial [6] concluded that ATP for FVT detected in the VF zone might safely reduce the morbidity of painful shocks. Reducing the shocks could increase patient quality of life, and increase device longevity.

The PainFREE Rx II Study [7] was a prospective, randomised, multi-centre trial that compared the safety and utility of empirical ATP (one burst sequence, eight pulses at 88% coupling interval) with shocks for FVT in a broad ICD population. PainFREE Rx II showed that the first ATP attempt terminated 229 of 284 (81%) FVT episodes. Forty out of 47 patients (85%) with FVT episodes presumably had at least one FVT shock prevented by ATP. ATP resulted in a 71% relative reduction in the proportion of shocked episodes. ATP programming did not lengthen FVT episode duration, its median value was 10.0 s in the ATP arm and 9.7 s in the shock arm. Acceleration of FVT was similarly low between treatment groups: it occurred in 4 of 273 monomorphic VT episodes (2%) in the ATP arm versus 2 of 145 (1%) in the shock arm. Syncope during FVT was rare: it occurred in 2 patients in the ATP group and 1 patient in the shock group.

The process of establishing the clinical role of a new therapeutic strategy, after its feasibility, safety, and efficacy as compared with the conventional therapy have been shown, comprises the conduction of an observational study to confirm results of previous randomised studies in general clinical practice. The main objective of the PITAGORA ICD trial, therefore, is to confirm the PainFREE II results in Italian clinical practice and to compare, in a randomised design, the termination efficacy of two different ATP sequences (burst eight pulses at 88% and ramp eight pulses starting at 91%).

Methods

Study Design

The PITAGORA ICD trial is a multi-centre, prospective, randomised, single blind study. At least 220 patients will be enrolled in about 24 Italian cardiological centres between January 2004 and December 2005. All patients enrolled will give written informed consent according to a protocol approved by local institutional review boards. Commercially available ICDs capable of being programmed for ATP for FVT via VF will be used. Following enrolment, patients will be randomised to treatment. ATP will be programmed in a burst configuration for half of them and in a ramp configuration for the other half.

Study Objectives

The main objective is to test the application in Italian clinical practice of two empirical ATP strategies on spontaneous FVT episodes. The primary end-point is quantification of the termination efficacy of two different sequences (burst eight pulses at 88% and ramp eight pulses starting at 91%). Secondary objectives are: estimation of the acceleration or syncopal rates associated with ATP treatment of spontaneous FVT episodes; estimation of the percentage reduction in the number of shocks delivered per patient; evaluation of different possible predictors of ATP success (VT rate, underlying disease, anti-arrhythmic drug treatment); evaluation of quality of life and hospitalisations; evaluation of circadian patterns of ventricular arrhythmias.

Patient Selection

The inclusion criteria comprise ICD indications (class I–IIA) according to the guidelines and implantation of an ICD capable of ATP for FVT via VF. Exclusion criteria are: patient life expectancy less than 1 year due to a non-cardiac chronic disease; patient on heart transplant list which is expected within 1 year; patient's age less than 18 years; unwillingness or inability of patient to provide written informed consent; patient's enrolment in, or intention to participate in, another clinical study during the course of this study; patient's inaccessibility for follow-up at the study centre; presence of ventricular tachyarrhythmias associated with reversible causes; presence of Brugada syndrome, long QT syndrome, or hypertrophic cardiomyopathy; presence of other electrical implantable devices, such as neurostimulators or others; mechanical tricuspid valve.

Study Size and Duration

The study will enrol a minimum of 220 patients within 2 years. The study will continue for a period of 12 months after the enrolment of the last patient; total study duration will thus be approximately 3 years.

The sample size has been chosen in order to have a collection of episodes comparable with those in the PainFREE Rx trial [6].

Device Programming

The device will be programmed according to the randomisation as shown in Table 1. Since only the FVT are considered for analysis, type and programming of VT therapies are left to the investigators' discretion. FVT and VF detection zones will be identical for all patients (Fig. 1):
- VF detection zone < 320 ms
- Optional VT detection zone > 320 ms
- FVT detection zone > 240 ms and < 320 ms

Table 1. First FVT therapy programming in the two study arms

	Burst ATP arm	Ramp ATP arm
Group treatment	ATP 8 pulses	ATP 15 pulses
Therapy no. 1		
Amplitude	8 V	8 V
Pulse width	1.6 ms	1.6 ms
Therapy type	Burst	Ramp
Number of initial pulses	8	8
R–S1 interval (%RR)	88%	91%
Interval decrement	10 ms	10 ms
Minimum interval	200 ms	200 ms
Number of sequences	1	1
NID VF	18/24	18/2
RNID VF	9/12	9/12
FVT therapies nos. 2–6	Shock	Shock

FVT, fast ventricular tachycardia; NID, number of interval detection; RNID, redetection

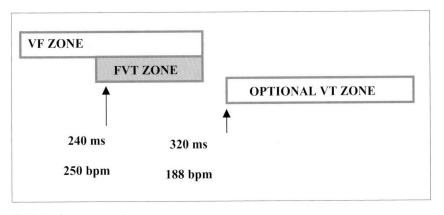

Fig. 1. Study programming

Data Collection Before Device Implantation

Baseline clinical data will be collected at study enrolment. These data include a complete clinical history particularly designed to capture cardiopulmonary symptoms and the occurrence and characteristics of ventricular arrhythmias before randomisation.

Follow-Up

Patients will be evaluated at follow-up visits as per clinical practice. Whenever the patients have episodes, an unscheduled follow-up visit will be performed as soon as possible. At each visit, the patient's clinical status will be recorded and the ICD interrogated; each stored arrhythmic event will be analysed and collected by save-to-disk procedures.

For patients not showing up at scheduled follow-up visits, they or their relatives will be contacted to know some about their life status.

Anti-arrhythmic Drug Therapy

Anti-arrhythmic drug therapy is left to the physician's discretion.

Data Analysis

Only the first ATP therapy will be considered as the basis for determining treatment success or failure. Success rates will be determined by episode. They will be corrected to take into account multiples episodes using the generalised estimating equations (GEE) method.

Appendix

Active study sites and investigators of PITAGORA ICD study are:
S. Luigi–S. Currò – Catania: Michele Gulizia, Giuseppina Francese; Garibaldi – Catania: Salvatore Mangiameli, Giuseppe Doria; S Sebastiano – Caserta: Franco Mascia, Pasquale Golino; Pugliese Ciaccio – Catanzaro: Vincenzo Antonio Ciconte, Roberto Ceravolo; ASL 10 – Polistena: Rocco Mario Polimeni, Giuseppe Meduri; Civico – Palermo: Stefano Sammartano, Umberto Giordano; Cannizzaro – Catania: Francesco Lisi, Francesco Liberti; Civile – Milazzo: Ludovico Vasquez, Francesco Badessa; Umberto I – Enna: Vasco Calogero, Carmelo Battaglia; Villa Sofia – Palermo: Orazio Pensabene; S. Giovanni di Dio – Agrigento: Ignazio Vaccaro, Calogero Catalano; Papardo – Messina: Giuseppe Busà, Santina Patané; S. Antonio Abate – Trapani: Calogero Puntrello; Muscatello – Augusta: Giacomo Chiarandà, Gianfranco Muscio; S. Elia – Caltanissetta: Salvatore Giglia; Vittorio Emanuele – Catania: Alfredo Virgilio, Antonio Circo; Civile – Ragusa: Vincenzo Spadola, Guglielmo Piccione; Iazzolino – Vibo Valentia: Michele Comito; Ferrari – Castrovillari: Giovanni Bisignani, Giovanni Sanpasquale; G. Rummo – Benevento: Marino Scherillo, Domenico Capobianco; Moscati – Avellino: Giuseppe De Fabrizio, Francesco Rotondi; Clinica Mediterranea – Napoli (Naples): Pasquale Nocerino; Monaldi – Napoli (Naples): Lucio Santangelo, Cavallaro; Perrino – Brindisi: Maria Cristina Scianaro, G. Ignone; Civile – Piacenza: Alessandro Capucci, Giovanni Quinto Villani.

References

1. Raitt MH, Dolack GL, Kudenchuk PJ et al (1995) Ventricular arrhythmias detected after transvenous defibrillator implantation in patients with a clinical history of only ventricular fibrillation. Implications for use of implantable defibrillator. Circulation 91:1996–2001
2. Swerdlow CD, Peter CT, Kass RM et al (1997) Programming of implantable cardio-

verter-defibrillators on the basis of the upper limit of vulnerability. Circulation 95:1497–1504

3. Schaumann A, von zur Muhlen F, Herse B et al (1998) Empirical versus tested anti-tachycardia pacing in implantable cardioverter defibrillators: a prospective study including 200 patients. Circulation 97:66–74

4. Nasir N Jr, Pacifico A, Doyle TK et al (1997) Spontaneous ventricular tachycardia treated by antitachycardia pacing. Cadence Investigators. Am J Cardiol 79:820–822

5. Fromer M, Brachmann J, Block M et al (1992) Efficacy of automatic multimodal device therapy for ventricular tachyarrhythmias as delivered by a new implantable pacing cardioverter-defibrillator. Results of a European multicenter study of 102 implants. Circulation 86:363–374

6. Wathen M, Sweeney M, DeGroot P et al (2001) Shock reduction using antitachycardia pacing for spontaneous rapid ventricular tachycardia in patients with coronary artery disease. Circulation 104:796–801

7. Wathen M, DeGroot P, Sweeney M et al (2004) Prospective randomized multicenter trial of empirical antitachycardia pacing versus shocks for spontaneous rapid ventricular tachycardia in patients with implantable cardioverter-defibrillators. Circulation 110:2591–2596

MADIT II/SCD-HeFT Results: Have They Already Achieved an Impact in Europe?

A. Arenal, M. Ortiz

Sudden cardiac death (SCD) is among the most common causes of death in developed countries, and even though there has been a reduction in total cardiac mortality, the percentage of deaths that are sudden has increased. This has resulted primarily from an increase in out-of-hospital sudden deaths. Moreover, SCD is the first presentation of cardiac disease in 33–50% of patients. Coronary artery disease is the most common underlying disease, being responsible for approximately 75% of all SCDs. The two most important risk factors for SCD are a left ventricular ejection fraction (LVEF) less than 40% and clinical congestive heart failure. The risk of mortality related to ejection fraction increases markedly when the LVEF falls below 40%. Interestingly, the incidence of SCD decreases from NYHA functional class I to class IV. It is most frequent in class II patients: in this setting, more than half of patients will die suddenly. As result of these epidemiological characteristics, primary prevention of SCD has targeted patients with coronary artery disease and congestive heart failure and significant depression of LVEF, which means mainly patients in functional classes II and III [1–4].

The MADIT II study included patients with a LVEF of less than 30% with a prior infarct (more than 1 month before enrollment) and no other risk stratification criteria. The study enrolled 1232 patients, 60% of whom received ICDs versus 40% who received conventional therapy. MADIT II was stopped before its completion after a follow-up period of 20 months, when a 30% relative reduction in mortality was demonstrated. However, the absolute reduction was only 5.6%. Although the MADIT II inclusion criteria have been accepted as a class IIA indication for ICD implantation, there is significant controversy regarding costs and applicability to the general population [5]. Like most ICD studies, MADIT II mainly enrolled patients who were hos-

Cardiology Department, Hospital General Universitario Gregorio Marañón, Madrid, Spain

pitalised, i.e. they were high-risk patients undergoing treatment. The mortality rate of the control group in MADIT II is probably higher than the mortality rate of patients who meet the enrollment criteria but who are found in a different setting.

The SCD-HeFT study randomised patients with clinical heart failure on stable medical therapy to (1) ICD plus optimal pharmacological therapy, (2) optimal pharmacological therapy plus amiodarone, or (3) optimal pharmacological therapy. This study included patients with heart failure with or without ischaemic heart disease in NYHA classes II–III and LVEF of 35% or less. To avoid the deleterious effect of right ventricular pacing, back-up pacing was not triggered until the heart rate dropped to 34 bpm and was set to pace at only 50 bpm. The mean LVEF of the 2521 patients enrolled was 25%, 70% of patients were in NYHA class II and the remainder were in class III, 52% of patients had ischaemic heart disease, and the mean QRS duration was 112 ms. With a median follow-up of 45.5 months, the mortality rate in the placebo group was 36.1% at 5 years or 7.2% per year. ICD therapy reduced all-cause mortality by 23% at 5 years.

As a result of these trials and other primary prevention trials, as occurred after MADIT I and MUSTT, the rate of ICD implantation is expected to increase significantly in the United States. However, in Europe the impact of these studies is still questionable. Although the incidence of SCD and survival rates are similar in the US and in Western Europe, the implantation rate in Europe is still markedly lower: whereas in 2001 the implantation rate was 208 per 1 million inhabitants in USA, in Europe it was 44 per million. According to the Medtronic Implantation Register, 50% of implants in the US and 23% of implants in Germany were for primary prevention. Undoubtedly the publication of the MADIT II trial has modified the indication for ICD implantation, but, if we compare the percentage of implantations between US and Europe, the impact seems to be geographically variable.

The next data must be considered with some caution since owing to the lack of national and transnational databases only partial information is available. In Germany only 8% of ICDs were implanted on the basis of a MADIT II indication (Guidant Implantation Records). In 2003, primary prevention, including patients fulfilling the MADIT II criteria, represented 10% of a total of 1500 ICD implantations reported to the National ICD Database in Spain. In our institution only 12% of implants performed during 2004 were due to MADIT II indications.

Detailed screening of postinfarction patients suggests that more than 1000 patients per year should meet the MADIT II criteria just in Spain [6]. According to these data only a minority of patients who fulfill the MADIT II criteria are receiving an ICD. Why this imbalance between suitable candidates and treated patients? There are several possible reasons:

1. Current guidelines do not consider a single trial, such as MADIT II, enough evidence for a class I indication.

2. Although MADIT II scores over MADIT I and MUSTT by avoiding complex, time-consuming, and expensive screening processes for candidates, the results of the latter two trials were markedly superior. Both showed a 55% reduction in total mortality and a 75% reduction in SCD. In MUSTT, there was an absolute reduction of SCD of 23%. This meant that three devices had to be implanted to save one life. Cost-effectiveness analyses of these studies suggested a cost of $16 000 to $22 000 per year of life saved – an extremely cost-effective result. In MADIT II there was no significant effect on mortality during the first year of follow-up; moreover, the absolute risk reduction was 5.6%. Therefore, in this trial around 18 ICDs are needed to save a life. In agreement with these observations, we have reported that despite their having a lower LVEF, MADIT II patients have a lower incidence of ventricular tachycardia (VT) and sustained VT than do MUSTT/MADIT I patients. No differences were found between MUSTT patients and secondary prevention patients [7].

3. In the SCD-HeFT trial all-cause mortality at 5 years was reduced by only 23% in the ICD group compared with placebo. The trial suggests that only about one patient in 10 will benefit from an ICD over 3–5 years. Moreover, the ICD benefit seems to be concentrated in patients from Canada and New Zealand, who had a 63% reduction in mortality, compared to an 18% reduction in mortality in US patients.

Conclusions

The MADIT II study and the SCD-HeFT studies suggest that the ICD reduces total mortality in patients with patients with LV dysfunction. However, the cost-effectiveness of this treatment makes it far from affordable. Better selection of patients that could benefit from an ICD might increase the cost-effectiveness and decrease the percentage of patients in whom an ICD will only produce inappropriate discharges and other undesirable effects. Subgroup analysis has demonstrated a progressive increase in effectiveness of the ICD as QRS duration increases. Little benefit was derived in patients with a QRS of less than 0.12 s, whereas if a QRS duration of 0.15 s was used as a cut-off, a marked reduction in SCD was observed, comparable to that in MUSTT and MADIT I. Similarly, in the SCD-HeFT trial the relative benefits of ICD therapy appeared greater in patients with NYHA class II heart failure, the group in which sudden death is expected to predominate. There seemed to be no benefit in patients with NYHA class III heart failure.

References

1. Moss AJ, Hall WJ, Cannom DS et al (1966) Improved survival with an implanted defibrillator in patients with coronary artery disease at high risk for ventricular arrhythmia. N Engl J Med 335:1933–1940
2. Buxton AE, Lee KL, Fisher JD et al (1999) A randomized study of the prevention of sudden death in patients with coronary artery disease. N Engl J Med 341:1882–1890
3. Moss AJ, Zareba W, Hall WJ et al, for the Multicenter Automatic Defibrillator Implantation Trial II Investigators (2002) Prophylactic implantation of a defibrillator in patients with myocardial infarction and reduced ejection fraction. N Engl J Med 346:877–883
4. Bardy GH, Lee KL, Mark DB et al (2004) Sudden Cardiac Death–Heart Failure Trial (SCD-HeFT). Paper presented at American College of Cardiology Annual Scientific Sessions, New Orleans 2004–Late Breaking Trial; 7–10 March 2004, New Orleans, LA
5. Reynolds MR, Josephson ME (2003) MADIT II (second Multicenter Automated Defibrillator Implantation Trial) debate: risk stratification, costs, and public policy. Circulation 108:1779–1783
6. Marti Almor J, Delclos Baulies M, Delclos Urges J et al (2004) Prevalence and clinical course of patients in Spain with acute myocardial infarction and severely depressed ejection fraction who meet the criteria for automatic defibrillator implantation. Rev Esp Cardiol 57:705-708
7. Ortiz M, Arenal A, González-Torrecilla E et al (2004) El desfibrilador automático implantable en la prevención primaria de la muerte súbita. ¿Existen diferencias entre los pacientes según los criterios de selección? Rev Esp Cardiol 57 (Suppl 2):141

Short QT: The Novel Gaita Syndrome?

F. Gaita[1], C. Giustetto[1], F. Di Monte[1], R. Schimpf[2], C. Wolpert[2], M. Borggrefe[2]

Ventricular fibrillation is the main cause of sudden death. It may occur in subjects with known heart disease, but also in subjects with an apparently normal heart. In the last 50 years inherited heart conditions have been described which may cause sudden death in the absence of heart disease. They share the common feature of being caused by genes encoding defective ion channel proteins. In most of the cases the diagnosis may be made from the 12-lead electrocardiogram. The most studied is long QT syndrome, described for the first time by Jervell and Lange-Nielsen [1] at the end of the 1950s and characterised by a long QTc interval at 12-lead ECG. During the last few decades the literature on long QT has constantly increased (even if in the first 10 years only 25 cases were described), while short QT has been substantially ignored. Algra et al. [2], however, in 1993 reported that in a group of 6693 patients who underwent 24-h Holter monitoring, a mean QTc < 400 ms was related to a two-fold risk of sudden death compared to an intermediate QTc value (400–440 ms) and similarly to patients with a mean QTc > 440 ms.

Only recently has the association between short QT interval and sudden death [3] on the one hand and atrial fibrillation [4] and short QT interval on the other been recognised and short QT syndrome identified as a genetic disorder [5, 6]. In 2003 our group established the relation between short QT and sudden death with the description of two families having a short QT interval at ECG and several cases of sudden death in the family history [3]. Factors that shorten the QT interval include an increase in heart rate, hyperthermia, increased calcium or potassium plasma levels, acidosis, and alterations of the autonomic tone. Secondary causes of transient QT interval

[1]Divisione di Cardiologia, Ospedale Civile, Asti, Italy; [2]1st Department of Medicine, University Hospital Mannheim, University of Heidelberg, Germany

reduction were ruled out in these patients. This alteration of the repolarisation was documented in all available ECGs recorded at different time points and ages, with a QT interval always less than 300 ms (Fig. 1), without significant dynamic changes during heart rate variations or on exertion. A QT interval constantly below 300 ms was proposed to define short QT.

Patients with short QT syndrome present with a wide spectrum of clinical manifestations, ranging from mild symptoms such as palpitations and dizziness to syncope and sudden death. Sudden death may occur at any time during life, sometimes in children in the first months of life. Sudden death is often the first clinical presentation. Syncope and palpitations with documentation of atrial fibrillation even at a young age and of ventricular extrasystoles are other symptoms related to short QT syndrome. In the observed patients invasive and non-invasive evaluation confirmed structurally normal hearts, and autopsies did not reveal any cardiac disease.

To understand how a short QT interval may be related to life-threatening arrhythmias, we have to consider that QT interval is the electrocardiographic expression of ventricular repolarisation, and there is a constant relationship between the ventricular effective refractory period (ERP) and the QT interval. At electrophysiological study these patients show very short atrial and ventricular ERPs. The duration of the refractory periods of the myocardium is known to be an important parameter for the vulnerability of the heart to fibrillation at both atrial and ventricular levels.

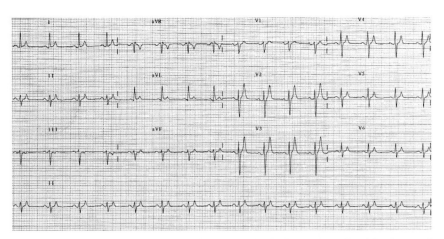

Fig. 1. Twelve-lead ECG of a 31-year-old patient who had experienced palpitations and presyncope. Sinus rhythm; heart rate 96 bpm; normal atrioventricular conduction; left axis deviation; narrow, tall, and peaked T waves in V2–V3; QT interval 220 ms; QTc 270 ms

Sudden death in the presence of short QT interval occurred in several generations in the described families, in both male and female subjects, suggesting an autosomal dominant mode of inheritance. Ventricular repolarisation is determined by the properties and the equilibrium of the inward sodium and calcium currents and of the outward potassium currents. The molecular substrate of short QT interval and related arrhythmic events should thus be either a factor that reduces sodium or calcium inward currents or a factor that increases potassium outward currents. Two different missense mutations were first identified in HERG (KCNH2), the gene encoding for the rapidly activating delayed rectifier potassium channel, I_{Kr}, causing a gain of function in the channel [5]. Subsequently, congenital short QT was linked also to a mutation in KCNQ1 (KvLQT1), causing a gain of function in I_{Ks}, the slowly activating delayed rectifier potassium current [6].

Because of the high incidence of sudden cardiac death and the absence of known drug therapy, placement of an implantable cardioverter–defibrillator (ICD) is presently the first-choice therapy [2, 7]. ICD implantation, however, is not feasible in every patient. For this reason we administered various anti-arrhythmic drugs to patients with short QT syndrome to evaluate whether they could prolong the QT interval into the normal range and thus potentially prevent symptoms and arrhythmia recurrences [8]. As the mutations found in our first families increase the activity of I_{Kr}, leading to heterogeneous abbreviation of action potential duration and refractoriness, the first drugs we administered were the class III anti-arrhythmic agents sotalol and ibutilide, which are selective I_{Kr} blockers. However, these drugs did not prolong the QT interval. The mutation must cause the loss of some of the physiological regulatory mechanisms, and I_{Kr} become no longer sensitive to drugs that normally have a specific action on it. Quinidine, on the other hand, produced a marked prolongation of the QT interval, which then entered the normal range, and of ventricular ERPs, preventing induction of ventricular fibrillation. Furthermore, quinidine treatment produced the appearance of an obvious ST segment and of broader T waves. The effect of quinidine may be explained by the fact that this drug has a widespread effect of blocking the potassium currents; besides acting on I_{Kr}, it also blocks the slow component of the delayed rectifier potassium current (I_{Ks}), the inward rectifier (I_{Ki}), the ATP-sensitive potassium channel (I_{KATP}), and the transient outward potassium current (I_{to}). This finding is particularly important because these patients are at risk of sudden death from birth, and ICD implant is not feasible in very young children. Moreover, quinidine therapy could be proposed to patients who refuse an ICD or to those who are getting frequent shocks from the device to limit ICD intervention, and in the prevention of atrial fibrillation episodes. Long-term follow-up of patients with ICD who receive quinidine, however, is needed to clarify whether this drug may be an alternative to ICD implantation.

In conclusion, short QT syndrome is an autosomal dominant genetic disorder with a high incidence of sudden death. Short QT should always be considered in the presence of a family history of sudden death, but also in patients with idiopathic atrial fibrillation and in patients with syncope and a structurally normal heart.

References

1. Jervell A, Lange-Nielsen F (1957) Congenital deaf-mutism, functional heart disease with prolongation of the QT interval and sudden death. Am Heart J 54:59–68
2. Algra A, Tijssen JGP, Roelandt JRTC et al (1993) QT interval variables from 24 hour electrocardiography and the two year risk of sudden death. Br Heart J 70:43–48
3. Gaita F, Giustetto C, Bianchi F et al (2003) Short QT syndrome. A familial cause of sudden death. Circulation 108:965–970
4. Gussak I, Brugada P, Brugada J et al (2000) Idiopathic short QT interval: a new clinical syndrome? Cardiology 94:99–102
5. Brugada P, Hong K, Dumaine R et al (2004) Sudden death associated with short QT syndrome linked to mutations in HERG. Circulation 109:30–35
6. Bellocq C, van Ginneken A, Bezzina C et al (2004) Mutation in the KCNQ1 gene leading to the short QT-interval syndrome. Circulation 109:2394–2397
7. Schimpf R, Wolpert C, Bianchi F et al (2003) Congenital short QT syndrome and implantable cardioverter defibrillator. Inherent risk for inappropriate shock delivery. J Cardiovasc Electrophysiol 14:1273–11277
8. Gaita F, Giustetto C, Bianchi F et al (2004) Short QT syndrome: pharmacological treatment. J Am Coll Cardiol 43:1294–1299

Remote Patient Management of ICD: Of What Value Is It in Clinical Practice?

S. SERMASI, M. MARCONI, M. MEZZETTI, G. PIOVACCARI

Introduction

The benefits of the implantable cardioverter-defibrillator (ICD) have been established in the primary and secondary prevention of ventricular arrhythmias and sudden cardiac death. Patients with ICDs require regular monitoring to ensure that the implanted device is working appropriately. At present monitoring is undertaken at a pacemaker centre with equipment and experienced staff. The number of ICD implantations is growing rapidly, underlining the necessity of developing new methods for patient- and doctor-friendly control of their function. The standard follow-up protocol for patients who have received ICDs includes a first outpatient check-up 1 month after implantation and a quarterly device interrogation by radiotelemetry [1]. If patients experience any problems between check-up visits that may be related to the device, they generally have to return to the device clinic.

Most published studies demonstrated a cumulative incidence of adequate ICD-delivered therapy ranging from 20% to over 60% depending on the duration of follow-up (6 months to 4 years) [2–4]. In our experience, 73% of ICD patients implanted in secondary prevention and 42% in primary prevention received appropriate ICD therapy during a 5-year and 4-year follow-up respectively. The Canadian Implantable Defibrillator Study (CIDS), during an 11-year follow-up, showed that 70% of the ICD group had appropriate therapy [appropriate shock or appropriate antitachycardia pacing (ATP)] and 50% received inappropriate therapy, including ATP, one shock or more inappropriate shocks [5]. This cause a high number of event-related or symptom-related visits to add to routinely scheduled follow-up visits.

Operative Unit of Cardiology, Infermi Hospital, Department of Cardiovascular Diseases, AUSL Rimini, Italy

Based on the manufacturer's analysis and/or device interrogation, 72% of death events in ICD patients were associated with malfunctioning ICDs, leads, or both [6]. ICD follow-up systems should include methods that can identify defects before they cause catastrophic events.

In addition, patients who have received ICDs often need to be re-programmed several times on the basis of changes in their clinical status or concomitant anti-arrhythmic therapy that successfully modifies the frequency and recurrence of ventricular arrhythmias.

Efforts are being made to introduce remote device-based monitoring systems that can wirelessly transmit device information from the patient to the pacemaker clinic. Besides the money saving in healthcare costs by reducing outpatient visits and emergency admissions, the opportunity to follow the patient over an uninterrupted time period should improve patient care [7]. In addition, so much information, significantly increasing the communication between physician and patient, is useful for patients who may have concerns about the device or their cardiac health: this too contributes to improving patients' quality of life.

Available Technologies

Home Monitoring (HM) Service

Chiodi has described technical characteristics and some clinical benefits of the HM Service (Biotronik GmbH & Co., Berlin, Germany) [8]. This system uses an implanted chip that transmits diagnostic data from the ICD to a modified GSM mobile phone unit. The ICD is able to send the data over a distance of about 2.5 m to the receiver. The receiver, which is battery powered, can be placed in the loading tray beside the patient or can be carried around with him. The information transmitted includes the number of ventricular tachyarrhythmias detected in each different monitor zone and ATP and shock therapies delivered, besides data about battery voltage, pacing and shock impedance, and device status. The message is then forwarded as an encrypted short message via the standard SMS procedure to the remote Service Centre, i.e. the central data processing unit to which all implant data are sent. Data are generated and transmitted either at set times (automatically every 24 h), following an event (the termination detection after treatment), or as a patient-triggered message. At the Service Centre incoming messages are automatically decrypted, the contents are collected into a database, and a Cardio Report is then sent to the physician in charge of the patient. The entire process takes a few minutes and requires no involvement on the patient's part.

Several studies have been performed to explore the clinical benefits of

HM technology in patients who have received Biotronik ICDs [9–11]. Elsner et al. published an interim analysis of the collected data from 177 ICD patients followed for 232 ± 109 days [12]. On the basis of daily HM information, ventricular tachyarrhythmias were detected in 39% of patients, 36% of whom received ICD therapy. Detected arrhythmias included 550 ventricular tachycardia (VT) and 239 ventricular fibrillation (VF) episodes. Nine hundred and eighty-five ATP attempts were documented in 34 patients, with a mean success rate of 70.2% (one or more attempts). Three hundred and thirty-two shock therapies were initiated in 53 patients, 200 of which were aborted. The preliminary report from the WAMMI study [13] provided interim data analysis in 180 ICD patients who were followed for a mean of 9 months. Two hundred and fifty-two episodes of VT or VF were detected via HM, 98 of which were terminated by programmed ATP and 58 by shock. Additional reports have focused on the use of the HM Service to evaluate effects of drugs or to detect supraventricular tachyarrhythmias or lead/device defects [14–16].

Continuous monitoring of device-delivered therapies as soon as they occur, appropriate or inappropriate, their success rate, and the incidence of relevant tachyarrhythmias may contribute to optimising how the device can work to help modifying programming and drug therapy. Furthermore, the HM Service may allow prompt detection of lead- or ICD-related technical failures which can be catastrophic to the patient [17].

CareLink Patient Management Network

The CareLink (CL) monitoring and software package (Medtronic Inc., Minneapolis, Minn., USA) allows the physician to collect data via a website from patients with implanted Medtronic ICDs. The CL includes a portable monitor used by patients to self-interrogate their ICD. The data are automatically downloaded by the monitor and sent through a standard telephone connection, directly to the secure Medtronic CL Network where doctors view and analyse patient device data stored on the server [18]. The transmission includes all data within the device memory: stored episodes, device parameters, and diagnostics. A 10-s rhythm electrogram is available at the time of the interrogation. Clinicians access their patients' data by logging onto the clinician website from any internet-connected PC, and patients can also view information about their device and condition on their own personal website [19].

In the CareLink trial 59 patients from 10 follow-up clinics across the United States completed 119 transmissions [18]. Review of the data transmissions revealed several clinically relevant findings such as asymptomatic episodes of paroxysmal atrial fibrillation, atrial sensing failures, and VT. The quality of the web-accessed data was comparable to that of in-office device interrogation. As a result, patients enjoy a timely and convenient connection to their care team and physicians may offer better patient care besides an improvement in the cost-effectiveness of clinic operations.

Housecall Plus Remote Patient Monitoring System

The Housecall Plus (HP; St. Jude Medical Co., Sylmar, Calif., USA) is a monitoring system to transmit complex ICD data: a full, in-office, programmer-based interrogation (electrograms, surface ECGs, delivered therapies and stored electrogram, etc.) in real time over standard telephone lines directly from patient to medical professional [20]. The patient must hold a transmitter over the ICD and the telephone is placed in a special cradle. Information is transmitted to a processing centre and then compiled and sent to the physician. During a 12-month study [21], 570 transmissions were received, revealing 54 delivered ICD therapies, 22 aborted therapies, and 30 episodes of non-sustained ventricular arrhythmias. In addition, 32 instances of trouble with the ICD or with the leads connected to the heart were revealed. Patients consider the transtelephonic ICD follow-up provided by HP satisfactory and easy to use, reducing the number of device clinic visits for routine follow-up and unwarranted trips to the emergency department.

Comment

All studies found high patient and physician satisfaction with the methods delivering remote monitoring of implanted devices. The ability to transmit information from any telephone connection means that patients have the comfort of knowing that their condition can be monitored wherever they are. Positive benefits include better use of resources including hospital-based staff, improved patient care, and the economic benefits associated with fewer unnecessary hospital admissions and patient transport costs [7]. The next step will be for these systems to allow the doctor to program the device without having the patient present [22].

References

1. Gregoratos G, Abrams J, Epstein AE et al (2002) ACC/AHA/NASPE 2002 guideline update for implantation of cardiac pacemaker and arrhythmia devices: summary article: a report of the American College of Cardiology/American Heart Association Task Force on Practice Guidelines. Circulation 106:2145–2161
2. Bunch TJ, White RD, Gersh BJ et al (2003) Long-term outcomes of out-of-hospital cardiac arrest after successful early defibrillation. N Engl J Med 348:2626–2633

3. Wolpert C, Kuschyk J, Aramin N et al (2004) Incidence and electrophysiological characteristics of spontaneous ventricular tachyarrhythmias in high risk coronary patients and prophylactic implantation of a defibrillator. Heart 90:667–671

4. Whang W, Mittleman MA, Rich DQ et al (2004) Heart failure and risk of shocks in patients with implantable cardioverter defibrillators. Results from the Triggers Of Ventricular Arrhythmias (TOVA) Study. Circulation 109:1386–1391

5. Bokhari F, Newman D, Greene M et al (2004) Long-term comparison of implantable cardioverter defibrillator versus amiodarone. Eleven-year follow-up of a subset of patients in the Canadian Implantable Defibrillator Study (CIDS). Circulation 110:112–116

6. Hauser R (2004) Implantable cardioverter defibrillator failure associated with death in the US. Food and Drug Administration database. In: ESC Congress, Munich, abstract vol 2, p 254

7. The National Horizon Scanning Center (2003) New and emerging technology briefing. Remote monitoring of implantable cardiac devices. July 2003. Dept of Public Health and Epidemiology. University of Birmingham, Birmingham, England, www.publichealth.bham.ac.uk/horizon

8. Chiodi L (2002) The home monitoring technology in implantable-cardioverter defibrillator therapy. In: M. Santini (ed) Progress in clinical pacing. CEPI-AIM Group, Rome (CD-ROM)

9. Wallbruck K, Stellbink C, Santini M et al (2002) The value of permanent follow-up of implantable pacemakers. First results of an European trial. Biomed Tech 47(Suppl 1):950–953

10. Stellbrink C, Gill S, Santini M et al (2003) Feasibility of remote monitoring of pacemakers with the help of home monitoring. Pacing Clin Electrophysiol 26(2 Part II):S444 (abstract)

11. Barbaro V, Bartolini P, Calcagnini G et al (2003) Evaluation of electromagnetic interference between wireless home monitoring pacemakers and GSM mobile phones: in-vitro and in-vivo studies. Pacing Clin Electrophysiol 26 (2 Part II):S447 (abstract)

12. Elsner CH, Dorszewsky A, Kottkamp H et al (2003) Can telemetric home monitoring of implantable defibrillators increase the treatment's cost-effectiveness ratio? IEEE J Comput Cardiol 30:193–197

13. Sauberman RB, Hsu W, Machado CB et al (2004) Technical performance and clinical benefit of remote wireless monitoring of implantable cardioverter defibrillators. Heart Rhythm 1(Suppl 1): S215 (abstract)

14. Brugada P et al (2003) Home monitoring technology for improved patient management in ICD therapy. Pacing Clin Electrophysiol 26(2 Part II):S126 (abstract)

15. Igidbashan D, Gill S, Santini M et al (2003) Remote documentation of effects of medication in patients with implantable home monitoring pacemakers. Pacing Clin Electrophysiol 26 (2 Part II):S63 (abstract)

16. Scholten MF, Thornton AS, Theuns DA et al (2004) Twiddler's syndrome detected by home monitoring device. Pacing Clin Electrophysiol 27:1151–1152

17. Theuns DA, Jordaens LJ (2003) Home monitoring in ICD therapy: future perspectives. Europace 5:139–142

18. Schoenfeld MH, Compton SJ, Mead RH et al (2004) Remote monitoring of implantable cardioverter defibrillators: a prospective analysis. Pacing Clin Electrophysiol 27:747–763

19. Medtronic News Release, April 2003. http://www.medtronic.com

BLSD Prevention of Sudden Death: What Is the Difference Between Lay People and Medical Professionals?

M. Santomauro[1], N. Monteforte[1], C. Riganti[2], E. Febbraro[1], C. Liguori[1], A. Costanzo[1], L. D'Agostino Di Salvatore[1], A. Casafina[1], M. Chiariello[1]

Sudden death (SD) is a real concern for medicine today, especially as it can occur in people with no signs of disease at all. It can be the first symptom of an underlying problem. The substrate for cardiac arrest is ventricular fibrillation (VF) or tachycardia (VT) in about 75% of cases, bradyarrhythmias in 20%, and atrioventricular dissociation in 5%. In the United States, more than 350 000 new cases of cardiac arrest are recorded annually, while in Italy it strikes more than 60 000 people every year, with a 10% overall mortality, 20% of this in people with no signs of disease at all. Survival to hospital discharge after out-of-hospital cardiac arrest (OHCA) remains poor, generally only in the 5% to 20% range, from the best of emergency response centres. The chances of surviving a cardiac arrest are strongly dependent on the speed of intervention and, especially, on correct execution of the four fundamental operations that represent the 'chain of survival'. The first step is activation of the emergency system, if the patient is unconscious, immediately followed by basic cardiopulmonary resuscitation known as 'basic life support' (BLS) [1–4], which consists of sequences of chest compression and artificial ventilation. Defibrillation, the third step (BLSD), is the only treatment that can stop VF/VT, while advanced cardiac life support (ACLS) is the last step, all according the ILCOR and AHA Guidelines 2000 [2, 5].

Since its discovery, external defibrillation has been the cornerstone of emergency cardiac care (ECC) and the principal intervention in most successful resuscitations from full cardiac arrest. The most effective intervention for VF is rapid defibrillation. In certain environments, survival rates can approach 80–100% when defibrillation is achieved within the first few minutes of a cardiac arrest. Despite efforts to bolster emergency medical care by

[1]Department of Cardiology, University Federico II, Naples; [2]Health Management, University Federico II, Naples, Italy

broadening training in defibrillation to include emergency medical technicians in addition to paramedics, response times for OHCA remain unacceptably long. The development in Italy of semi-automatic external defibrillators (AEDs) is due to Monteleone's law promulgated on 3 April 2001, which allows non-medical personnel to use semi-automatic defibrillators if trained. Further technological developments in recent years have made these devices more portable and simpler to use. With these improvements and the recognition that time to defibrillation is one of the most critical, if not the most important, factors in clinical outcome, AED use by laypersons has developed widespread support [6, 7]. More widespread use of AEDs may significantly affect response times to OHCA and therefore affect survival.

The AED identifies VF in cardiac arrest victims and provides the means to deliver defibrillation shocks. The operator is required neither to make judgements regarding the cardiac rhythm nor to confirm the need for defibrillator shocks. Recent advances have enhanced the ease of use of AEDs, including instructional verbal prompts, simplified displays, and icons to help in proper pad placement. An emphasis on human-factors design has simplified the steps that the user has to perform. In addition, the application of more effective low-energy biphasic waveforms to these devices as a means of energy delivery has significantly reduced their size and enhanced their portable nature. The clinical utility of biphasic waveform use in victims of OHCA has been well demonstrated. More efficient use of energy by biphasic waveform AEDs leads to smaller capacitors and batteries. This contributes to the significantly smaller overall size of the newest AEDs.

The impetus for support of the broader use of AEDs derives from observations that the single most important factor determining outcome from cardiac arrest is time to defibrillation. Providing defibrillation to a cardiac arrest victim improves survival by about 10% per minute during the first 10 min of the arrest. Use of AEDs by trained lay people has been shown to improve survival from OHCA. Likewise, use of AEDs in OHCA by medical professionals has significantly improved response times and yielded survival rates as high as 58%. Even if lay people can be trained effectively to the use of AED, they cannot use the manual defibrillator as the medical practitioner does, and showed a longer time of utilisation for the defibrillation than the time spent by the medical practitioner (Fig. 1). Moreover, recently a completely automatic trainer defibrillator has been introduced that allows us to train lay people in the use of the new device. Anyway Monteleone's law mentions only the use of AEDs and not about the automatic one, which by contrast can be used by the medical practitioner. Moreover, the AHA has recently approved the use of defibrillator even for children between 1 and 8 years, using the specific paediatric patches.

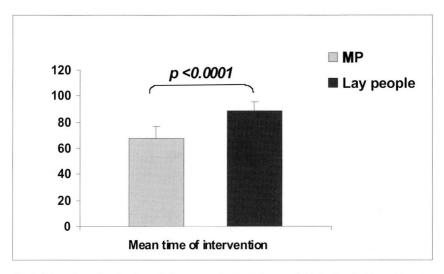

Fig. 1. Time from beginning of the scenario to delivery of AED shock. Mean time to defibrillation was 88 ± 7 s for lay people and 67 ± 9 s for the medical professionals (MP)

Undoubtedly, many public arenas exist in which response times by trained medical personnel may be unacceptably long. The AHA estimates that wider use of AEDs by first-line responders could avert 20 000 to 100 000 deaths per year. Several studies show that AEDs can be used safely and effectively by rescuers with minimal or no previous training in their use, although speed, compliance, and safety can still be improved. These studies support the idea that the use by citizens of publicly accessible AEDs is feasible, and that organised AED training should also focus on community responders and on-site responders. The initial programmes on the use of AEDs by people other than medical professionals involved community responders such as police officers and fire-fighters [8–11]. More recently data have become available from studies based on on-site schemes in which AEDs have been placed in strategic locations such as airports and casinos, or a hybrid approach with on-site AED location plus involvement of community responders [12–15]. Several studies suggest that a tiered response system increases survival rates even if it reduces the time to shock only by 1 or 2 min [16, 17]. Overall survival rates in the various studies vary from less than 3% to over 50%. Time to shock varies remarkably among studies, ranging approximately from an estimated 2 to 11 min.

In seeking a reduction of the time from the onset of VF to defibrillation, deployment of AEDs in public places is a very attractive option. Two large-scale observational studies involving airlines have been carried out [13–17].

Both studies reported remarkable results for treatment of witnessed VF, with greater than 55% survival, and confirmed that time to shock is a major determinant of success. However, a high incidence of unwitnessed cardiac arrest and non-shockable rhythms also occur. Identification and training of the medical practitioner, community, on-site, and home responders should be guided by analysis of the local environment.

A new area of debate centres on whether cardiopulmonary resuscitation (CPR) is an important component of training for rescuers who are not healthcare professionals. Some studies indicate that survival can increase when rescuers use an AED without delivery of BLS [18]. However, other studies show that BLS can increase survival significantly if combined with early defibrillation [19]. Some authors, however, have not questioned the potential value but rather the feasibility of CPR undertaken by lay people. Concern has been raised about reluctance among lay people to perform CPR on a stranger using mouth-to-mouth ventilation due to aversion or fear of infection. Therefore concern exists that linking CPR administration to defibrillation may limit the acceptance of AEDs. The use of chest compressions only as a substitute for CPR may represent an acceptable alternative for lay people, but this needs further research.

In conclusion, AEDs have developed concurrently with our understanding of time to defibrillation as a crucial factor determining the outcome of cardiac arrest [20–23]. Historically, the complexity and size of AEDs dictated that they could be used only by trained medical professionals. Recent technological developments and emphasis on human-factors design have made these devices much more portable and straightforward to use. These factors have supported the notion of a broader use of AEDs, including by lay persons. The absolute differences between lay people and medical professionals, however, were small and may be of little clinical relevance. Furthermore, lay subjects demonstrated proficiency in electrode placement and safety precautions with the AED system used. These findings suggest that use of this AED by untrained lay people may be feasible. The utility of a simplified training program may be in helping a user perform under the pressure and anxiety of an actual emergency rather than learning a complex operational task. Otherwise it is very important that a BLSD course also includes CPR technique.

References

1. American Heart Association (1992) Guidelines for cardiopulmonary resuscitation and emergency cardiac care, part I: Introduction. JAMA 268:2171–2183
2. American Heart Association in collaboration with the International Liaison Committee on Resuscitation (ILCOR) (2000) Guidelines 2000 for cardiopulmonary

resuscitation and emergency cardiovascular care. An international consensus on science. Circulation 102(Suppl I):I-l-I-384

3. Handley JH, Monsieurs KG, Bossaert LL (2001) European Resuscitation Council guidelines 2000 for adult basic life support. Resuscitation 48:199–205

4. Monsieurs KG, Handley JH, Bossaert LL (2001) European Resuscitation Council guidelines 2000 for automated external defibrillation. Resuscitation 48:207–209

5. Robertson C, Steen P, Adgey J et al (1998) The European Resuscitation Council guidelines for advanced life support. Resuscitation 37:81–90

6. Cummins RO, Doherty A, Hein K et al (1997) Teaching citizens to use an AED during the AHA HeartSaver course: active vs passive learning and long-term retention of skills. Circulation 96(Suppl I):I365

7. Priori SG, Bossaert LL, Chamberlain DA et al (2004) Policy conference: ESC–ERC recommendations for the use of automated external defibrillators (AEDs) in Europe. Eur Heart J 3:1–9

8. Cummins RO, Hazinski MF, Kerber RE et al (1998) Low-energy biphasic waveform defibrillation: evidence-based review applied to emergency cardiovascular care guidelines. Circulation 97:1654–1667

9. Tunstall-Pedoe H, Bailey L, Chamberlain DA et al (1992) Survey of 3765 cardiopulmonary resuscitations in British hospitals (the BRESUS study): methods and overall results. BMJ 304:1347–1351

10. Fromm RE Jr, Varon J (1997) Automated external versus blind manual defibrillation by untrained lay rescuers. Resuscitation 33:219–221

11. Myerburg RJ, Fenster J, Velez M et al (2002) Impact of community-wide police car deployment of automated external defibrillators on survival from out-of-hospital cardiac arrest. Circulation 106:1058–1064

12. Caffrey SL, Willoughby PJ, Pepe PE et al (2002) Public use of automated external defibrillators. N Engl J Med 347:1242–1247

13. Page RL, Joglar JA, Kowal RC, et al (2000) Use of automated external defibrillators by a US airline. N Engl J Med 343:1210–1216

14. Davies CS, Colquhoun M, Graham S et al (2002) Defibrillators in public places: the introduction of a national scheme for public access defibrillation in England. Resuscitation 52:13–21

15. Valenzuela TD, Roe DJ, Nichol G et al (2000) Outcomes of rapid defibrillation by security officers after cardiac arrest in casinos. N Engl J Med 343:1206–1209

16. Van Alem AP, Vrenken RH, de Vos R et al (2004) Use of automated external defibrillator by first responders in out-of-hospital cardiac arrest: prospective controlled trial. BMJ 328:396

17. Stotz M, Albrecht R, Zwicker G et al (2003) EMS defibrillation-first policy may not improve outcome in out-of-hospital cardiac arrest. Resuscitation 58:277–282

18. Capucci A, Aschieri D, Piepoli MF et al (2002) Tripling survival from sudden cardiac arrest via early defibrillation without traditional education in cardiopulmonary resuscitation. Circulation 106:1065–1070

19. Wik L, Hansen TB, Fylling F et al (2003) Delaying defibrillation to give basic cardiopulmonary resuscitation to patients with out-of-hospital ventricular fibrillation: a randomized trial. JAMA 289:1389–1395

20. Santomauro M, Ottaviano L, D'Ascia C et al (2002) Sudden cardiac death prevention through hospital early defibrillation: Naples experience. Ital Heart J 1(Suppl 1):92–95

21. Santomauro M, Ottaviano L, Borrelli A et al (2002) Organization Project for Early

Semiautomatic in Hospital Defibrillation (Heart Project). Progress in Clinical Pacing, Rome, 3–6 December 2002, p 46

22. Santomauro M, Ottaviano L, Borrelli A et al (2003) Sudden cardiac death prevention through hospital early defibrillation. Naples experience. Pacing Clin Electrophysiol 26:S186

23. Santomauro M, Ottaviano L, Borrelli A et al (2003) Organization Project for Precocious Semiautomatic in Hospital Defibrillation (Naples Heart Project). In: Gulizia M (ed), New Advances in Heart Failure and Atrial Fibrillation, Springer Milan, pp 139–149

ACC/ESC Recommendations for the Clinical Management of Hypertrophic Cardiomyopathy: A Practical Perspective

P. Delise, M. Bocchino, L. Sciarra, E. Marras, N. Sitta, L. Coro', E. Moro

In November 2003 the American College of Cardiology (ACC) and the European Society of Cardiology (ESC) published in the *Journal of the American College of Cardiology* an expert consensus document on hypertrophic cardiomyopathy (HCM) to inform practitioners about the state of the art in managing this particular disease [1]. HCM is a genetic disease which can cause sudden cardiac death (SCD), particularly in young people (including athletes). As HCM is uncommon (1:500 in the general population) [2], many cardiologists do not see many patients with this disease, and may therefore have some difficulty in managing the cases of the patients they do see.

This document has been written by specialists with extensive experience of managing HCM. However, the statements and treatment strategies put forward by the panel are very cautious owing to the considerable difficulties involved in reaching conclusions: (1) because the disease is uncommon, the available data are relatively limited; (2) HCM has a broad disease spectrum, so individual patients may have very different risk profiles; (3) large-scale controlled and randomised study designs (as in coronary artery disease) are not available. Consequently most information derives from non-randomised and retrospective studies.

Genetics and Phenotypic Expression of the Disease

HCM is inherited as a mendelian autosomal dominant trait and is caused by mutations in any one of 10 genes, each encoding protein components of cardiac sarcomere composed of thick or thin filaments with contractile, struc-

Division of Cardiology, Hospital of Conegliano (Treviso), Italy

tural, or regulatory functions [3]. This genetic diversity is compounded by intragenic heterogeneity, with about 200 mutations now identified, most of which are missense, with a single amino acid residue substituted by another [4]. The molecular defects responsible for HCM are usually different in unrelated individuals. The phenotypic expression of HCM is the product not only of the mutation itself but also of modifier genes and environmental factors [5]. These factors account for the phenotypic variability of affected individuals even in the same family, carrying identical disease-causing mutations.

There is increasing recognition of the role of genetics in the genesis of the electrophysiological abnormalities associated with left ventricular hypertrophy (LVH) such as atrial fibrillation (AF) [6], Wolf-Parkinson-White (WPW), or heart block [7]. Furthermore, particular mutant genes seem to be associated with a particularly high risk of sudden death [3].

Not all individuals harbouring a genetic defect will express the clinical features of HCM at all times during life. In fact there is no minimal LV wall thickness required to be consistent with the presence of an HCM-causing mutant gene [2, 8]. It is common for children less than 13 yeas old to be 'silent' mutation carriers without evidence of LVH on an echocardiogram. Most commonly the spontaneous appearance of LVH occurs during the adolescent years, with the morphological expression usually complete at the time of physical maturity, about 17-18 years of age [9]. Finally, some studies have demonstrated age-related penetrance and late onset of the phenotype, in which delayed and de novo appearance of LVH occurs in mid-life and even later [10].

Laboratory DNA analysis for mutant genes is the most definitive method for establishing the diagnosis of HCM. At present, however, even in the USA [1], there are several obstacles to the translation of genetic research into practical clinical applications and routine clinical strategy.

Clinical Characteristics and Natural History of HCM

The diagnosis of HCM is easily established echocardiographically by demonstrating LVH, which is typically asymmetrical in distribution. Left ventricular wall thickening is associated with a non-dilated and hyperdynamic chamber in the absence of any other cardiac or systemic disease (e.g. hypertension).

The usual clinical diagnostic criterion for HCM is a maximum LV thickness greater than or equal to 15 mm. However, genotype–phenotype correlations have shown that virtually any wall thickness (including those within normal range) may be compatible with the presence of a HCM mutant gene [10, 11].

Patients with HCM may present with outflow obstruction under resting conditions or develop dynamic subaortic gradients in response to provocative manoeuvres (Valsalva manoeuvre, effort) or agents (isoproterenol) [11]. Obstruction may be either subaortic (caused by systolic anterior motion of the mitral valve leaflets) or mid-cavity in location. It is generally recognised that a subaortic gradient of 30 mmHg or more reflects true mechanical impedance to outflow.

The clinical course of HCM is variable; patients may remain stable over long periods of time, with up to 25% of a HCM cohort achieving normal longevity (> 75 years) [11, 12]. However, for many patients the course may be punctuated by adverse clinical events. The main adverse events are the following: (1) sudden cardiac death (SCD); (2) progressive symptoms (angina, dyspnoea, syncope) in the presence of preserved systolic function; (3) progressive congestive heart failure; (4) embolic stroke, mainly attributable to atrial fibrillation (AF).

Recent reports from non-tertiary centres, not subject to referral bias, cite annual mortality rates in the region of about 1% per year [10, 11]. For patients aged over 50 years at diagnosis, the probability of survival for 5, 10, and 15 years is 85%, 74%, and 57%, which is not significantly different from that in the general population [12]. However, there are subgroups of patients within the broad HCM spectrum with annual mortality rates exceeding 1%, in some studies as high as 6% per year [13–15].

Risk Stratification for Sudden Cardiac Death

Sudden cardiac death (SCD) may be the initial manifestation of HCM, most frequently in asymptomatic or mildly symptomatic young people [11, 16, 17]. In the USA, HCM is the most common cause of cardiovascular SCD in young athletes [18].

This devastating complication, however, is infrequent and high-risk HCM patients constitute only a minority of the overall disease population [10–15].

SCD is most frequent in adolescent and young adults (less than 35 years old). However, the risk of SCD also extends through mid-life and beyond [18, 19]. The basis of this particular predilection of SCD for the young is unresolved. The available data suggest that SCD in HCM is related to malignant ventricular arrhythmias.

Many risk markers have been identified. The highest risk for SCD has been associated with a number of factors [16, 20] (Table 1). Major factors are: (1) Prior cardiac arrest or (2) spontaneously occurring and sustained ventricular tachycardia (VT); (3) family history of premature HCM-related SCD, particularly in a close relative or multiple in occurrence; (4) unexplained syncope, particularly in the young or exertional or recurrent; (5) wall thickness > 30 mm, particularly in adolescent and young adults; (6)

Table 1. Risk factors for sudden cardiac death in HCM (ACC/ESC consensus document)

Major
Cardiac arrest (ventricular fibrillation)
Spontaneous sustained ventricular tachycardia
Family history of premature sudden death
Unexplained syncope
LV thickness ≥ 30 mm
Abnormal exercise blood pressure
Non-sustained ventricular tachycardia

Possible in individual patients
Atrial fibrillation
Myocardial ischaemia
Left ventricular outflow tract obstruction
High-risk mutation
Intense physical exertion

---

abnormal blood pressure response during upright exercise; (7) non-sustained VT on Holter monitoring of at least 120/min. Minor factors (possible in individual patients) are: (1) AF; (2) myocardial ischaemia; (3) LV outflow obstruction; (4) identification of a high-risk mutant gene; (5) intense physical exertion.

Syncope. Syncope can be a premonitory symptom of SCD. However, the sensitivity and specificity of syncope or presyncope as a predictor of SCD is low, possibly because most such events in this disease are probably not in fact secondary to arrhythmias or related to outflow obstruction. There are many potential causes of syncope in HCM, such as vagal, neurally mediated syndromes, etc. [11, 15].

Extreme LVH (>30 mm). This is observed in about 10% of patients [21]. Paradoxically, most patients with extreme LVH do not experience marked symptomatic disability. Although most patients who die suddenly have a wall thickness of less than 30 mm, extreme LVH is associated with a higher risk of SCD. Some authors suggest a substantial long-term risk in patients with a wall thickness greater than 30 mm: 20% over 10 years and 40% over 20 years (annual mortality 2%) [21]. Other investigators, however, have maintained that extreme hypertrophy is a predictor of SCD only when associated with other risk factors such as unexplained syncope, etc. [22]. On the basis of such data the ACC/ESC panel [1] suggests that, 'although it is not resolved as to whether extreme hypertrophy as a sole risk factor is sufficient to justify a recommendation for prevention of SCD with an ICD, serious consideration for such an intervention should be given to young patients'.

NSVT. Ventricular arrhythmias are a frequent feature in patients with HCM. About 90% of adults present with premature ventricular beats, which are often frequent or complex, ventricular couplets in about 40%, and NSVT in 20–30% [23]. Some authors suggest a prognostic value only for NSVT encountered in young patients, but not in adults [24].

Atrial fibrillation. AF is the most common sustained arrhythmia in HCM, occurring in 20–25% of patients [25]. AF is well tolerated in about one-third of patients and is not considered an independent determinant of SCD [26]. However, it is possible that in certain susceptible patients AF may trigger malignant ventricular arrhythmias [27]. Furthermore, paroxysmal AF may also be responsible for acute clinical deterioration with syncope or heart failure resulting from reduced diastolic filling and cardiac output. AF is independently associated with heart-failure-related death and the occurrence of fatal and non-fatal stroke [26].

Myocardial ischaemia. Chest pain may be reported both by young and adult patients. In the latter coronary artery disease may coexist with HCM. In any case, chest discomfort in HCM is probably due by bursts of myocardial ischaemia. In fact scars are frequently found at autopsy in HCM [28], while in living patients fixed or reversible myocardial perfusion defects can be documented [29]. Myocardial ischaemia is probably a consequence of abnormal microvasculature, consisting of intramural coronary arterioles with thickened walls and narrow lumen. One report suggests that short-tunnelled (bridged) intramyocardial segments of the left anterior descending coronary artery independently convey increased risk for cardiac arrest, probably mediated by myocardial ischaemia [30].

LV outflow obstruction (gradient > 30 mmHg). It is generally accepted that LV outflow obstruction can only be regarded as a minor risk factor for SCD. In fact the impact of gradient on SCD risk is not sufficiently strong to merit a role as the predominant deciding clinical parameter and the primary basis for decision to intervene with an implantable cardioverter–defibrillator (ICD) [31].

High risk mutation. It has been proposed, on the basis of genotype–phenotype correlations, that the genetic defects responsible for HCM could represent the primary determinant and stratifying marker for SCD, with specific mutations conveying either favourable or adverse prognosis [3, 4, 10]. For example, it has been suggested that some cardiac β-myosin heavy chain mutations (such as Arg403Gln and Arg719Gln) and some troponin-T mutations are associated with a higher incidence of SCD [1, 3]. However, some authors suggest that routine clinical testing has low yield [32], and the ACC/ESC panel of experts [1] state that at present 'it is premature to draw definite conclusions regarding gene-specific clinical outcomes based solely on the presence of a particular mutation'.

Electrophysiological study (EPS). Programmed ventricular stimulation is of limited value in stratifying the risk of SCD in HCM [11, 15, 33]. In contrast with post acute myocardial infarction patients, monomorphic VT is rarely induced. On the contrary, polymorphic VT and ventricular fibrillation (VF) are frequently induced by aggressive stimulation protocols even in low-risk subjects [33]. As in coronary artery disease and in dilated cardiomyopathy, the induction of polymorphic VT and/or VF is considered a non-specific finding. In sum, EPS is generally not indicated in HCM. It may have a value in patients with unexplained syncope or sustained palpitations to detect supraventricular re-entrant tachycardias or monomorphic VT.

In conclusion, several risk factors have been identified in HCM. However, most of the clinical markers of SCD risk are limited by a relatively low positive predictive value, due in part to relatively low event rates. On the other hand, these markers have a high negative predictive value (> 90%). Therefore the absence of risk factors can be used to identify patients who have a low likelihood of SCD.

Prevention of Sudden Cardiac Death

Historically, treatment strategies to reduce the risk of SCD have been predicated on the administration of drugs such as beta-blockers [11, 15, 34], verapamil [11, 34], type IA anti-arrhythmic agents (quinidine, disopyramide) [35] and, more recently, amiodarone [36, 37]. However, there is no evidence that this practice is effective in mitigating the risk of SCD. Other therapies targeted to reduce LV outflow tract obstruction have been employed, such as surgical septal myectomy, percutaneous alcohol septal ablation, and pacemaker implantation. Despite their clinical benefit, no single one of these procedures has demonstrated a favourable effect in reducing the risk of sudden death. Finally, ICD implantation has been proposed, which certainly has the ability to interrupt malignant ventricular arrhythmias, but the indications for which, owing to the difficulty of identify accurately the patients at highest risk, are in part questionable.

Beta-blockers. Beta-blockers are a preferred drug treatment strategy for symptomatic patients with outflow gradients present only during exertion. In fact there is little evidence that they reduce LV obstruction at rest. These agents lessen LV contractility and possible reduce microvascular myocardial ischaemia. They should be closely monitored in young patients because even moderate doses can affect growth, impair school performance, or trigger depression in children and adolescents [11].

Verapamil. Verapamil has been widely used empirically in the past with a reported benefit for many patients [11]. However, this drug may also harbour a potential for adverse consequences. It has been reported to cause death in a few HCM patients with severe disabling symptoms related to marked outflow obstruction [34]. Adverse haemodynamic effects are presumably the result of the vasodilating properties predominating over negative inotropic effects, causing a worsening of outflow obstruction and pulmonary hypertension up to the point of cardiogenic shock. SCD has been reported in infants as a result of intravenous administration of the drug [34].

Disopyramide. This drug was introduced for its negative inotropic effect, producing a benefit in severely limited patients by decreasing outflow obstruction and mitral regurgitant volume [35]. Disopyramide may prolong the QT interval, possibly increasing the risk of malignant ventricular arrhythmias.

Amiodarone. Some reports suggest a favourable effect of this drug on the risk of SCD [36, 37]. Amiodarone has been suggested for use as a bridging treatment in very young high-risk children intended to receive an ICD later, after sufficient growth and maturation has occurred [1]. However, its efficacy has not been proved in randomised controlled studies.

Surgical septal myectomy. Persistent, long-lasting improvement in disabling symptoms and exercise capacity has been demonstrated for this procedure [11, 15, 34, 38, 39]. The effect of surgery per se on longevity is unresolved due to the lack of controlled randomised studies. However, there is some suggestion in retrospective non-randomised studies that surgical relief of outflow obstruction in severely symptomatic patients may reduce long-term mortality and possibly SCD [40].

Percutaneous alcohol septal ablation. This treatment reduces LV outflow obstruction, although to a lesser degree than surgery [41]. The long-term effect of this procedure is unknown, because to date only relatively short follow-ups are available. As alcohol ablation produces a scar, a facilitating effect on re-entrant arrhythmias cannot be excluded. In any case, the impact of this procedure on the incidence of SCD is unresolved.

Dual-chamber pacing. A favourable effect of pacing in HCM with LV outflow obstruction has been demonstrated in randomised, cross-over, double-blind studies, although this favourable effect was less than suggested by the observational studies [42, 43]. However, there is no evidence that pacing reduces the risk of SCD.

Implantable cardioverter–defibrillator. According to the ACC/ESC expert panel [1], when the risk of SCD is judged to be unacceptably high, the ICD is the most effective and reliable treatment. Randomised controlled studies in HCM (such as in post acute myocardial infarction or heart failure patients) are not available. Only one multi-centre retrospective study is available, conducted in high-risk patients who underwent ICD implantation for secondary or primary prevention of SCD [44]. In this study, appropriate device interventions occurred at a rate of 11% per year in secondary prevention and 5% per year for primary prevention. In the latter case, it must be emphasised that patients were generally asymptomatic or mildly symptomatic and were implanted on the basis of common non-invasive risk factors (syncope, family history of SCD, LVH > 30 mm, etc.).

The ICD is strongly warranted for secondary prevention of SCD in patients with spontaneous episodes of cardiac arrest and/or VT (class I according to ACC/AHA/NASPE and ESC guidelines) [20, 45].

Because of the low positive predictive value of any single risk factor, ICD implantation for primary prevention is questionable. The ACC/AHA/NASPE 2002 guidelines designated the ICD for primary prevention of SCD as a class IIb indication [45]. In 2001, the ESC Task Force on Sudden Cardiac Death [20] suggested categorising ICD for primary prevention as a class IIa indication in the presence of multiple major risk factors.

The ACC/ESC expert panel [1] suggests managing patients on an individual basis in clinical practice, taking into account the overall clinical profile including age, the strength of the risk factor identified, and the potential complications, largely related to lead systems and to inappropriate device discharges. Among risk factors, a family history of SCD in close relatives and LVH > 3 mm in subjects less than 35 years old are suggested to be strongly considered in deciding about ICD implantation.

References

1. Maron BJ, McKenna WJ, Danielson GK et al (2003) ACC/ESC clinical expert consensus document on hypertrophic cardiomyopathy: a report of the American College of Cardiology Task Force on Clinical Experts Consensus Documents and the European Society of Cardiology Committee for Practice Guidelines. J Am Coll Cardiol 42:687–713
2. Maron BJ, Gardin JM, Flack JM et al (1995) Prevalence of hypertrophic cardiomyopathy in a general population of young adults. Echocardiographic analysis of 4111 subjects in the CARDIA Study. Circulation 92:785–789
3. Maron BJ, Moller JH, Seidman CE et al (1998) Impact of laboratory molecular diagnosis on contemporary diagnostic criteria for genetically transmitted cardiovascular diseases: hypertrophic cardiomyopathy, long-QT syndrome, and Marfan syndrome. Circulation 98:1460–1471
4. Seidman JG, Sidmn CE (2001) The genetic basis for cardiomyopathy: from mutation identification to mechanistic paradigms. Cell 104:557–567
5. Lechin M, Quinones MA, Omran A et al (1995) Angiotensin-I converting enzyme genotypes and left ventricular hypertrophy in patients with hypertrophic cardiomyopathy. Circulation 92:1808–1812
6. Gruver EJ, Fatkin D, Dodds GA et al (1999) Familial hypertrophic cardiomyopathy and atrial fibrillation caused by Arg663His betacardiac myosin heavy chain mutation. Am J Cardiol; 83: H13-H18

7. Arad M, Benson DW, Peez-Atayde AR et al (2002) Constitutively active AMP kinase mutations cause glycogen storage disease mimicking hypertrophic cardiomyopathy. J Clin Invest 109:357–362

8. Spirito P, Maron BJ (1987) Absence of progression of left ventricular hypertrophy in adults patients with hypertrophic cardiomyopathy. J Am Coll Cardiol 9:1013–1017

9. Maron BJ, Spirito P, Wesley Y et al (1986) Development and progression of left ventricular hypertrophy in children with hypertrophic cardiomyopathy. N Engl J Med 315:610–614

10. Niimura H, Bachinski, Sangwatanaroj S et al (1998) Mutations in the gene for cardiac myosin-binding protein C and late-onset familial hypertrophic cardiomyopathy. N Engl J Med 338:248–257

11. Maron BJ (2002) Hypertrophic cardiomyopathy: a systematic review. JAMA 287:1308–1320

12. Maron BJ, Casey SA, Hauser RG et al (2003) Clinical course of hypertrophic cardiomyopathy with survival to advanced age. J Am Coll Cardiol 42:882–888

13. McKenna W, Deanfield J, Faruqui A et al (1981) Prognosis in hypertrophic cardiomyopathy: role of age and clinical, electrocardiographic and hemodynamic features. Am J Cardiol 47:532–538

14. Krikler DM, Davis MJ, Rowland E et al (1980) Sudden death in hypertrophic cardiomyopathy: associated accessory pathways. Br Heart J 43:245–251

15. Spirito P, Seidman CE, McKenna WJ et al (1997) The management of hypertrophic cardiomyopathy. N Engl J Med 336:775–785

16. Maki S, Ikeda H, Muro A et al (1998) Predictors of sudden cardiac death in hypertrophic cardiomyopathy. Am J Cardiol 82:774–778

17. Elliott PM, Poloniecki J, Dickie S et al (2000) Sudden death in hypertrophic cardiomyopathy: identification of high risk patients. J Am Coll Cardiol 36:2212–2218

18. Maron BJ, Shirani J, Poliac LC et al (1996) Sudden death in young competitive athletes. Clinical, demographic, and pathological profiles. JAMA 276:199–204

19. Maron BJ, Olivotto I, Spirito P et al (2000) Epidemiology of hypertrophic cardiomyopathy-related death: revisited in a large non-referral-based patient population. Circulation 102:858–864

20. Priori S, Aliot E, Bolmstrom-Lundquist C et al (2001) Task force on sudden cardiac death of the European Society of Cardiology. Eur Heart J 22:1374–1450

21. Spirito P, Bellone P, Harris KM et al (2000) Magnitude of left ventricular hypertrophy and risk of sudden death in hypertrophic cardiomyopathy. N Engl J Med 342:1778–1785

22. Elliott PM, Gimeno B Jr, Mahon NG et al (2001) Relation between severity of left ventricular hypertrophy and prognosis in patients with hypertrophic cardiomyopathy. Lancet 357:420–424

23. Adabag AS, Casey SA, Maron BJ (2002) Sudden death in hypertrophic cardiomyopathy: patterns and prognostic significance of tachyarrhythmias on ambulatory Holter ECG. Circulation 106:710

24. Monserrat L, Elliott PM, Gimeno JR et al (2003) Non-sustained ventricular tachycardia in hypertrophic cardiomyopathy: an independent marker of sudden risk in young patients. J Am Coll Cardiol 42:873–879

25. Cecchi F, Olivotto I, Montereggi A et al (1995) Hypertrophic cardiomyopathy in Tuscany: clinical course and outcome in an unselected regional population. J Am Coll Cardiol 26:1529–1536

26. Olivotto I, Cecchi F, Case SA et al (2001) Impact of atrial fibrillation on the clinical

course of hypertrophic cardiomyopathy. Circulation 104:2517–2524

27. Stafford WJ, Trohman RG, Bilskr M et al (1996) Cardiac arrest in adolescent with atrial fibrillation and hypertrophic cardiomyopathy. J Am Coll Cardiol 7:701–704

28. Davies MJ, McKenna WJ (1995) Hypertrophic cardiomyopathy, pathology and pathogenesis. Histopathology 26:493–500

29. Choudhoury L, Marholdt H, Wagner A et al (2002) Myocardial scarring in asymptomatic or mildly symptomatic patients with hypertrophic cardiomyopathy. J Am Coll Cardiol 40:2156–2164

30. Yetman AT, McCrindle BW, MacDonald C et al (1998) Myocardial bridging in children with hypertrophic cardiomyopathy – a risk factor for sudden death. N Engl J Med 339:1201–1209

31. Maron MS, Olivotto I, Betocchi S et al (2003) Effect of left ventricular outflow tract obstruction on clinical outcome in hypertrophic cardiomyopathy. N Engl J Med 348:295–303

32. Ackerman MJ, VanDriest SL, Ommen SR et al (2002) Prevalence and age-dependence of malignant mutations in the beta-myosin heavy chain and troponin T genes in hypertrophic cardiomyopathy: a comprehensive outpatient perspective. J Am Coll Cardiol 39:2042–2048

33. Fananapazir L, Chang AC, Epstein SE (1992) Prognostic determinants in hypertrophic cardiomyopathy. Perspective evaluation of a therapeutic strategy based on clinical, Holter, hemodynamic, and electrophysiologic findings. Circulation 86:730–740

34. Wigle E, Rakowski H, Kimball BP et al (1995) Hypertrophic cardiomyopathy. Clinical spectrum and treatment. Circulation 92:1680–1692

35. Sherid MV, Pearle G, Gunsburg DZ (1998) Mechanism of benefit of negative inotropes in obstructive hypertrophic cardiomyopathy. Circulation 97:41–47

36. McKenna WJ, Oakley CM, Krikler DM et al (1985) Improved survival with amiodarone in patients with hypertrophic cardiomyopathy and ventricular tachycardia. Br Heart J 53:412–416

37. Cecchi F, Olivotto I, Montereggi et al (1998) Prognostic value of non-sustained ventricular tachycardia and the potential role of amiodarone treatment in hypertrophic cardiomyopathy: assessment in an unselected non-referral based patient population. Heart 79:331–336

38. Maron BJ, Merrill WH, Freier PA et al (1978) Long-term clinical course and asymptomatic status of patients after operation for hypertrophic subaortic stenosis. Circulation 57:1205–1213

39. Merrill WH, Friesinger GC, Graham TP J et al (2000) Long-lasting improvement after septal myectomy for hypertrophic obstructive cardiomyopathy. Ann Thorac Surg 69:1732–1735

40. Theodoro DA, Danielson GK, Feldt RH et al (1996) Hypertrophic obstructive cardiomyopathy in pediatric patients: results of surgical treatment. J Thorac Cardiovasc Surg 112:1589–1597

41. Quin JX, Shiota T, Lever HM et al (2001) Outcome of patients with hypertrophic obstructive cardiomyopathy after percutaneous transluminal septal myocardial ablation and septal myectomy surgery. J Am Coll Cardiol 38:1994–2000

42. Maron BJ, Nishimura RA, McKenna WJ et al (1999) Assessment of permanent dual-chamber pacing as a treatment for drug-refractory symptomatic patients with obstructive hypertrophic cardiomyopathy. A randomized, double-blind, cross-over study (M-PATHY). Circulation 99:2927–2933

43. Nishimura RA, Trusty JM, Hayes DL et al (1997) Dual-chamber pacing for hypertrophic cardiomyopathy: a randomized, double-blind, cross-over trial. J Am Coll Cardiol 29:435–441

44. Maron BJ, Shen W-K, Link MS et al (2000) Efficacy of implantable cardioverter-defibrillators for the prevention of sudden death in patients with hypertrophic cadiomyopathy. N Engl J Med 342:365–373

45. Gregoratos G, Abrams J, Epstein AE et al (2002) ACC/AHA/NASPE 2002 guideline update for implantation of cardiac pacemakers and antiarrhythmia devices. Circulation 106:2145–2161

Risk Identification in Arrhythmic Athletes with Fatal or Resuscitated Cardiac Arrest

F. Furlanello[1], A. Bertoldi[2], C. Furlanello[3], G. Galanti[10], P. Manetti[10], F. Fernando[4], F. Terrasi[5], M. Dallago[2], L. Gramegna[2], M. Barbareschi[9], A. Biffi[6], G. Vergara[7], G. Inama[8], G. Butera[1], C. Esposito[1], M. Marangoni[12], G. Thiene[11], R. Cappato[1]

Although rare and uncommon, sudden cardiac death (SCD) in young competitive athletes is a devastating event [1–18]. The identification of potential mechanisms precipitating SCD may help to prevent future events in athletes with similar conditions [1, 3, 13, 16].

Methods

We report on 30 years of continuous monitoring (see Table 1) of a population of 2640 young competitive athletes identified with important arrhythmias (2286 males; mean age 21.5 years), 345 (13%) competing at the international elite level (298 males; mean age 24.4 years). The arrhythmic athletes were evaluated with a codified individualised study protocol [1, 3, 7, 16].

Study subjects

Two categories of athlete are considered:
1. Athletes in whom cardiac arrest (CA) may be considered predictable:
    a) Those with exertional premonitory cardiac symptoms that may indicate significant cardiac abnormality: syncope, prolonged palpitations, dyspnoea, and chest pain;

[1]Department of Clinical Arrhythmia and Electrophysiology, Policlinico San Donato, Milan; [2]Department of Cardiology, S.Chiara Hospital, Trento; [3]ITC / Irst, Trento; [4]Sport Medicine Centre, S.Andrea Hospital, Rome; [5]Villa Bianca Hospital, Trento; [6]Sports Science Institute, Italian National Olympic Committee, Rome; [7]Division of Cardiology-Ospedale S.Maria del Carmine, Rovereto; [8]Department of Cardiology, Maggiore Hospital, Crema; [9]Department of Pathology, S.Chiara Hospital, Trento; [10]Sport Medicine Centre University, Florence; [11]Institute of Pathology, University of Padua Medical School, Padua; [12]University of Verona, Italy

b) Those with a cardiac risk, i.e. identified as having life-threatening arrhythmias by cardiological screening, according to the current recommendations for athletic eligibility (26th Bethesda Conference 1996, NASPE Consensus Conference 2001 [15], Italian COCIS 2003). This population included athletes not compliant with treatment and/or banned athletic activity.

2. Athletes in whom CA occurred as a 'first cardiac symptom'.

Diagnostic Screening

For each athlete, the risk assessment, if necessary, included: family and past history, clinical evaluation, routine blood tests (including thyroid tests), resting and stress test ECG, Holter recording, also during intense physical activity, cardiac events recorder, implantable loop-recorder, 2D–Doppler echocardiography, stress echocardiography (baseline and during exercise), transoesophageal echocardiography, CT, MRI, 3D MR angiography, signal-averaged ECG, head-up tilt-test, specific blood test (i.e. for viral agents, vector-borne pathogens), pharmacological testing (flecainide administration, isoproterenol infusion), genetic studies, transoesophageal electrophysiological (EP) study (until 1996), endocavitary EP study also with new mapping methods, cardiac catheterisation and angiography, endomyocardial biopsy, (as of 2001) microvolt T-Wave Alternans (mTWA) before EP study [16]. Necropsy was performed in all athletes who died and the pathological investigation of the heart was carried out in the majority of the cases at the Institute of Pathology, University of Padua, according to methods previously reported [16, 19–21].

Results

During 30 years of monitoring, 62 major events were reported in 58 athletes, 24 of which (0.9%) were SD (4 with prior CA on field), while 38 (1.4%) were CA. In the subset of elite athletes, the major events were 13 (22.4%), made up of 6 SD (1.7%) and 7 (2.0%) CA (Table 1).

Table 1. Competitive athletes with arrhythmias (summary of the population studied from 1974 to April 2004)

Athletes	N	Male	Female	Average age (years)	Follow-up (months, min.–max.)	N with SD	N with CA
All athletes	2640	2286	354	21.5	3-190	24 (0.9%)	38 (1.4%)
Elite athletes	345	298	47	24.4	3-180	6 (1.7%)	7 (2.0%)

Underlying Condition

Underlying conditions among victims of CA and SD were: arrhythmogenic right ventricular dysplasia (ARVD) 15 (9 CA, 6 SD), Wolff–Parkinson–White syndrome (WPW) 9 (7, 2), myocarditis 9 (3, 6), coronary artery disease 7 [3 (1 congenital), 4], dilated cardiomyopathy 7 (4, 3), mitral valve prolapse 3 (1, 2), Lev-Lenègre disease 4, hypertrophic cardiomyopathy 3, primary electrical heart disease 1, long QT syndrome 1, commotio cordis 2 (1, 1) non compact myocardium with catecholaminergic polymorphic VT (CPVT) [1] (Table 2). CA/SD were observed in competitive arrhythmic athletes regardless of ranking; 13 of the 58 (22.4%) were elite professional athletes.

Table 2. Underlying condition among young competitive athletes with fatal and resuscitated cardiac arrest (CA)

	Fatal CA		Resuscitated CA		Total CA	
	Events	%	Events	%	Events	%
ARVD	6	25	9	23.6	15	24.2
WPW	2	8.3	7	18.4	9	14.5
Myocarditis	6	25	3	7.9	9	14.5
Coronary artery disease	4	16.6	3a	7.97	7	11.3
Dilated cardiomyopathy	3	12.5	4	0.6	7	11.3
Lev-Lenègre disease	-	-	4	10.6	4	6.4
Hypertrophic cardiomyopathy	-	-	3	7.9	3	4.8
Commotio cordis	1	4.16	1	2.6	2	3.2
Non-compact myocardium with catecholaminergic polymorphic VT	-	-	1	2.6	1	1.6
Mitral valve prolapse	2	8.3	1	2.6	3	4.8
Long QT syndrome	-	-	1	2.6	1	1.6
Primary electrical heart disease	-	-	1	2.6	1	1.6
Total	24[b]		38		62	

ARVD, arrhythmogenic right ventricular dysplasia; WPW, Wolff–Parkinson–White syndrome; VT, ventricular tachycardia

[a] 1 congenital

[b] 4 with prior CA

CA/SD were exercise-related in the majority of cases (90%), occurring either during practice (51.8%) or during competition (48.2%) (Table 3). The mechanisms responsible for SCD on the athletic field were mostly represented by destabilisation of an arrhythmogenic substrate. Ventricular tachycardia/fibrillation was the most frequent final event (~90% of the cases), with asystole in the remaining patients (Table 4). The majority of athletes (> 60%) suffered CA/SD after warning symptoms during exertion and/or with an arrhythmic risk already identified. The remaining athletes had CA/SD as the first, unpredictable presentation.

Table 3. Relationship between CA/SD and exercise activity

Activity	CA	SD	Total
At rest	2	4	6 (9.6%)
Exertion	36	20	56 (90.4%)
Practice	19	10	29 (51.8%)
Competition	17	10	27 (48.2%)

Table 4. Risk identification in athletes with CA/SD: documented or induced decisive arrhythmic events

VT/VF	44
Torsades de pointes	2
Pre-excited AF	11
Total VF	57 (91.9%)
Paroxysmal AV block	4
Asystolic commotio cordis	1
Total asystole	5 (8.1%)

VT, ventricular tachycardia; VF, ventricular fibrillation; AF, atrial fibrillation; AV, atrioventricular

Clinical Outcome and Management

The follow-up ranged from 12 to 208 months. At the last clinical control, 24 subjects had deceased and 34 were alive. Among these, 7 are active in sports after successful radiofrequency catheter ablation (WPW), 3 are alive with complete recovery (1 commotio cordis, 2 myocarditis). In 5, a cardiac pacemaker was implanted. In 15, an implantable cardioverter–defibrillator (ICD) was implanted, with hybrid therapy in all. The ICD discharges happened in all but two. The time from implantation to first discharge ranged from 2 to

40 months. In 5, radiofrequency catheter ablation for refractory VT was performed. Four subjects are on long-term anti-arrhythmic drug treatment. One young subject underwent surgical correction of congenital coronary artery anomaly.

Summary

An unpredictable fatal and/or resuscitated CA occurred as first symptom only in 37% of the competitive athletes, independently of ranking (30% were in elite athletes). The underlying diseases were mainly myocarditis, coronary artery disease, WPW, and commotio cordis. CA/SD were observed in competitive arrhythmic athletes regardless of their ranking and was exercise-related in the majority of cases, occurring during either practice or competition; only in few cases occurred at rest (in subjects with WPW, coronary artery disease, myocarditis, or dilated cardiomyopathy).

Warning symptoms such as exertional syncope and severe palpitations and/or an already identified risk with arrhythmological work-up occurred in 63% of cases, independently of ranking (70% in elite athletes with CA/SD). Twenty-five percent of the athletes were totally non-compliant with treatment and/or banned from athletic activity.

Conclusions

Competitive athletes, including those at elite level, identified as being at high risk of arrhythmias must be forbidden athletic activity until the risk is still present in the individual subject. Additional measures should include a periodical clinical check-up, an appropriate life-style, anti-arrhythmic drug administration, interventional and/or hybrid therapies with special regard to ICD implantation, and, when possible, RFCA (i.e. in subjects with WPW, ventricular tachycardia recurrences, storm of ICD interventions). Every effort must be made to continuously add in to the arrhythmological clinical approach to the competitive athlete the newest non-invasive (genetic studies, T wave alternans study [16], etc.) and invasive risk stratifiers (electrophysiological testing and mapping), together with the newest cardiac imaging investigation tools.

This long-term ongoing arrhythmological study of a large population of young competitive athletes offers an opportunity of making known in the sport world any information that can realise an early diagnosis as well as strong clinical management of subjects at high risk of CA/SD, particularly in those with exertional premonitory cardiac symptoms or with a cardiac risk already identified.

Aknowledgements: The authors wish to thank the secretary Anna Stenghel for her helpful cooperation.

References

1. Furlanello F, Bertoldi A, Fernando F et al (2000) Competitive athletes with arrhythmias. Classification, evaluation and treatment. In: Bayes de Luna A, Furlanello F, Maron BJ, Zipes DP (eds) Arrhythmias and sudden death in athletes. Kluwer Academic, Dordrecht, pp 89–105

2. Thiene G, Basso C, Corrado D (2000) Pathology of sudden death in young athletes: European experience. In: Bayes de Luna A, Furlanello F, Maron BJ, Zipes DP (eds) Arrhythmias and sudden death in athletes. Kluwer Academic, Dordrecht, pp 49–69

3. Furlanello F, Fernando F, Galassi A et al (2001) Ventricular arrhythmias in apparently healthy athletes. In: Malik M (ed) Risk of arrhythmia and sudden death. BMJ Books, London, pp 316–324

4 Corrado D, Basso C, Rizzoli G et al (2003) Does sports activity enhance the risk of sudden death in adolescents and young adults? J Am Coll Cardiol 42:1959–1963

5. Furlanello F, Bentivegna S, Cappato R et al (2003) Arrhythmogenic effects of illicit drugs in athletes. Ital Heart J 4:829–837

6. Furlanello F, Bertoldi A, Bentivegna S et al (2004) Atrial fibrillation and illicit drugs in athletes. Ital Heart J 5(Suppl 1):44–46

7. Bertoldi A, Furlanello F, Fernando F et al (2002) Risk stratification in elite athletes with arrhythmias. In: Furlanello F, Bertoldi A, Cappato R (eds) Proceedings of The New Frontiers of Arrhythmias 2002. Ital Heart J, 5(Suppl 1): 218–219

8. Furlanello F, Bertoldi A, Esposito C et al (2004) Illicit drugs and cardiac arrhythmias in athletes. In: Adornato E (ed) Cardiac Rhythm Control in 2004, Proceedings of the IXth Southern Symposium on Cardiac Pacing. Taormina September 29–October 2, Rome, L. Pozzi, pp 8–20

9. Al Sheikh T, Zipes D (2000) Guidelines for competitive athletes with arrhythmias. In: Bayes de Luna A. Furlanello F, Maron BJ, Zipes DP (eds) Arrhythmias and sudden death in athletes. Kluwer Academic Dordrecht, pp 119–151

10. Maron BJ (2000) The paradox of exercise. N Engl J Med 343:1409–1411

11. Maron BJ (2000), Cardiovascular causes and pathology of sudden death in athletes: the American experience. In: Bayes de Luna A, Furlanello F, Maron BJ, Zipes DP (eds) Arrhythmias and sudden death in athletes. Kluwer Academic, Dordrecht, pp 31–48

12. Maron BJ (2003) Sudden death in young athletes. N Engl J Med 349:1064–1075

13. Maron BJ (1993) Sudden death in young athletes: lessons from the Hank Gathers affair. N Engl J Med 329:55–57

14. Maron BJ, Mitten MJ, Quandt EK et al (1998) Competitive athletes with cardiovascular disease: the case of Nicholas Knapp. N Engl J Med 339:1632–1635

15. Estes NAM, Link MS, Cannom D et al (2001) Report of the NASPE policy conference on arrhythmias and the athlete. J Cardiovasc Electrophysiol 12:1208–1219

16. Thiene G (2004) Sudden cardiac death and apparently intact heart: pathological examination. Ital Heart J 5(suppl 1):S88–S89

17. Cerrone M, Priori S (2004) Arrhythmic competitive athletes with apparently 'intact heart': genetic molecular bases. Ital Heart J 5(Suppl 1):S90–S92

18. Furlanello F, Galanti G, Manetti P et al (2004) Microvolt T-wave alternans as predictors of electrophysiological testing results in professional competitive athletes. ANE, July 2004, vol 9 no 3, pp 201-206

19. Thiene G, Basso C, Corrado D (2001) Cardiovascular causes of sudden death. In: Silver MD, Gotlieb AI, Schoen FJ (eds) Cardiovascular pathology. Churchill Livingstone, Philadelphia, PA, pp 326–374

20. Basso C, Calabrese F, Corrado D et al (2001) Postmortem diagnosis in sudden cardiac death victims: macroscopic, microscopic and molecular findings. Cardiovasc Res 50:290–300

21. Basso C (2004) Arrhythmic competitive athletes with apparently 'intact heart': silent myocarditis. Ital Heart J 5(Suppl 1):S92–S94

NEW TRENDS IN PHYSIOLOGICAL PACING AND OPTIMAL PACING SITES

Physiological Pacing: Perspective

I.E. Ovsyshcher

Does Physiological Pacing Exist?

When introduced about 25 years ago, dual chamber pacing (DDD) was declared a 'universal' or 'physiological' mode of pacing. Lately, another definition of DDD pacing has emerged: 'true physiological pacing.' If there is 'true physiological pacing', logically there should also be 'false' or 'spurious' physiological pacing.

Physiological pacing 'may be achieved only by preserving, or, if that is impossible, by restoring or attempting to imitate the normal electrophysiological characteristics of the heart [i.e. normal chronotropism of cardiac rhythm with normal sino-atrial and atrioventricular (AV) activation] [1]. This paper will discuss current data regarding both kinds of 'physiological' pacing for patients with sinus node dysfunction.

The available 'true' physiological pacemaker is equipped with modern sophisticated diagnostic and therapeutic systems and features. However, even these sophisticated systems cannot support the requirements listed above for physiological pacing and provoke prolonged intra-atrial and intraventricular, interatrial and interventricular conduction time. This alternation in conduction time may significantly modify synchronisation in the activation and contraction of the right and left heart and especially the left ventricle (LV) [1]. From the electrophysiological (EP) and haemodynamic points of view, a patient with DDD pacing is identical to the patient with ectopic right atrium (RA) rhythm originating from the location of the atrial lead and ectopic ventricular rhythm originating from the right ventricle (RV) apex. Consequences of permanent alterations in atrial conduction may lead to atrial arrhythmias such as atrial fibrillation (AF); RV apical pacing

Electrophysiology Laboratory, Faculty of Health Sciences, Ben Gurion University of the Negev, Beer-Sheva, Israel

leads to abnormal, retrograde depolarisation comparable with left bundle branch block (LBBB). As a result, DDD pacing leads to a combination of EP patterns of ectopic atrial and ectopic ventricular rhythm. When heart rate increases to more than 100 bpm, these rhythms should be classified as ectopic atrial tachycardia and ectopic ventricular tachycardia [1]. These EP alternations may lead to haemodynamic consequences. However, up to 10 years ago there was no solid evidence regarding adverse outcomes of 'physiological' pacing and the central subject for discussion was dual chamber versus ventricular single chamber pacing (VVI/R). The initial assumption that DDD was superior to VVI was based on the intuition that the maintenance of AV synchrony afforded by DDD pacing is very important and is adequate to imitate normal EP patterns; later there were numerous retrospective studies which presented a significant body of evidence regarding the lower morbidity and mortality associated with atrial-based versus ventricular pacing [1–4]. Over the last 10 years the results of several prospective trials have been published where, surprisingly, no difference in mortality appeared between physiological and non-physiological pacing (VVI/R), and the difference in morbidity was significantly less [6–12]than had been previously believed [2–4]. The next period which significantly changed the credibility of 'physiological' pacing, was the beginning of the twenty-first century. In this period the studies tested the hypothesis that, even when AV synchrony is preserved, ventricular desynchronisation imposed by RV apical pacing increased the risk of congestive heart failure (CHF) and AF [13–17].

Physiological Pacing for Sinus Node Dysfunction

Sinus node dysfunction (SND) is the dominant indication for cardiac pacing in many countries [5]. The optimal pacing mode for treatment of symptomatic SND has been debated for long time. A large number of observational studies have indicated that selection of pacing mode may be a factor in the clinical outcome for patients with symptomatic bradycardia in terms of development of AF, thromboembolism, CHF, mortality, and quality of life [2–4]. These retrospective studies were criticised for selection bias, and it was suggested that the only way to avoid this bias was to perform randomised controlled trials of pacing mode selection [2, 4]. The recent data from six randomised trials on mode selection in patients with SND will be discussed below.

The AAI vs VVI Trial

Ten years ago the AAI vs VVI trial, the first randomised trial comparing AAI and VVI pacing in 225 consecutive patients with SND and normal AV conduction, was published by Andersen et al. [6]. After a mean follow-up of 40 months, 23% of the patients in the VVI group had AF compared with 14% in the AAI group ($P = 0.12$). Three years later, after an extended follow-up to a mean of 5.5 years, the differences in occurrence of AF between the AAI (24%) and VVI (35%) groups had increased substantially in favour of AAI pacing ($P = 0.012$) [7]. The Kaplan–Meier curves of freedom from AF diverged after 3 years of follow-up, indicating a delay after pacemaker implantation before the deleterious effect of VVI or the beneficial effect of AAI pacing becomes evident. In the VVI group NYHA functional class increased during follow-up ($P < 0.001$), and the use of diuretics increased. These findings were associated with a decrease in LV fractional shortening and an excess dilatation of the left atrium (LA) in the VVI group as compared with the AAI group [8]. Total mortality was significantly less in the AAI group ($P = 0.045$), and the excess mortality in the VVI group was due to cardiovascular deaths [7].

The PASE Trial

In 1998 the Pacemaker Selection in the Elderly (PASE) Trial, the first randomised trial of VVIR versus DDDR pacing, was published [9, 10]. A total of 407 patients with SND, AV block, or other indications were included. Crossover from VVIR to DDDR pacing because of pacemaker syndrome occurred in 26% of patients. The primary end-point was health-related quality of life, which did not differ between the two treatment groups at the end of follow-up. There was no significant difference in the incidence of AF between treatment groups.

The Italian Trial

At the same time Mattioli et al. reported a randomised trial [11] which included 210 patients with AV block and SND and with no history of prior AF. Patients received either VVI/VVIR, or a 'physiological pacemaker' (AAI/DDD/DDDR/VDD). Follow-up was up to 5 years. An increase in the incidence of chronic AF was observed in patients with SND who received VVI/VVIR pacing ($P < 0.02$).

The CTOPP Trial

This was the first large-scale randomised trial of pacing mode selection in patients with SND and AV block, published in the year 2000 [12]; it included 1474 patients with VVI/VVIR pacemakers and 1094 patients with physiological pacing (DDD/DDDR or AAI/AAIR). Mean follow-up was 3 years (range 2–5 years). No significant difference was observed in the primary end point (stroke or cardiovascular death) between treatment groups. The Kaplan–Meier curves of AF diverged after 2 years of pacing and an 18% risk reduction was observed in the physiologically paced group (P = 0.05). After an extended follow-up, (up to 6 years) still no significant difference between treatment groups was observed in regard to the primary end-point. AF remained more frequent in the VVIR group while the difference between groups significantly increased (P = 0.009) [13].

The MOST Trial

In the MOST trial, published in 2002 [14], 2010 patients with SND were included. All patients were implanted with a DDDR pacemaker, and afterwards the programming was randomly assigned to VVIR or DDDR pacing mode. A total of 313 patients (31%) crossed over from VVIR to DDDR. Pacemaker syndrome was the reason for cross-over in 16% of VVIR patients. At the end of follow-up AF was more frequent in the VVIR than in the DDDR group (P = 0.008). No differences were observed between groups in the primary end-point death or non-fatal stroke or in the end-points all-cause mortality, cardiovascular death, stroke, or 'death-stroke-or-hospitalisation for CHF'. Recently the MOST investigators have reported a correlation between cumulative percentage of ventricular pacing (Cum%VP) and an increasing risk of hospitalisation for heart failure [15]. Increasing Cum%VP was found to be clearly associated with an increasing incidence of AF both during VVIR and during DDDR pacing.

The AAIR vs DDDR Trial

In another Danish study [16], a total of 177 consecutive patients with SND, normal AV conduction, and no bundle branch block were randomised to treatment with AAIR and DDDR pacemakers programmed with a short AV interval (DDDR-s) or DDDR pacemaker programmed with a long AV interval (DDDR-l). Mean follow-up was 2.9 ± 1.1 years. In the AAIR group no significant changes were observed in such echocardiographic parameters as LA and LV diameter and LV fractional shortening (LVFS) from baseline to last follow-up (primary end-points). In both DDDR groups, LA diameter increased significantly (P < 0.05), and in the DDDR-s group, LVFS also decreased significantly (P < 0.01). AF was significantly less common in the AAIR group, 7.4% vs. 23.3% in the DDDR-s group vs 17.5% in the DDDR-l group (P = 0.03). The proportion of RV pacing was 90% in the DDDR-s group and 17% in the DDDR-l group. The risk of developing AF in the AAIR group compared to the DDDR-s group was significantly decreased after adjustment for brady-tachy syndrome [relative risk 0.27 (95% CI 0.09–0.83), P = 0.02]. Mortality and CHF did not differ between groups.

Ongoing Trials

Two randomised trials of mode selection in SND are ongoing [18]. The DAN-PACE trial, comparing AAIR and DDDR pacing in 1900 patients, was started in 1999 in Denmark. Inclusion is expected to be completed in 2007. Mean follow-up will be 5.5 years. The primary end-point is all-cause mortality; AF is a secondary outcome event.

The Systematic Trial Of Pacing for Atrial Fibrillation (STOP-AF) [18] is designed to test VVI pacing vs. DDD or AAI pacing in 350 patients with regard to the incidence of chronic and paroxysmal AF.

Discussion

According to data available from randomised trials, VVI/R pacing is an unattractive therapy for patients with SND, increasing the incidence of AF, CHF, thromboembolism, and death compared with AAI/R pacing. DDDR also increased LA and LV size and decreased LV function, and probably as a result of these changes, patients with DDDR had increased incidence of CHF and AF compared with those with AAIR pacing. The lack of ventricular desynchronisation in the AAI/R mode may explain the remarkable benefit of atrial pacing compared with VVI/R and DDD/R pacing obtained by the Danish group in patients with SND, in a protocol where the investigation focused only on the role of AV synchrony. These findings are supported by data from the recent DAVID trial (The Dual Chamber and VVI Implantable Defibrillator trial) comparing ICDs with DDDR (70 bpm) and VVI (40 bpm) respectively [17]. Higher mortality and hospitalisation for new or worsened CHF were significantly more common in the DDDR group, most likely due to ventricular desynchronisation caused by RV pacing. The harmful consequences of RV pacing in the MOST trial also appeared related to non-physiological LV contraction [15]. The MOST study found a correlation between the cumulative percentage of RV pacing index and the development of AF.

The same mechanism probably explains the higher incidence of new or worsened CHF in the ICD group than in the conventionally treated group in the MADIT II trial [19]. The effect of RV apical pacing on LV activation patterns and times is similar to that observed during LBBB [20, 21]. RV apical pacing results in asynchronous ventricular activation and delayed LV activation time due to slow initial propagation of the electrical wavefront through ventricular myocardium rather than through the His–Purkinje system. The greater the mass of ventricular myocardium activated by muscle-to-muscle conduction prior to activation of the Purkinje system, the longer the QRS duration and the greater the ventricular asynchrony. It is therefore not surprising that apical RV pacing is pathological and imposes acute and chronic adverse effects on ventricular haemodynamic function, myocardial perfusion, and cellular structure [20, 21]. These experimental data are validated by the above-mentioned clinical observations that chronic ventricular pacing in both the VVI/R and the DDD/R modes causes increased left heart size and reduced LV function compared with normal heart activation and atrial pacing, which presumably explains the adverse outcomes in the clinical trials cited previously. Furthermore, ventricular desynchronisation may explain why the difference between DDD/R and VVIR in the PASE, MOST, and CTOPP trials only was modest; the beneficial effect of preserving AV synchrony was partly outweighed by the harmful effect of ventricular desynchronisation. It should be emphasised that in *none* of the studies mentioned was AV interval optimised, which may compensate harmful outcome of RV pacing [1].

Conclusions

Significant outcomes of adverse effects of RV apical pacing are established. In patients with SND, AAI/R pacing is preferable and its adverse effects are not yet widely accepted. This mode of pacing can be presently recognised as closest to physiological. Only in this pacing mode did outcomes of a randomised trial [6–8] support previous observational studies regarding morbidity and mortality. Despite this, the use of atrial pacing has been limited [22] by concern about the development of AV block. In patients with conduction system disease and AV block, alternatives to RV apical pacing are needed to address the issue of ventricular synchrony [23].

Obviously, there is no *one* available physiological pacemaker for patients who need ventricular pacing. In patients with LV dysfunction, interventricular synchrony is possibly more important than AV synchrony and can be restored by biventricular pacing. There is *no* study that demonstrates that optimal AV synchrony may neutralise ventricular asynchrony due to apical RV pacing. Meanwhile, for the patient who needs ventricular pacing, apical RV pacing should be minimised as much as clinically possible. The role of optimisation of AV interval and/or alternate site(s) for atrial and ventricular pacing have yet to be established. An alternative site may be at any location in the endocardium as well as in epicardium of one or both of the atria and the ventricles [21, 23].

Late note

In the January issue of *Circulation* (2005, 111:174–181) a paper by Rinfret et al. advocating the use of DDDR in patients with SND was published. Data in the paper are based on 4-year follow-up of MOST patients. The authors concluded that for treating patients with SND, dual-chamber pacing is cost-effective in comparison with single chamber ventricular pacing.

So, for patients with SND, VVI/R is worst; dual chamber is better and AAI/R (if possible) is better than both.

References

1. Ovsyshcher IE (1997) Toward physiological pacing: optimization of cardiac hemodynamics by AV delay adjustment. Pacing Clin Electrophysiol 20:861–865
2. Connolly SJ, Kerr C, Gent M et al (1996) Dual-chamber versus ventricular pacing: critical appraisal of current data. Circulation 94:578–583
3. Ovsyshcher I (1995) Matching optimal pacemaker to patient: do we need a large scale clinical trial of pacemaker mode selection? Pacing Clin Electrophysiol 18:1845–1852
4. Ovsyshcher IE, Hayes DL, Furman S (1998) Dual-chamber pacing is superior to ventricular pacing: fact or controversy? Circulation 97:2368–2370
5. Ovsyshcher IE, Furman S (2003) Determinants of geographic variations in pacemakers and implantable cardioverter defibrillators implantation rates. Pacing Clin Electrophysiol 26:474–478
6. Andersen HR, Thuesen L, Bagger JP et al (1994) Prospective randomised trial of atrial versus ventricular pacing in sick-sinus syndrome. Lancet 344:1523–1528
7. Andersen HR, Nielsen JC, Thomsen PE et al (1997) Long-term follow-up of patients from a randomised trial of atrial versus ventricular pacing for sick sinus syndrome. Lancet 350:1210–1216
8. Nielsen JC, Andersen HR, Thomsen PE et al (1998) Heart failure and echocardiographic changes during long-term followup of patients with sick sinus syndrome randomized to single chamber atrial or ventricular pacing. Circulation 97:987–995
9. Lamas GA, Orav J, Stambler BS et al (1998) Quality of life and clinical outcomes in elderly patients treated with ventricular pacing as compared with dual chamber pacing. N Engl J Med 338:1097–1104
10. Ellenbogen KA, Stambler BS, Orav EJ et al (2000) Clinical characteristics of patients intolerant to VVIR pacing. Am J Cardiol 86:59–63
11. Mattioli AV, Vivoli D, Mattioli G (1998) Influence of pacing modalities on the incidence of atrial fibrillation in patients without prior atrial fibrillation. A prospective study. Eur Heart J 19:282–286
12. Connolly SJ, Kerr CR, Gent M et al (2000) Effects of physiologic pacing versus ventricular pacing on the risk of stroke and death due to cardiovascular causes. Canadian Trial of Physiologic Pacing Investigators. N Engl J Med 342:1385–1391
13. Kerr CR, Connolly SJ, Abdollah H et al (2004) Canadian Trial of Physiological Pacing: effects of physiological pacing during long-term follow-up. Circulation 109:357–362
14. Lamas GA, Lee KL, Sweeney M et al (2002) Ventricular pacing or dual-chamber pacing for sinus-node dysfunction. N Engl J Med 346:1854–1862
15. Sweeney MO, Hellkamp AS, Ellenbogen KA et al (2003) Adverse effect of ventricular pacing on heart failure and atrial fibrillation among patients with normal baseline QRS duration in a clinical trial of pacemaker therapy for sinus node dysfunction. Circulation 107:2932–2937

16. Nielsen JC, Kristensen L, Andersen HR et al (2003) A randomized comparison of atrial and dual-chamber pacing in 177 consecutive patients with sick sinus syndrome: echocardiographic and clinical outcome. J Am Coll Cardiol 42:614–623

17. Wilkoff BL, Cook JR, Epstein AE et al (2002) Dual-chamber pacing or ventricular backup pacing in patients with an implantable defibrillator: The Dual chamber and VVI Implantable Defibrillator (DAVID) Trial. JAMA 288:3115–3123

18. Albertsen AE, Nielsen JC (2003) Selecting the appropriate pacing mode for patients with sick sinus syndrome: evidence from randomized clinical trials. Card Electrophysiol Rev 7:406–410

19. Moss AJ, Zareba W, Hall WJ et al (2002) Prophylactic implantation of a defibrillator in patients with myocardial infarction and reduced ejection fraction. N Engl J Med 346:877–883

20. Vernooy K, Verbeek XAAM, Peschar M et al (2005) Left bundle branch block induces ventricular remodelling and functional septal hypoperfusion. Eur Heart J 26:91–98

21. Vanagt WY, Verbeek XA, Delhaas T et al (2004) The left ventricular apex is the optimal site for pediatric pacing: correlation with animal experience. Pacing Clin Electrophysiol 27:837–843

22. Ector H, Ovsyshcher IE, Oto A et al (2003) The registry of the European Working Group on cardiac pacing: 2000–2001 (abstract). Europace 4:B100

23. Lieberman R, Grenz D, Mond HG et al (2004) Selective site pacing: defining and reaching the selected site. Pacing Clin Electrophysiol 27(6 Pt 2):883–886

Optimal Pacing Site in the Atrium and the Ventricle for Patients with Sino-Atrial Disease

G. Senatore, C. Amellone, G. Donnici, B. Giordano, G. Trapani, J.I. Rocanova, M. Fazzari

Patients with sick sinus syndrome (SSS) present symptoms due to bradycardia and chronotropic incompetence. Pacemaker implantation is indicated in these patients because it eliminates symptoms and improves quality of life. Besides, many patients with sino-atrial disease have a high incidence of atrial arrhythmias, mainly atrial fibrillation (AF; brady–tachy syndrome) [1]. In 1983, Coumel et al. were the first to observe the efficacy of overdrive atrial pacing to prevent recurrences of vagally mediated AF [2]. In the following years many studies were performed to investigate alternative pacing strategies to reduce the incidence of AF.

Atrial Pacing

Retrospective uncontrolled studies have yielded concordant results suggesting that AAI/R or DDD/R (physiological pacing) is associated with a lower incidence of chronic AF [3, 4]. Connolly et al. provided the first substantial evidence that atrial or dual-chamber pacing was useful in reducing progression to permanent AF as compared to ventricular pacing in patients with SSS (2.6% vs 6.8%, respectively) [5]. Other studies confirmed a modest benefit offered by physiological pacing, significant after at least 2 years from implant [6–9]. Conclusions from these trials suggested that a history of AF and sinus node dysfunction represent major risk factors of recurrent chronic AF after pacemaker implantation. No difference was observed in the incidence of AF in patients paced for atrioventricular (AV) block according to pacing mode. These beneficial effects of dual-chamber pacing in reducing AF recurrences may involve both mechanical and electrophysiological factors. Atrial or dual-

Division of Cardiology, Hospital of Cirie' (Turin), Italy

chamber pacing provides synchronised filling patterns and ventricular contraction, prevents consistent retrograde conduction, and reduces atrial overload and stretch. In addition, atrial pacing can prevent AF by eliminating pauses caused by bradycardia and by suppressing atrial ectopic beats. In conclusion, these studies proved a certain benefit conferred by atrial pacing in preventing AF in patients with SSS, and great interest was aroused in investigating the optimal pacing site.

The rationale for alternative site pacing is derived from the fundamental premise that conduction delays in the atrium are essential to the initiation of intra-atrial re-entrant mechanisms that underlie AF. These conduction delays may be in part anatomical and in part functional [10–12]. Besides, in patients with prolonged interatrial conduction time, a standard atrial lead position in the right appendage may produce deleterious left heart timing intervals, reducing the benefits provided by physiological pacing. Based on these observations, different pacing strategies were attempted in order to improve the modest benefit from right appendage pacing in patients with SSS.

-   *Biatrial pacing.* This approach utilises synchronous atrial pacing from the high right atrium and the coronary sinus. The aim is to reduce prolonged interatrial delay. D'Allones et al. reported a series of 86 patients with remarkable interatrial delay. After biatrial pacing, P wave duration was significantly reduced (187 ± 29 ms vs 106 ± 14 ms, $P < 0.01$) and 64% of patients were in stable sinus rhythm [13].

-   *Dual-site right atrial pacing.* Pacing is obtained from a first lead in the high right atrium and a second screw-in active fixation lead positioned at the coronary sinus ostium. Saksena et al. [14] reported a first experience with 30 patients. At 3-year follow-up 56% of patients were free from AF. The DAPPAF investigators [15] enrolled 120 patients with recurrent AF and bradycardia requiring pacing. Dual-site pacing tended to prolong the time to first AF recurrence and to improve quality of life. The SYNBIA-PACE study [16] investigated 42 patients with a history of AF, prolonged duration of P wave, and intra-atrial conduction. At 9-month follow-up, dual-site pacing was shown to have increased the time to first AF recurrence and reduced the AF burden.

-   *Bachmann's bundle.* Bachmann's bundle (BB) serves to conduct cardiac impulses from the right to the left atrium. Some studies of acute BB pacing observed reduced P wave duration, increased symmetry of atrial activation, and decreased inducibility of AF [17, 18]. A multi-centre prospective randomised study compared the efficacy of BB regional pacing in 120 patients (57 patiens with pacing from atrial right appendage and 67 patients with pacing from BB). Investigators observed significant shortening of P wave duration. At 1-year follow-up 75% of the patients paced at BB were free from chronic AF, compared with 47% paced at the traditional site [19].

- *Interatrial septum.* Pacing at the interatrial septum is intended to achieve simultaneous pacing of both atria. Various approaches to atrial pacing have been evaluated. In 1997 Spencer et al. presented a initial experience with the atrial lead (Medtronic 4058) positioned in the most anterior region of the right interatrial septum. This approach allowed both atria to be paced simultaneously [20]. In patients with standard indications for pacemaker implantation and episodes of AF, the atrial septum was paced at the posterior triangle of Koch. This approach was safe and feasible and significantly reduced mean P wave duration and symptomatic episodes of AF [21]. Other reports, and our own experience, confirm the observation of clinical benefits in terms of reduction of AF recurrences in patients with a septal atrial lead [22, 23].

Besides alternative pacing sites, other strategies have been attempted in order to improve the efficacy of pacing in preventing AF recurrences. Several prospective studies have demonstrated that a faster atrial pace results in a higher percentage of paced beats and a reduction of AF recurrences. In order to increase the percentage of atrial pacing and to reduce sudden rate changes after premature beats, new algorithms have been proposed. These algorithms provide atrial pacing at a rate which is maintained only slightly higher than the intrinsic rate and reduces the dispersion of refractoriness. Many studies have evaluated the role of these algorithms in patients with AF recurrences. Benefit derived from pacing at an alternative site could be increased with the use of algorithms, and several authors evaluated this combined strategy. The ASPECT trial evaluated the combined role of an atrial septal lead location and atrial pacing algorithms in the prevention of atrial tachyarrhythmias in 298 patients. The algorithms did not succeed in reducing AF burden and frequency, regardless of atrial lead position; however, prevention pacing was associated with a reduced frequency of premature atrial contractions and with a reduced frequency of symptomatic atrial tachyarrhythmia only in patients with atrial septal leads [24].

Finally, these studies demonstrated that interatrial septum pacing is safe and feasible, avoids the technical problems due to the use of two atrial leads, and permits simultaneous activation of both atria. Compared to the traditional right appendage pacing, septal pacing reduces AF recurrences and progression to chronic AF. Patients with SSS and paroxysmal AF could be suitable candidates for septal atrial lead pacing.

Ventricular Pacing

Although theoretically very attractive, atrial pacing for the prevention of AF has proved to be of quite modest benefit. A possible cause of this is the high percentage of ventricular pacing achieved in all studies, with a detrimental effect that could be reducing benefits from atrial pacing.

Four major clinical trials have been unable to demonstrate a clear benefit of DDDR pacing over VVIR pacing for the clinical endpoints of total mortality, cardiovascular mortality, and stroke. The Danish Study [25] enrolled 225 patients with symptomatic bradycardia, randomised to undergo AAI pacing or VVI pacing, with long-term follow-up. Significantly, overall survival was higher in the AAI group, with fewer cardiovascular deaths, less AF, fewer thromboembolic complications, and less heart failure than in the VVI group. However, AAI stimulation cannot be suitable for all patients with SSS: it requires stable long-term AV conduction and sinus rhythm, whereas SSS is a spectrum of electrical disorders including AF and AV block. For these reasons, other studies have considered the role of atrial pacing in DDD pacemaker versus ventricular pacing. In the CTOPP study [26] more than 2500 patients with all-cause bradycardia were randomised to undergo ventricular-based pacing or physiological pacing and followed for 3 years. The pacing mode did not produce a significant difference in the primary endpoint of stroke or cardiovascular death. Physiological pacing significantly reduced the cumulative risk of any AF and of chronic AF. In this study DDD pacemakers were not provided with algorithms to minimise ventricular pacing, with consequently a high cumulative percentage of ventricular pacing that could offset benefits from atrial pacing. Another large randomised study (MOST) [27] investigated more than 2000 patients with SSS randomised to receive DDDR or VVIR pacemakers, with as primary endpoint death from any cause or non-fatal stroke. At a median follow-up of 33 months no difference in relation to total mortality or stroke was found; but dual-chamber pacing reduce newly diagnosed and chronic AF and progression to heart failure. A strong relation between the percentage of ventricular pacing (in both the DDDR and the VVIR group) and the risk of progression to heart failure was observed. Ventricular pacing in DDDR mode for more than 40% of the time conferred a 2.6-fold increased risk of heart failure. Other interesting suggestions come from the DAVID trial [28], which has enrolled 506 implantable cardioverter–defibrillator (ICD) patients with no indication for antibradycardia pacing and left ventricular dysfunction (EF < 40%). Patients were randomly assigned to receive an ICD with back-up VVI at 40 beats/min versus DDDR at 70 beats/min, with as primary endpoint a combination of death and heart-failure-related hospitalisation. At 18 months VVI 40 was associated with a 16% rate of heart-failure hospitalisation or death, versus 26.7% for DDDR 70 ($P = 0.03$).

In conclusion, in patients with SSS, ventricular pacing should be minimised in order to maintain benefit produced by atrial pacing. Different strategies have been proposed to optimise right ventricular pacing: a novel right ventricular pacing site, manipulation of DDDR timing cycles to minimise unnecessary right ventricular pacing, and the use of novel pacing algorithms.

Alternative pacing sites, such as right ventricular outflow tract or ventricular septum, are supposed to improve synchronous activation of the ventricle and thus avoid impairment of ventricular function. New active fixation leads guarantee feasibility, good thresholds, adequate sensing, and stability. Initial experience with these new tools should be supported by large, long-term, randomised studies in order to demonstrate an advantage on the right ventricular apex.

A long AV delay did not succeed in reducing total ventricular pacing time.

The current generation of devices have new features to minimise ventricular pacing. The Search AV (SAV+, Medtronic EnPulse) offers the capability to search out longer AV intervals, up to 320 ms, in patients with intact or intermittent AV conduction. A prospective, multi-centre, non-randomised trial evaluated the ability of SAV+ ON to preserve intrinsic ventricular activation in 194 patients with intact AV conduction. At 1-month follow-up patients with SAV+ ON had 76.3% ventricular sensing vs 2.8% in those with SAV+ OFF [29].

Another new algorithm is the minimal ventricular pacing mode (MVP, Medtronic, Minneapolis) implemented in a dual-chamber ICD. This provides AAI/R pacing with ventricular monitoring and back-up DDD/R pacing only as needed during episodes of AV block. Single dropped ventricular beats are permitted (Wenckebach behaviour), while higher-level AV conduction failure causes mode switching to DDD/R to prevent asystole. Tests for a return to normal AV conduction are made, and if AV conduction is detected, the ICD returns to AAI/R mode. A randomised study with MVP was performed on 30 patients with DDD/R ICDs. Each patient spent a week in DDD/R mode and a week in MVP. The cumulative percentage of ventricular pacing was significantly lower during MVP than during DDD/R pacing (3.79% vs 80.6%, $P < 0.0001$). Three patients (10%) presented transient AV block with switch to DDD/R, confirming that a ventricular back-up could be opportune even in patients without a history of AV block.

Conclusions

Patients with SSS should be implanted with a dual-chamber pacemaker. Alternative sites appear superior to the traditional right appendage site since they improve atrial synchrony and may reduce AF recurrences. The hig percentage of ventricular pacing in DDD mode in all studies is a common pitfall comparing physiological pacing and VVI mode is characteristic of a common pitfall: ventricular pacing has a deleterious effect on both atrial and ventricular function that may mask the real beneficial entity of atrial pacing. New pacing site in the right ventricle and use of algorithms to minimise ventricular pacing is likely to lead to more consistent positive results. In conclusion, data from the literature suggest that in patients with SSS atrial pacing from an alternative site should be used, employing algorithms to attain the highest possible percentage of atrial pacing and to reduce ventricular pacing as much as possible.

References

1. Wolf PA, Abbott RD, Kannel WB (1991) Atrial fibrillation as an independent risk factor for stroke: The Framingam Study. Stroke 22:983–988
2. Coumel P, Friocourt P, Mujica J (1983) Long-term prevention of vagal atrial arrhythmias by atrial pacing at 90/minute: experience with 6 cases. Pacing Clin Electrophysiol 6:552–560
3. Lamas GA, Estes NM, Schneller S (1992) Does dual chamber pacing prevent atrial fibrillation? The need for a randomized controlled trial. Pacing Clin Electrophysiol 15:1109–1113
4. Frielingsdorf J, Gerber AE, Hess OM (1994) Importance of maintained atrioventricular synchrony in patients with pace-makers. Eur Heart J 15:1431–1441
5. Connolly SJ, Kerr C, Gent M et al (1996) Dual chamber versus ventricular pacing: critical appraisal of current data. Circulation 94:578–583
6. Andersen HR, Nielsen JC, Thomsen PE (1994) Prospective randomized trial of atrial versus ventricular pacing in sick sinus syndrome. Lancet 344:1523-1528
7. Andersen HR, Nielsen JC, Thomsen PE et al (1997) Long-term follow-up of patients from a randomized trial of atrial versus ventricular pacing in sick sinus syndrome. Lancet 350:1210–1216
8. Lamas GA, Orav J, Strambler BS et al (1998) Quality of life and clinical outcomes in elderly patients treated with ventricular pacing as compared with dual chamber pacing. N Engl J Med 338:1097–1104
9. Connolly SJ, Kerr CR, Gent M et al (2000) Effects of physiologic pacing on the risk of stroke and death due to cardiovascular causes. Canadian Trial of Physiologic Pacing Investigators. N Engl J Med 342:1385–1391
10. Papageorgiou P, Monahan K, Boyle NG et al (1996) Site-dependent intra-atrial conduction delay: relationship to initiation of atrial fibrillation. Circulation 94:384–389
11. Saksena S, Giorgberidze I, Prakash A et al (1996) Endocardial mapping during induced atrial fibrillation (abstract). Circulation 94 (Suppl I):I555

12. Platonov PG, Yuan S, Hertervig E et al (2001) Further evidence of localized posterior interatrial conduction delay in lone paroxysmal atrial fibrillation. Europace 3:100–107

13. Revault d'Allones G, Favin D, Leclercq C et al (2000) Long term effects of biatrial synchronous pacing to prevent drug-refractory atrial tachyarrhythmia: a nine-year experience. J Cardiovasc Electrophysiol 11:1081–1091

14. Saksena S, Delfaut P, Prakash A et al (1998) Multisite electrode pacing for prevention of atrial fibrillation. J Cardiovasc Electrophysiol 9:S155-S162

15. Saksena S, Prakash A, Ziegler P et al for the DAPPAF Investigators (2002) The Dual Site Atrial Pacing for Prevention of Atrial Fibrillation (DAPPAF) trial: improved suppression of atrial fibrillation with dual-site atrial pacing and antiarrhythmic drug therapy. J Am Coll Cardiol 40:1140–1150

16. Mabo P, Daubert JC, Bouhour JB et al (1999) Biatrial synchronous pacing for atrial arrhythmia prevention: the SYNBIA-PACE study (abstract). Pacing Clin Electrophysiol 22:755

17. Bailin SJ, Johnson WB, Hoyt R (1995) Differential atrial pacing: implications for atrial activation (abstract). Circulation 92:I405

18. Yu WC, Tsai CF, Hsieh MH et al (2000) Prevention of the initiation of atrial fibrillation: mechanism and efficacy of different atrial pacing modes. Pacing Clin Electrophysiol 23:373–379

19. Bailin SJ, Adler S, Giudici M (2001) Prevention of chronic atrial fibrillation by pacing in the region of Bachmann's bundle: results of a multicenter randomized trial. J Cardiovasc Electrophysiol 12:912–917

20. Spencer W, Zhu D, Markowitz T et al (1997) Atrial septal pacing: a method for pacing both atria simultaneously. Pacing Clin Electrophysiol 20:2739–2745

21. Padeletti L, Porciani MC, Michelucci A et al (1999) Interatrial septum pacing: a new approach to preventing recurrent atrial fibrillation. J Interv Cardiac Electrophysiol 3:35–43

22. Kale M, Bennett DH (2002) Atrial septal pacing in the prevention of paroxysmal atrial fibrillation refractory to antiarrhythmic drugs. Int J Cardiol 82:167–175

23. Senatore G, Fazzari M, De Simone A et al (2001) Dynamic atrial pacing (DAO) and multisite atrial pacing for prevention of atrial fibrillation: the STADIM trial. In: Bloch Thomsen PE (ed) Proceedings of Europace 2001, Monduzzi, Bologna, pp 413-417

24. Padeletti L, Purerfellner H, Adler S et al (2003) Combined efficacy of atrial septal lead placement and atrial pacing algorithms for prevention of paroxysmal atrial tachyarrhythmia. J Cardiovasc Electrophysiol 14:1189–1195

25. Andersen HR, Nielsen JC, Thomsen PE et al (1997) Long-term follow-up of patients from a randomized trial of atrial versus ventricular pacing for sick sinus syndrome. Lancet 350:1210–1216

26. Connolly SJ, Kerr CR, Gent M et al (2000) Effects of physiologic pacing versus ventricular pacing on the risk of stroke and death due to cardiovascular causes. N Engl J Med 342:1385–1391

27. Sweeney M, Hellkamp A, Ellenbogen K et al (2003) Adverse effect of ventricular pacing on heart failure and atrial fibrillarion among patients with normal baseline QRS duration in a clinical trial of pacemaker therapy for sinus node dysfunction. Circulation 107:2932–2937

28. Wilkoff B, Dual Chamber and VVI Implantable Defibrillator trial investigators (2002) Dual-chamber pacing or ventricular backup pacing in patients with an

implantable defibrillator. The Dual Chamber and VVI Implantable Defibrillator (DAVID) trial. JAMA 288:3115–3123

29. Milasinovic G, Sperzel J, Compton S et al (2004) Preserving intrinsic ventricular activation with a novel pacemaker algorithm: Search AV+. Heart Rythm 1:S277 (abtracts)

Role of His-Bundle Pacing: Reliability and Potential to Avoid Ventricular Dyssynchrony

F. Zanon, E. Baracca, S. Aggio, G. Boaretto, G. Pastore, P. Zonzin

Increasing clinical evidence shows that conventional right ventricular pacing is detrimental to left ventricular function. Recent studies in canines [1] showed that right ventricular apical (RVA) pacing causes abnormal contraction patterns due to abnormal activation of the left ventricle during RVA pacing compared to normal sinus rhythm. Moreover, these studies gave evidence that sustained RVA pacing is associated with histological and structural changes that cause left ventricular function to deteriorate. In humans, short- and long-term studies [2, 3] have confirmed the adverse effects of RVA pacing.

A theoretical pacing system that could preserve the normal Purkinje activation should be considered the ideal pacing approach, because the ventricular dyssynchrony would be prevented and the normal activation pattern maintained. However, the traditional pacing tools do not allow an easy approach to the His bundle, and therefore few clinical reports of this pacing mode exist in the literature.

Deshmukh et al. [4, 5] reported the results of direct His-bundle pacing (DHBP) in patients with chronic heart failure and atrial fibrillation who were candidates for ablate-and-pace strategy because of a rapid and pharmacologically uncontrolled ventricular rate. According to Deshmukh et al., the criteria for verification of the DHBP were the following: (1) recording of His bundle potential with the permanent pacing lead; (2) pace-ventricular interval equal to His-ventricular interval ± 15 ms; (3) paced QRS morphology and duration equal to the intrinsic QRS in all 12 ECG leads.

Twelve out of 18 patients in the first study and 39 out of 54 patients in the second study were successfully paced. In a long-term follow-up (42 months) the

Division of Cardiology, General Hospital, Rovigo, Italy

mean NYHA class improved from 3.5 to 2.2 and the ejection fraction increased from 0.23 ± 0.11 to 0.33 ± 0.15. In these studies by Deshmukh et al. the total procedure time was 3.7 ± 1.6 h and a standard screw-in lead (helix 1.5 mm) with modified J-shaped stylet was used to reach the His bundle.

Vázquez et al. [6] attempted DHBP in 12 patients without structural heart disease selected for AV nodal ablation due to uncontrolled paroxysmal atrial fibrillation or for pacemaker implantation because of supra-His conduction disturbances with a normal conduction system. DHBP was successfully achieved in 8 out of 12 patients. Acute and 3-month electrical performances were acceptable and the authors reported a procedure time of 192 min using an approach similar to that of Deshmukh et al.

DHBP is really difficult to achieve with a standard lead with a modified stylet, extending implant time and causing recurrent acute dislodgements. The tools for biventricular stimulation, designed to facilitate the insertion of leads into the coronary sinus and from there to the lateral distal cardiac vein, suggested the idea that new active-fixation leads guided by steerable catheters could allow right ventricular selective sites to be reached.

The first dedicated tool is the Medtronic SelectSecure system, composed by a steerable catheter (SelectSite – Model C304, Medtronic Inc.) and a 4.1-Fr no stylet, active fixation, bipolar, steroid-eluting lead (Model 3830, Medtronic Inc.). Recently, we started using this new pacing approach in our centre. DHBP was attempted in 25 patients (17 male, mean age 77 ± 8 years) with standard pacemaker indication and a narrow QRS. All patients underwent implantation using the SelectSecure system. DHBP was achieved in 23 patients (92%); two patients were paced in the His area, but the QRS morphology and duration under pacing were different from the native ones.

In DHBP pacing, the acute pacing threshold was 2.4 ± 1.2 V at a pulse width of 0.5 ms, whereas sensed potentials were 3.0 ± 2.0 mV. No major complications were observed.

In conclusion, our preliminary experience with this new tool shows that DHBP is feasible. However, future studies will be necessary to confirm the real benefits of this new pacing technique.

References

1. Amitani S, Miyahara K, Somara H et al (1999) Experimental His-bundle pacing: histopathological and electrophysiological examination. Pacing Clin Electrophysiol 22[Pt. I]:562–566
2. Gomes JA, Damato AN, Akhtar N et al (1977) Ventricular septal motion and left ventricular dimensions during abnormal ventricular activation. Am J Cardiol 39:641–650

3. Tse H, Lau CP (1997) Long term effects of right ventricular pacing on myocardial perfusion and function. J Am Coll Cardiol 29:744–749

4. Deshmukh P, Casavant D, Romannyshyn M et al (2000) Permanent, direct His-bundle pacing – a novel approach to cardiac pacing in patients with normal His-Purkinje activation. Circulation 101:869–877

5. Deshmukh P, Romannyshyn M (2004) Direct His-bundle pacing: present and future. Pacing Clin Electrophysiol 27[Pt. II]:862–870

6. Vázquez P, Pichardo R, Gamero J et al (2001) Estimulación permanente del haz de His tras ablación medianteradiofrecuencia del nodo auriculoventricular en pacientes con trastorno de la conducción suprahisiano. Rev Esp Cardiol 54:1385–1393

Pacemaker for Vasovagal Syncope: Good for the Few

M. BRIGNOLE

The decision to implant a pacemaker needs to be kept in the clinical context of a benign condition which frequently affects young patients. Thus, cardiac pacing should be limited as the last-resort choice to a very selected small proportion of patients affected by severe vasovagal syncope. How to select these patients still remains partly uncertain.

Background

The term 'vasovagal syncope' refers to a reflex response that, when triggered, gives rise to vasodilation and bradycardia, although the contribution of both of these to systemic hypotension and cerebral hypoperfusion may differ considerably. It is valuable to assess the relative contribution of cardioinhibition and vasodepression before embarking on treatment as there are different therapeutic strategies for the two entities. The triggering events may vary considerably over time in any individual patient. 'Classical' vasovagal syncope is mediated by emotional or orthostatic stress and can be diagnosed by history taking. 'Non-classical' presentations are frequent, and these forms are diagnosed by minor clinical criteria, exclusion of other causes of syncope (absence of structural heart disease), and positive response to tilt testing or carotid sinus massage. Examples of non-classical vasovagal syncope include episodes without clear triggering events or premonitory signs.

Criteria for Selection of Patients

In general, initial 'treatment' of all forms of neurally-mediated reflex syncope consists of reassurance as to the benign nature of the syndrome, educa-

Department of Cardiology and Arrythmologic Centre, Ospedali del Tigullio, Lavagna (Genua), Italy

tion regarding avoidance of triggering events and predisposing factors, recognition of premonitory symptoms and manoeuvres to abort the episode, and avoidance of volume depletion and prolonged upright posture. The above measures are sufficient for the vast majority of patients affected by vasovagal syncope. Additional treatment may be necessary in the high risk or high frequency settings defined by the ESC Task Force on Syncope [1] when syncope:

- is very frequent, e.g. alters the quality of life
- is recurrent and unpredictable (absence of premonitory symptoms) and exposes patients to 'high risk' of trauma
- occurs during participation in a 'high risk' activity (e.g. driving, machine operator, flying, competitive athletics, etc.).

Among these settings, cardiac pacing may be reserved for those patients with cardioinhibitory vasovagal syncope with a frequency of more than five attacks per year or severe physical injury or accident and age above 40 years [1]. In order to limit the vasodepressor component of the vasovagal reflex, dual-chamber pacemakers with rate hysteresis features are usually preferred, although formal comparison studies among modes of pacing have not yet been performed.

Results from Randomised Controlled Trials

Pacing for vasovagal syncope has been the subject of five major multicentre randomised controlled trials [2–6], of which three gave positive and two gave negative results. Putting together the results of the five trials, 318 patients were evaluated; syncope recurred in 21% (33/156) of the paced patients and in 44% (72/162) of non-paced patients ($P < 0.000$). However, all the studies have weaknesses, and further follow-up studies addressing many of these limitations (particularly the pre-implant selection criteria for patients who might benefit from pacemaker therapy) need to be completed before pacing can be considered an established therapy.

Future Perspectives

It seems that pacing therapy might be effective in some but not in all patients. This is not surprising if we consider that pacing is probably efficacious for asystolic reflex but has no role in combating hypotension, which is frequently the dominant reflex in vasovagal syncope. How to stratify the patients is still uncertain. A recent study using the implantable loop recorder as reference standard [7] showed that only about half of the patients had an asystolic pause recorded at the time of spontaneous syncope which might eventually benefit from a pacemaker. In the other patients a pacemaker is unlikely to be effective. The role of the implantable loop recorder for selecting patients who may benefit from cardiac pacing is actually under evaluation.

A widely used method for selecting patients suitable for cardiac pacing is the finding of a cardioinhibitory form of syncope during tilt testing. However, recent data showed that the mechanism of tilt-induced syncope was frequently different from that of the spontaneous syncope recorded with the Implantable Loop Recorder [7]. These data show that the use of tilt testing for assessing the effectiveness of different treatments has important limitations and its use is now disregarded in the ESC Guidelines [1].

References

1. Brignole M, Alboni P, Benditt D et al (2004) Guidelines on management (diagnosis and treatment) of syncope. Update 2004 – Executive summary and recommendations. Eur Heart J 25:2054–2072
2. Connolly SJ, Sheldon R, Roberts RS et al (1999) The North American vasovagal pacemaker study (VPS): a randomised trial of permanent cardiac pacing for the prevention of vasovagal syncope. J Am Coll Cardiol 33:16–20
3. Sutton R, Brignole M, Menozzi C et al (2000) Dual-chamber pacing in treatment of neurally-mediated tilt-positive cardioinhibitory syncope. Pacemaker versus no therapy: a multicentre randomized study. Circulation 102:294–299
4. Ammirati F, Colivicchi F, Santini M (2001) Permanent cardiac pacing versus medical treatment for the prevention of recurrent vasovagal syncope. A multicenter, randomized, controlled trial. Circulation 104:52–57
5. Connolly SJ, Sheldon R, Thorpe KE et al (2003) Pacemaker therapy for prevention of syncope in patients with recurrent severe vasovagal syncope: Second Vasovagal Pacemaker Study (VPS II). JAMA 289:2224–2229
6. Giada F, Raviele A, Menozzi C et al (2003) The vasovagal syncope and pacing trial (Synpace). A randomized placebo-controlled study of permanent pacing for treatment of recurrent vasovagal syncope. PACE 26:1016 (abstract)
7. Moya A, Brignole M, Menozzi C et al (2001) Mechanism of syncope in patients with isolated syncope and in patients with tilt-positive syncope. Circulation 104:1261–1267

Quality of Life of Patients with an Atrial Defibrillator: Does Optimal Programming Achieve the Goal of Maintaining Sinus Rhythm as Well as Improve Quality of Life?

A. Quesada, V. Palanca, J. Jiménez, O. Villalba, R. Payá, J.R. Balaguer, S. Villalba, J. Roda

Introduction

The quality of life (QoL) of patients with atrial fibrillation (AF) has been demonstrated to be worse than that of age-matched healthy subjects; either worse than or as impaired as that of patients either with a recent prior myocardial infarction or who have recently undergone coronary angioplasty; and the same as that of patients with heart failure [1, 2]. Limitations of current drug-based strategies for AF are leading to increasing use of non-pharmacological therapies. Although atrial defibrillators (stand-alone and dual chamber defibrillators with both atrial antibradycardia and antitachycardia pacing) have shown both safety and high efficacy in suppressing AF and other regular atrial tachycardias (AT), several concerns remain regarding shock tolerance and real improvement of QoL. Thus, the impact of this type of non-pharmacological therapy on QoL is far from well-established, especially when the long term is considered [3]. In this chapter we review the benefits and risks imposed to QoL both by the device and by AF itself, and how some programming strategies and psychological interventions can help us in the difficult management of patients with drug-refractory AF.

Quality of Life and Psychosocial Disturbances in AF-ICD Patients

Two fundamental premises should be emphasised. First of all, patients with AF, whether symptomatic or not, have impaired QoL. Secondly, QoL improves with treatment of AF, and at least some of these improvements are related to the restoration and maintenance of sinus rhythm [1–3]. Thus,

Cardiac Electrophysiology and Arrhythmias Section, Department of Cardiology, Hospital General Universitario de Valencia, Spain

when one looks for QoL changes in these patients, it is mandatory to distinguish between those due to the arrhythmia itself and those secondary to the presence of an implanted device, and even those following discontinuation of drug therapies.

Several studies have reported QoL modifications in patients with atrial defibrillators [3, 4]. Focusing on the dual devices (with atrial and ventricular capabilities), in the AF-only study two QoL instruments were used to assess the impact of implantation of the dual implantable cardioverter–defibrillator (ICD) on patients' QoL: the Medical Outcomes Study Short Form (SF-36), a standardised health survey instrument that has eight scales, and the Symptom Checklist, a disease-specific instrument. In the SF-36 there was a statistically significant improvement in Physical Function, Physical Role, Vitality, and Social Function scales from baseline to 3 months, which was sustained at 6 months' follow-up [4]. The Symptom Checklist measures patients' perceptions of the frequency and severity of 16 AF arrhythmia-related symptoms. A change in symptoms over time was discerned in 73 patients, and again they showed a significant decrease (improvement) from baseline to 3 months and from baseline to 6 months' follow-up.

Programming of atrial shocks remained constant during the follow-up, and programming of patient-initiated shocks, either alone or along with timed shocks, increased from 54% of patients at baseline to 72% at last contact. Sixty-seven patients (67/144, 47%) used the patient assistant to deliver patient-initiated shocks.

Using the Symptom Checklist/Frequency and Severity Scale for all items and the SF-36 questionnaire, we have reported the changes after dual ICD implantation in 40 patients with refractory AF [5]. Both instruments showed significant improvements in physical activities because of health problems, in limitations in usual role activities because of physical health problems and in perceived bodily pain. The patients assigned to early delivery of atrial shock after AF onset, compared with the patients who did not receive atrial shock, showed a significant reduction of AF burden, a greater reduction in number of hospitalisations, and greater improvement of QoL.

Thus, the defibrillator effectively counteracted the reduction of QoL imposed by the arrhythmia. Possible explanations for this could be the symptomatic characteristics of the population selected, the baseline high effectiveness of the shocks (the mean number of shocks per episode was 1.2 and more than 86% of episodes required only 1 shock), and the limited numbers of shocks during the follow-up.

The PASSAT study evaluated in 96 patients enrolled in the AF-Only Study, QoL, psychosocial distress, and acceptance of ICD therapy for atrial tachyarrhythmias (ICD-AT) over a mean follow-up period of 19 months, [6]. From implantation to survey, a significant change in AF symptoms and severity scores and QoL (SF-36) scores was registered. ICD-AT therapy acceptance was high, with 71.3% of patients scoring in the 75th percentile on the Florida Patient Acceptance Survey. ICD-AT acceptance was correlated with the Physical Component Scale and Mental Health Component Scale scores of the SF-36. ICD-AT acceptance correlated negatively with depressive symptomatology, trait anxiety, illness intrusiveness, and AF symptom and severity scores. ICD-AT acceptance did not correlate with preimplantation cardioversions, number of atrial shocks, AF episodes detected by the device, or device implant duration.

However, although QoL increases in many patients, in some patients psychological disturbances could result in reduced acceptance of atrial shocks. Several risk factors have been identified to predict poor toleration of living with an ICD. These include young patient age, multiple ICD discharges, low social support, female gender, premorbid psychological difficulties, poor understanding of the device and the disease, and more severe medical conditions. Although the number of shocks is very important (both the individual and the cumulative effects of each shock), as is the experience of suffering an ICD storm, the crucial role of psychological well-being and improved perceived AF symptom burden for the long-term acceptance of ICD-AT therapy has been stressed [6].

The shocks will affect both the patient and his/her relatives. In the patient, the pain from the electrical discharges can generate catastrophic thinking, leading to fear and anxiety. In the relatives, shocks generate avoidance behaviour that increases the catastrophic thinking. In our experience, symptoms of depression and anxiety are common following the implantation, arising from concerns about both the device and the disease itself. The clinical outcome and the confrontation strategies that the patients adopt will determine the psychological outcome and the acceptance of the therapy. Adaptive, positive strategies lead to good patient–ICD coexistence, the most frequently used being spiritual or social-type strategies based on religious belief or on the confidence and support of the family or physician. Non-adaptive, negative strategies, especially avoidance and non-acceptance of the disease and device, will originate eventually lead to rejection of the treatment, with the catastrophic thinking dominated by irrational belief. Psychologically, these irrational beliefs can be treated with cognitive therapy, such as cognitive restructuring.

Dual ICD 'Optimal' Programming for AF Patients

The optimisation of several programming parameters can increase the efficacy of the device, especially those aimed at both reducing the number of shocks and improving their efficacy, achieving higher therapy/device acceptance.

1. *Apical ventricular pacing may be avoided.* Apical right ventricular pacing alters the normal cardiac activation sequence, and there is cumulative evidence that it may induce a depression of left ventricular function. The results of several trials suggest strongly that loss of ventricular synchrony may result in increasing incidence of AF, heart failure, and death. In the MOST sub-study [7], ventricular pacing was associated with an increased risk of AF, and the risk of AF increased linearly with the cumulative percentage of ventricular pacing (approximately 1% for each 1% increase in the latter).

   Although intrinsic ventricular activation was preserved with AAI pacing, low-rate VVI pacing, fixed long AV intervals, and DDI pacing, each of these approaches has disadvantages or modest effectiveness. Recently, new atrioventricular (AV) algorithms have been developed to achieve minimal ventricular pacing. A randomised pilot study with 30 patients using one of these (MVP, Medtronic) showed an impressive reduction in cumulative percentage of ventricular pacing (3.8% vs 80.6%), maintaining AV synchrony [8]. More studies are required to demonstrate whether this reduction in ventricular pacing can reduce the incidence of AF.

2. *Preventive and antitachycardia pacing.* Some preventive algorithms are available in dual ICD defibrillators, such as atrial pacing preference and atrial rate stabilisation (provides pacing to eliminate long pauses following atrial premature beats). In the AF-only study, no effect on burden or number of episodes was observed [9], whereas in the ADOPT study [10], with a similar algorithm for atrial overdrive pacing but in a pacemaker population with associated bradycardia, a significant reduction in burden was encountered. Interestingly, it has been communicated [11] that a high percentage of ventricular pacing can counterbalance the benefits of the algorithm.

   Atrial pacing therapies (ATP) have a high efficacy in suppressing many of the atrial tachycardia (AT) episodes (the most prevalent arrhythmia in this type of patients) [12–14] and might be delivered early, within or immediately after the first minute, and programmed in AT and AF zones. Although many episodes of AF/AT last less than 1 min, the probability of inducing sustained AF with ATP is low when it is delivered in stable rhythms. In addition to ramp and burst ATP, we usually activate atrial 50-Hz burst pacing because it has a low but additive efficacy (over 5–10% episodes in total, after the conventional ATP has been delivered).

3. *Shocks, pathway, and programming.* Three possible cardioversion strategies are available in the atrial ICD: patient self-activated, automatic, and in-hospital manually administered shocks [13, 15]. Whatever method is

used, it is mandatory to limit the number of shocks per episode and day (only one is advisable) and to try to increase their success rate. We reported a greater reduction of burden with automatic versus in-hospital manually delivered shocks, suggesting that early delivery of atrial shock after AF onset may be the best strategy [5]. Early restoration of sinus rhythm could reduce the electrophysiological remodelling process, increasing the periods of sinus rhythm and decreasing the AF burden in the long-term follow-up. Similar reductions have been observed with patient-activated shocks. However, to avoid treating self-limited episodes, a certain duration of the arrhythmia is required; the investigators of the Jewel AF, AF-only study reported a longer duration of AF prior to shock > 3 h as one of the determinants of first-shock success [16]. Usually 6 h of sustained atrial tachyarrhythmia are programmed before shock delivery.

The right-atrium-to-coronary-sinus electrode configuration significantly reduces the atrial defibrillation threshold [17]. This was also observed in the Jewel AF, AF-only study, in which the use of a coronary sinus electrode was accompanied by a higher success rate of shock [16]. Thus, a coronary sinus electrode should be considered in all patients undergoing evaluation for insertion of an atrial defibrillator.

4. *Close monitoring after implantation and use of adjuvant treatments.* Treatment of AT/AF episodes should be aggressive shortly after implantation (AF-only study, unpublished data); it results in a significant decrease in AT/AF burden, and this is accompanied by a decrease in the frequency of atrial cardioversion shocks. However, the risk of multiple shocks (even only one or two) does exist, leading to a psychological deterioration cascade and catastrophic and irrational thinking. Early comprehensive management of the patient, including not only medical support but also psychological, familial ,and social monitoring and assistance, can overcome the danger of therapy rejection.

Sedation with midazolam (15 mg, elixir) significantly increases the acceptability of atrial shock regardless of the cardioversion method. Shocks without sedation are significantly less acceptable in this type of patient [18]; if sedation is not used, automatic night cardioversion results in sleep disturbances as well as concerns about future pain or discomfort. It is advisable not to decrease (even to increase) anti-arrhythmics drug use, together with intensive treatment of heart failure (and left ventricular dysfunction). The synergistic effect of cardiac resynchronisation therapy is currently under investigation (RENEWAL 4 AVT study).

Thus, most drug-refractory AF-ICD patients (a heterogeneous population) accept the device and the shocks with improvement in their QoL. Optimisation of programming can help to achieve this goal. However, the presence of psychological disturbances in a subset of these patients make it necessary to view the hybrid therapy as a multidisciplinary task that may include not just pacing and shock therapies, drugs, and ablation techniques, but also early and intensive psychosocial monitoring and intervention.

References

1. Dorian P, Jung W, Newman D et al (2000) The impairment of health-related quality of life in patients with intermittent atrial fibrillation: implications for the assessment of investigational therapy. J Am Coll Cardiol 36:1303–1309

2. Luderitz B, Jung W (2000) Quality of life in atrial fibrillation. J Interv Card Electrophysiol 4:201–209

3. Engelmann DE, Pehrson S (2003) Quality of life in nonpharmacologic treatment of atrial fibrillation. Eur Heart J 15:1387–1400

4. Newman DM, Dorian P, Paquette M et al for Worldwide Jewel AF AF-Only Investigators (2003) Effect of an implantable cardioverter defibrillator with atrial detection and shock therapies on patient-perceived, health-related quality of life. Am Heart J 145:841–846

5. Ricci R, Quesada A, Pignalberi C et al (2004) Dual defibrillator improves quality of life and decreases hospitalizations in patients with drug refractory atrial fibrillation. J Interv Card Electrophysiol 10:85–92

6. Burns JL, Sears SF, Sotile R et al (2004) Do patients accept implantable atrial defibrillation therapy? Results from the Patient Atrial Shock Survey of Acceptance and Tolerance (PASSAT) Study. J Cardiovasc Electrophysiol 15:292–294

7. Sweeney MO, Hellkamp AS, Ellenbogen KA et al for MOde Selection Trial Investigators (2003) Adverse effect of ventricular pacing on heart failure and atrial fibrillation among patients with normal baseline QRS duration in a clinical trial of pacemaker therapy for sinus node dysfunction. Circulation 107:2932–2937

8. Sweeney M, Shea J, Fox V et al (2004) Randomized pilot study of a new atrial-based minimal ventricular pacing mode in dual-chamber implantable cardioverter-defibrillators. Heart Rhythm 1:160–167

9. Quesada A on behalf of AF investigators (2002) Dual defibrillator in patients with atrial fibrillation: clinical outcomes, quality of life and resource utilization. Mediterr J Pacing Electrophysiol 4:186–191

10. Carlson M, Ip J, Messenger J (2003) A new pacemaker algorithm for the treatment of atrial fibrillation: results of the Atrial Dynamic Overdrive Pacing Trial (ADOPT). J Am Coll Cardiol 42:627–633

11. Gold M, Fain E, Ip J et al (2004) Frequent ventricular pacing attenuates the benefit of dynamic atrial overdrive for the prevention of atrial fibrillation. NASPE, Heart Rhythm Society 2004, San Francisco, CA

12. Schoels W, Swerdlow CD, Jung W et al for the Worldwide Jewel AF Investigators (2001) Worldwide clinical experience with a new dual chamber implantable cardioverter defibrillator system. J Cardiovasc Electrophysiol 12:521–528

13. Gold MR, Sulke N, Schwartzman DS et al for the Worldwide Jewel AF-only Investigators (2001) Clinical experience with a dual chamber implantable cardioverter defibrillator to treat atrial tachyarrhythmias. J Cardiovasc Electrophysiol 12:1247–1253

14. Gillis A, Unterberg-Buchwald C, Schmidinger G et al for the GEM III AT worldwide investigators (2002) Safety and efficacy of advanced atrial pacing therapies for atrial tachyarrhythmias in patients with a new implantable dual chamber cardioverter-defibrillator. J Am Coll Cardiol 40:1653–1659

15. Wellens HJJ, Lau CP, Luderitz B et al (1998) Atrioverter: an implantable device for the treatment of atrial fibrillation. Circulation 98:1651–1656

16. Swerdlow CD, Schwartzman D, Hoyt R et al for the Worldwide Model 7250 AF-Only Investigators (2002) Determinants of first-shock success for atrial implantable cardioverter defibrillators. J Cardiovasc Electrophysiol 13:347–354

17. Mitchell AR, Spurrell PA, Kamalvand K et al (2002) What is the optimal electrode configuration for atrial defibrillators in man? Europace 4:41–46

18. Boodhoo L, Mitchell A, Ujhelyi M et al (2004) Improving the acceptability of the atrial defibrillator: patient-activated cardioversion versus automatic night cardioversion with and without sedation (ADSAS 2). Pacing Clin Electrophysiol 27:910–917

HAEMODYNAMIC SENSING IN THE CONTROL OF PACING FUNCTION

Haemodynamic Assessment by Transvalvular Impedance Recording

M.G. Bongiorni[1], E. Soldati[1], G. Arena[1], G. Giannola[1], C. Bartoli[1], A. Barbetta[2], F. Di Gregorio[2]

Full autoregulation of a pacing device is an important prospect in the advancement of cardiac stimulation, which is expected to integrate in a global controlling system several automatic functions such as mode switching, rate-responsive pacing, adaptation of sensitivity and pulse energy, AV delay tuning, and more. Since the final aim of cardiac pacing is ensuring a blood supply that properly matches the patient's functional conditions, haemodynamic sensors could be proposed as the best candidates for supervision of an implantable pacemaker. However, currently available haemodynamic sensors, such as peak endocardial acceleration (PEA) or unipolar ventricular impedance, have been designed to monitor processes and parameters correlated with the ventricular contraction strength [1–4], whereas adequate haemodynamic control of cardiac function would better be achieved through assessment of the ejected blood volume [5, 6].

Volume Information from Impedance Data

So far, no one has attempted to include a flowmeter in the design of a permanent stimulator, since such a sensor would be too complex and unreliable in the long run. On the other hand, suitable information on the stroke volume (SV) trend can be derived by measuring the electric impedance of the ventricle, which is proportional to the distance between the sampling points and inversely related to the cross-sectional area of the conducting medium [7]. Any change in ventricular blood volume should entail a corresponding change in intraventricular impedance. The ideal tool to correlate impedance and volume changes is a multipolar catheter, as currently used in acute

[1]CardioThoracic Department, University of Pisa; [2]Medico Clinical Research, Rubano (Padua), Italy

haemodynamic studies [8, 9]. However, impedance fluctuations induced by ventricular mechanical activity can be detected even with conventional pacing leads, in either unipolar or bipolar modality. Unipolar impedance, measured between the tip ventricular electrode and the pacemaker case, is thought to be modulated by structural modifications in the electrode's microenvironment. The main information extracted from the unipolar impedance signal is a score of the fluctuation steepness, which can be affected by the contraction strength [3, 10]. Bipolar intraventricular impedance, recorded between the tip and the ring ventricular electrode, has been suggested to be mainly dependent on the ventricular volume. In this case as well, the system should be sensitive just to local events in the ventricular apex, which is taken as a representative sample of the whole ventricle. The absolute values of minimum and maximum bipolar impedance in a cardiac cycle are sensitive to preload and contractility modifications, and the reported changes are consistent with the hypothesis of an inverse relationship between ventricular impedance and volume [5, 6, 11].

Indeed, impedance measurements are known to be affected by additional factors, including electrode position and movement. Special care in data management has been suggested to remove non-specific effects and maximise the impedance sensitivity to volume changes [6]. In addition, further advantages were produced by the development of an alternative method for cardiac impedance recording, i.e. the assessment of transvalvular impedance (TVI). TVI is measured between an atrial and a ventricular electrode, thus increasing the dipole length with respect to the intraventricular impedance while keeping both the poles inside the heart [12–14]. This virtually avoids the artefacts produced by thorax movement, which affect the unipolar ventricular impedance, allowing impedance recording without high-pass filtering. In the presence of a bipolar ventricular lead, TVI can be measured with either the tip or the ring ventricular electrode [15]. In the latter case, there is no close contact with the ventricular wall, and therefore cyclic impedance changes should better reflect pure volume modifications associated with the pump function.

Transvalvular Impedance as a Haemodynamic Indicator

The TVI waveform generally features high stability and signal-to-noise ratio, even with DC coupling. The absolute minimum and maximum TVI are recorded, respectively, in telediastole and telesystole, and are assumed to be inversely related to the maximum and minimum ventricular volume. Studies conducted with external devices connected to the pacing leads during pacemaker implantation or replacement procedures confirmed that end-diastolic

TVI (edTVI) depends on the preload, while end-systolic TVI (esTVI) is sensitive to cardiac contractility. In these experiments, preload modifications were produced by cardiac rate changes, while positive inotropic and chronotropic effects were induced by the administration of a beta-adrenergic drug. All the patients were lying supine and could not move during the test [15–17].

To overcome these limitations, we recorded TVI in patients undergoing the extraction of infected pacing leads. In such cases, it is normal practice to expose the lead connectors before the extraction procedure for pocket draining. This made possible connecting an external device with chronically implanted leads in patients free to move, in order to study the TVI response to postural changes and physiological autonomic stimulation during an ergometric stress test.

The transition from lying supine to standing upright is known to entail a reduction in ventricular filling due to the opposing action of gravity, with consequent blood accumulation in the leg veins and corresponding SV decrease imposed by the intrinsic regulation of the heart. This effect is physiologically counteracted by a positive chronotropic reaction, aimed at maintaining an adequate cardiac output. In these circumstances, we observed a reversible reduction in the peak-to-peak excursion of the TVI signal, resulting from an increase in edTVI (Fig. 1). Data were processed considering the peak-to-peak TVI amplitude as a SV indicator [5, 11]. The relationship between the two parameters was assumed to be approximately linear in the physiological range. Any change in edTVI or esTVI with respect to their baseline values was expressed as a percentage of the peak-to-peak TVI amplitude at rest and represented an equal and opposite volume change, expressed as a percentage of the baseline SV. According to this model, the TVI modifications induced by standing up indicated a 20% decrease in SV with respect to the supine position, ascribed entirely to a preload reduction (Fig. 2).

A physical stress test was performed on the ergometric bicycle, increasing the power by 20 W every 3 min. At the start of exercise, TVI measurements indicated an increase in SV, resulting from both an increase in end-diastolic volume (EDV) and a decrease in end-systolic volume (ESV). With increasing workload EDV was constant, whereas ESV kept on slowly decreasing. When the exercise was stopped, EDV and SV dropped quickly, whereas ESV remained reduced in the early recovery stage (Fig. 3). The results suggest that SV adaptation was achieved by the contribution of both intrinsic and extrinsic cardiac regulation. Skeletal muscle activity readily increased the venous return and the preload, which rapidly dropped at the end of exercise. On the other hand, the autonomic nervous system induced a progressive increase in both sinus rate and myocardial contractility. The enhanced con-

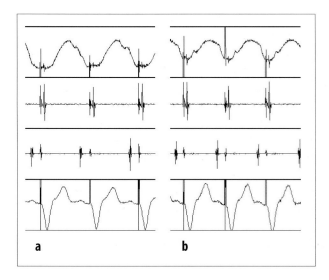

Fig. 1a, b. From *top* to *bottom:* transvalvular impedance (TVI), ventricular and atrial electrograms, surface ECG. An external recorder was connected with exposed chronic pacing leads, prior to lead extraction, while VDD pacing was performed by a new contralateral implant. This explains the double signal shown in the ventricular electrogram: the first deflection is the artefact produced by the spike delivered by the contralateral lead; the second is the R wave detected after a conduction delay. **a** Supine position. The sinus rate was 90 ± 4 bpm. End-diastolic TVI (edTVI), end-systolic (esTVI) and peak-to-peak TVI excursion averaged, respectively, 420 ± 3, 483 ± 1, and 63 ± 3 Ω. **b** Standing upright. The sinus rate increased to 116 ± 3 bpm. EdTVI, esTVI and peak-peak TVI were 432 ± 4, 483 ± 2, and 51 ± 5 Ω, respectively. The changes in edTVI and peak-to-peak TVI were highly significant ($P < 10^{-6}$, Student's t-test)

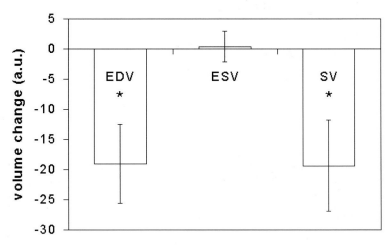

Fig. 2. Modifications in ventricular end-diastolic volume (EDV), end-systolic volume (ESV), and stroke volume (SV) induced by the transition from supine to upright standing, as inferred from TVI data. The *asterisks* indicate statistically significant variations. Volume changes are scaled in arbitrary units, corresponding to 1/100 of the reference SV, and are derived by expressing the changes in edTVI, esTVI, and peak-to-peak TVI as a percentage of the peak-to-peak TVI excursion recorded in the supine position. The variations in EDV and ESV are equal and opposite to the corresponding normalised TVI changes: an impedance increase represents an equivalent volume decrease, while an impedance decrease represents a volume increase

tractility entailed a reduction in the residual ESV, which lasted longer than sinus tachycardia when the exercise was stopped. This could be due to the different physiological regulation of ventricular myocytes and sinus node fibres, since the former are mainly sensitive to the sympathetic influence, while the latter are markedly dependent on both sympathetic and parasympathetic control.

In the case of either preload or contractility changes, the information derived from TVI was in agreement with the physiological expectation, suggesting the general reliability of the proposed haemodynamic model and supporting the hypothesised correspondence between TVI and ventricular volume. The TVI sensor can provide indications as to the inotropic state of the heart, which can be useful in patient follow-up and in the regulation of rate-responsive pacing. Indeed, the TVI-indicated rate closely reproduced the sinus rate trend during adrenergic challenge in patients with good chronotropic competence [17].

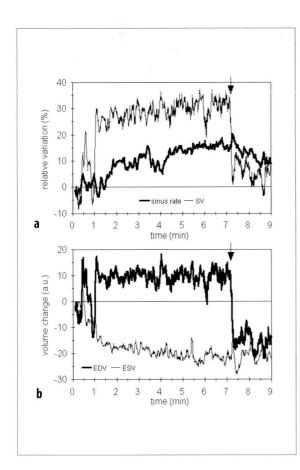

Fig. 3a, b. Stress test on the ergometric bicycle; the *arrows* indicate the end of the exercise. Changes in SV, EDV and ESV are derived from TVI data. **a** Relative variation in sinus rate and SV. **b** Relative changes in EDV and ESV. The modifications in minimum and maximum TVI values in each cardiac cycle were converted into corresponding volume changes, as described for Fig. 2

Haemodynamic Surveillance of Pacing and Sensing

An essential piece of information to be expected from a haemodynamic sensor concerns the occurrence of systolic ejection, whatever the SV or the myocardial contractility. Thanks to the excellent signal-to-noise discrimination, TVI proved reliable in the check for correct association of electrical and mechanical events at every heartbeat, in the case of either evoked or intrinsic activity. After ventricular pacing, a significant TVI increase detected in the systolic window allows confirmation of capture [12, 13, 18]. After ventricular sensing, a TVI response is expected as well: if it does not occur, the reality of the recorded electric event should be questioned. The application of the TVI sensor in ventricular pacing and sensing validation has been successfully tested with an external pacemaker, which reacted to capture loss by increasing the pulse energy and to TVI-indicated electric interference with the sensing function by switching over to a ventricular-triggered pacing mode [18]. The system proved equally sensitive to evoked or intrinsic ventricular activation, thus ensuring the prompt detection of possible fusion beats (Fig. 4).

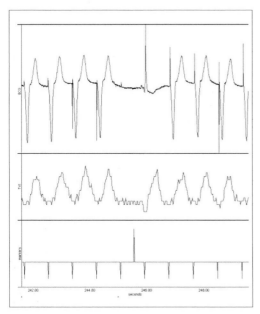

Fig. 4. Surface ECG (*upper tracing*) and corresponding TVI waveform (*middle*) and event markers (*lower tracing*), recorded by an external pacemaker. Threshold analysis in VVI pacing (downward markers). Ventricular capture entails clear-cut TVI responses, until an ineffective spike is delivered. In this case, the TVI signal remains at the baseline, allowing capture loss recognition (upward alarm marker) and automatic pulse energy increase. The following event is a fusion beat, producing a TVI fluctuation promptly detected by the pacemaker (no further alarm markers are released). Thereafter, effective overdrive pacing is regained. Note the different morphology of the TVI signal in case of VVI pacing (positive deflection) or intrinsic conduction (biphasic waveform, starting with a smaller negative deflection associated with the P wave on the surface ECG and indicating active ventricular filling). In this test, several episodes of capture loss were induced. After ineffective stimulation, the TVI noise never exceeded 20% of the reference signal. As a result, the capture validation algorithm based upon the TVI sensor showed 100% sensitivity and specificity

Conclusions

Effective haemodynamic sensing would open the way to the autoregulation of a number of pacemaker functions, which could thus be integrated into a single control system. The TVI sensor can be proposed to play this crucial role, allowing the assessment of systolic and diastolic modifications in ventricular volume by means of conventional pacing leads.

References

1. Pichlmaier AM, Braile D, Ebner E et al (1992) Autonomic nervous system controlled closed loop cardiac pacing. Pacing Clin Electrophysiol 15:1787–1791
2. Rickards AF, Bombardini T, Corbucci G et al (1996) An implantable intracardiac accelerometer for monitoring myocardial contractility. Pacing Clin Electrophysiol 19:2066–2071
3. Osswald S, Cron T, Gradel C et al (2000) Closed-loop stimulation using intracardiac impedance as a sensor principle: correlation of right ventricular dP/dt max and intracardiac impedance during dobutamine stress test. Pacing Clin Electrophysiol 23:1502–1508
4. Plicchi G, Marcelli E, Parlapiano M et al (2002) PEA I and PEA II based implantable haemodynamic monitor: pre clinical studies in sheep. Europace 4:49–54
5. Chirife R, Tentori MC, Mazzetti H, Dasso D (2001) Hemodynamic sensors: are they all the same? In: Raviele A (ed) Cardiac arrhythmias 2001. Springer, Milan, pp 566–575
6. Chirife R (2003) Hemodynamic assessment with implantable pacemakers. How feasible and reliable is it? In: Raviele A (ed) Cardiac arrhythmias 2003. Springer, Milan, pp 705–712
7. Arthur W, Kaye GC (2001) Clinical use of intracardiac impedance: current applications and future perspectives. Pacing Clin Electrophysiol 24[Pt I]:500–506
8. Applegate RJ, Cheng CP, Little WC (1990) Simultaneous conductance catheter and dimension assessment of left ventricular volume in the intact animal. Circulation 81:638–648
9. Kass D, Chen-Huan C, Curry C et al (1999) Improved left ventricular mechanics from acute VDD pacing in patient with dilatated cardiomyopathy and ventricular conduction delay. Circulation 99:1567–1573
10. Griesbach L, Gestrich B, Wojciechowski D et al (2003) Clinical performance of automatic closed-loop stimulation systems. Pacing Clin Electrophysiol 26[Pt I]:1432–1437
11. Chirife R, Ortega DF, Salazar A (1993) Feasibility of measuring relative right ventricular volumes and ejection fraction with implantable rhythm control devices. Pacing Clin Electrophysiol 16:1673–1683
12. Di Gregorio F, Morra A, Finesso M, Bongiorni MG (1996) Transvalvular impedance (TVI) recording under electrical and pharmacological cardiac stimulation. Pacing Clin Electrophysiol 19[Pt II]:1689–1693
13. Bongiorni MG, Soldati E, Arena G et al (1997) Trans valvular impedance as a marker of cardiac activity. In: Vardas PE (ed) Europace '97. Monduzzi, Bologna, pp 525–528

14. Morra A, Panarotto D, Santini P, Di Gregorio F (1997) Transvalvular impedance (TVI) sensing: a new way toward the hemodynamic control of cardiac pacing. In: Vardas PE (ed) Europace '97. Monduzzi , Bologna, pp 529–533

15. Gasparini M, Curnis A, Mantica M et al (2001) Hemodynamic sensors: what clinical value do they have in heart failure? In: Raviele A (ed) Cardiac arrhythmias 2001. Springer, Milan, pp 576–585

16. Di Gregorio F, Curnis A, Pettini A et al (2002) Trans-valvular impedance (TVI) in the hemodynamic regulation of cardiac pacing. In: Mitro P, Pella D, Rybár R, Valočik G (eds) Cardiovascular diseases 2002. Monduzzi, Bologna, pp 53–57

17. Gasparini G, Curnis A, Gulizia M et al (2003) Can hemodynamic sensors ensure physiological rate control? In: Raviele A (ed) Cardiac arrhythmias 2003. Springer, Milan, pp 725–731

18. Bongiorni MG, Soldati E, Arena G et al (2003) Transvalvular impedance: does it allow automatic capture detection? In: Raviele A (ed) Cardiac arrhythmias 2003. Springer, Milan, pp 733–739

Rate-Responsive Pacing Controlled by Transvalvular Impedance: Preliminary Clinical Experience

E. Occhetta[1], G. Gasparini[2], A. Curnis[3], M. Gulizia[4], M. Bortnik[1], A. Magnani[1], A. Corrado[2], L. Bontempi[3], G. Mascioli[3], G.M. Francese[4], F. Di Gregorio[5], A. Barbetta[5], A. Raviele[2]

Introduction

All the different sensors used to assess the patient's metabolic demand in rate-responsive pacing feature well-known advantages and disadvantages. Activity sensors are usually quick and highly sensitive, but lack specificity since they can be activated by either active or passive motion. Physiological sensors are more specific, but can be slow and only sensitive to intensive exercise conditions [1]. Haemodynamic sensors, aimed at regulating the pacing rate according to the inotropic tone [2–8], can be affected by preload modifications independently of the influence exerted by the autonomic nervous system on the cardiac function [9–12]. Preload monitoring is thus advisable to take into account the contribution of the intrinsic heart regulation to the actual haemodynamic performance.

A new haemodynamic sensor based on transvalvular impedance (TVI) has been proposed to assess relative preload and stroke volume (SV) changes at the same time, by using standard pacing leads [13–15]. TVI is recorded without high-pass filtering and impedance data are processed on the assumption of an inverse relationship with right-ventricular volume: an increase in the absolute TVI value in telediastole (edTVI) represents a decrease in diastolic ventricular volume (EDV), while a decrease in edTVI indicates an increase in EDV. Peak-to-peak TVI excursion from diastole to end-systole is proportional to SV, which is a function of EDV, according to Starling's law. The relationship between TVI-derived SV and EDV at any time defines the current inotropic index, which can be applied to drive a rate-responsive system following the modifications in ventricular contractility induced by the autonomic nervous system [9, 10, 16, 17].

[1]Division of Cardiology, School of Medicine, Università degli Studi del Piemonte Orientale, Novara; [2]Cardiology O.U., Ospedale Umberto I, Mestre (Venice); [3]Cardiology O.U. Spedali Civili, Brescia, Italy; [4]Cardiology O.U, Ospedale S. Luigi - S. Currò, Catania; [5]Medico Clinical Research, Rubano (Padua), Italy

The TVI sensor has been implemented in an external cardiac pacemaker, which automatically adapts the pacing rate according to the inotropic index. The aim of the present study was to check and evaluate the rate-responsive function of this device under pharmacological adrenergic stimulation.

Materials and Methods

Tests were performed in 30 patients, during the implantation of bipolar dual-chamber pacing systems for conventional indications. Permanent pacing leads from any manufacturer were temporarily connected with an external DDD-R pacemaker (Ext Sophòs, Medico, Padua, Italy), equipped for TVI recording. The TVI signal was sampled at 64 Hz with DC coupling, in order to work out the minimum diastolic and maximum systolic impedance in each cycle (edTVI and esTVI, respectively). Diastolic and systolic intervals were rate-adaptive time windows, triggered by each pacing or sensing ventricular event. EdTVI and esTVI were filtered for possible outliers, averaged over a programmable number of cycles, and converted into the corresponding inotropic index, which specified the TVI-indicated pacing rate (TVI rate) according to the relation:

TVI rate = basic rate + resting rate x inotropic index x rate gain,

where the rate gain is a programmable factor used for individual tuning of the rate-responsive system. The actual pacing rate applied by the stimulator corresponded to the current TVI rate after a smoothing process. The trends of cardiac rate (either intrinsic or paced) and TVI rate, as well as the TVI waveform and the associated event markers, were stored in the stimulator memory and optionally transmitted to a PC through an optically isolated serial cable, for real-time display.

The TVI recording configuration was chosen between two possible alternatives, i.e. using the ring atrial electrode and either the tip or the ring ventricular electrode. The ring-tip configuration usually provided higher signals, which could be sensitive, however, to possible artefacts generated by cardiac contraction at the electrode–myocardium interface. The ring–ring configuration provided smaller signals with the advantage of lower noise, since both the electrodes were directly in contact with the blood conducting volume. In both configurations, TVI was derived from the voltage generated by the application of subthreshold current pulses with amplitude programmable from 15 to 45 µA. The same electrodes were used for both current injection and voltage sampling.

After TVI signal acquisition in resting conditions, β-adrenergic stimulation was induced by intravenous administration of 2 µg/min isoproterenol (IPN), which was continued until the cardiac rate exceeded 90 bpm. Whenever possible, the stimulator basic rate and the rate gain were programmed so as to keep the TVI rate below the sinus rate, in order to avoid overdrive pacing and allow the comparison of TVI rate and sinus rate trends. The relationship between TVI inotropic index and sinus rate changes with respect to the resting rate in each patient was evaluated by linear regression analysis and expressed by the squared Pearson correlation coefficient.

Results

At the time of testing, stable intrinsic atrial activity was present in 28 cases at rest, while 2 patients received atrial pacing throughout the procedure. Sequential ventricular pacing was performed in 57% of the patients, while the remaining exhibited intrinsic AV conduction. The ring–ring and ring–tip TVI configurations were chosen, respectively in 67% and 33% of the cases. A representative example of the recorded TVI signal is shown in Fig. 1. The minimum impedance was recorded within 200 ms following the electrical ventricular activation, which was indicated by either R wave detection or pacing spike emission. Thereafter the impedance increased, reaching the maximum value at a time compatible with the end of the systole.

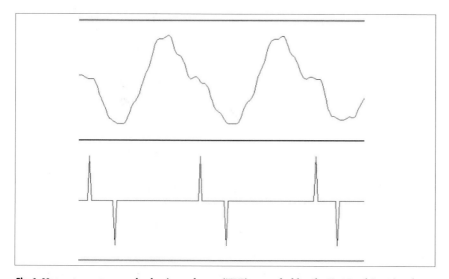

Fig. 1. *Upper trace:* transvalvular impedance (TVI) recorded by the Ext Sophòs stimulator in a patient at rest. Ring–tip TVI configuration; end-diastolic TVI = 482 ± 5 Ω, end-systolic TVI = 577 ± 3 Ω. *Lower trace:* pacemaker event markers, demonstrating intrinsic atrial (upward spike) and ventricular activity (downward spike). The sinus rate was 66 ± 1 bpm

All patients provided with intrinsic atrial activity showed positive chronotropic response to IPN. In addition, β-adrenergic stimulation enhanced myocardial contractility, as suggested by the trend of TVI-derived inotropic index, which increased from about 0 in resting conditions up to maximum values ranging from 0.4 to 3.4 in the patient group (mean ± SD = 1.2 ± 1.0). In 27 out of 28 patients, the time course of the inotropic index reflected the sinus rate trend, so that a linear correlation between the two parameters was demonstrated. The squared Pearson correlation coefficient averaged 0.81 ± 0.12, being higher than 0.7 in 93% of the cases. The reciprocal of the individual regression slope corresponded to the optimal rate gain to be applied in each patient, which ranged from 0.1 to 2 with a mean of 0.8 ± 0.6. The product of current inotropic index times the individual rate gain proved a good approximation of relative sinus rate changes observed during IPN-induced stimulation (Fig. 2). As a consequence, the TVI rate closely reproduced the sinus rate trend, as well as the maximum extent of the intrinsic chronotropic response. The highest sinus rate value reached in each patient is compared with the TVI rate derived at the same time in Fig. 3. Very

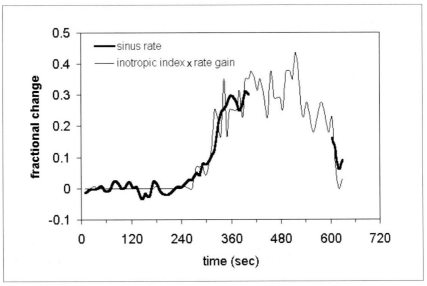

Fig. 2. Fractional change in sinus rate (defined as: (current rate – resting rate)/resting rate; *heavy line*) and product TVI inotropic index x rate gain (*light line*), during intravenous administration of 2 μg/ml isoproterenol. The rate gain was equal to the slope of the individual linear regression of fractional sinus rate on inotropic index. Positive chronotropic and inotropic effects started simultaneously and showed similar time courses, until the sinus rhythm was temporarily suppressed by overdrive pacing. Consequently, the TVI-indicated rate (given by: basic rate + resting rate x inotropic index x rate gain) paralleled the sinus rate trend

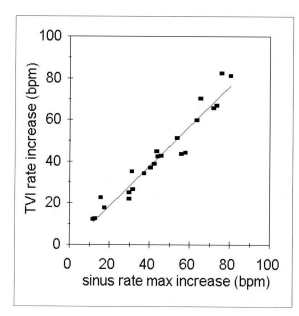

Fig. 3. Relationship between the maximum increase in sinus rate induced by β-adrenergic stimulation in each patient and the corresponding rate increase indicated by TVI at the same time. The regression line is described by the equation: $y = 0.96x - 0.56$, with $r^2 = 0.94$

good correspondence was demonstrated by a regression line featuring slope and squared correlation coefficient both close to 1.

The relationship between inotropic index and sinus response could not be assessed in the patients undergoing atrial pacing throughout the test. Nevertheless, in these cases as well IPN administration entailed a substantial increase in the inotropic index and a corresponding acceleration in the pacing rate.

Conclusions

The present study demonstrates that TVI data processing based on the inverse relationship with right ventricular volume provides an index of cardiac contractility that correlates closely with the simultaneous sinus rate modifications induced by adrenergic challenge. Similar progressive changes in the inotropic index are noticed even when the chronotropic adaptation is prevented. In contrast, a rate increase produced by overdrive pacing in the absence of contractility modifications does not affect the inotropic index [18].

TVI is sensitive to myocardial properties controlled by the sympathetic nervous system, is capable of discriminating the haemodynamic effects of intrinsic and extrinsic heart regulation, and is totally free of positive feedbacks from the cardiac rate. Therefore, this new sensor can be proposed as an advanced tool in the physiological regulation of rate-responsive pacing.

References

1. Lau CP (1993) Rate adaptive cardiac pacing: single and dual chamber. Futura, Mount Kisco, NY

2. Rickards AF, Bombardini T, Plicchi G et al (1996) An implantable intracardiac accelerometer for monitoring myocardial contractility. Pacing Clin Electrophysiol 19:2066–2071

3. Langenfeld H, Krein A, Kirstein M et al (1998) Peak endocardial acceleration based clinical testing of the "BEST" DDDR pacemaker. Pacing Clin Electrophysiol 21:2187–2191

4. Osswald S, Cron T, Gradel C et al (2000) Closed-loop stimulation using intracardiac impedance as a sensor principle: correlation of right ventricular dP/dt max and intracardiac impedance during dobutamine stress test. Pacing Clin Electrophysiol 23:1502–1508

5. Clementy J, Kobeissi A, Garrigue S et al (2000) Validation by serial standardised testing of a new rate-responsive pacemaker sensor based on variations in myocardial contractility. Europace 3:124–131

6. Occhetta E, Bortnik M, Francalacci G et al (2001) How reliable and effective are haemodynamic sensors to correct chronotropic incompetence? In: Raviele A (ed) Cardiac arrhythmias 2001. Springer, Milan, pp 586–594

7. Griesbach L, Gestrich B, Wojciechowski D et al (2003) Clinical performance of automatic closed-loop stimulation systems. Pacing Clin Electrophysiol 26(Pt I):1432–1437

8. Santini M, Ricci R, Pignalberi C et al (2004) Effect of autonomic stressors on rate control in pacemakers using ventricular impedance signal. Pacing Clin Electrophysiol 27:24–32

9. Chirife R, Tentori MC, Mazzetti H et al (2001) Hemodynamic sensors: are they all the same? In: Raviele A (ed) Cardiac arrhythmias 2001. Springer, Milan, pp 566–575

10. Chirife R (2003) Hemodynamic assessment with implantable pacemakers. How feasible and reliable is it? In: Raviele A (ed) Cardiac arrhythmias 2003. Springer, Milan, pp 705–712

11. Occhetta E, Magnani A, Bortnik M et al (2003) Hemodynamic sensors: their impact in clinical practice. In: Raviele A (ed) Cardiac arrhythmias 2003. Springer, Milan, pp 713–718

12. Cron TA, Hilti P, Schächinger H et al (2003) Rate response of a closed-loop stimulation pacing system to changing preload and afterload conditions. Pacing Clin Electrophysiol 26(Pt I):1504–1510

13. Di Gregorio F, Morra A, Finesso M, Bongiorni MG (1996) Transvalvular impedance (TVI) recording under electrical and pharmacological cardiac stimulation. Pacing Clin Electrophysiol 19(Pt II):1689–1693

14. Bongiorni MG, Soldati E, Arena G et al (1997) Transvalvular impedance as a marker of cardiac activity. In: Vardas PE (ed) Europace '97. Monduzzi, Bologna, pp 525–528

15. Morra A, Panarotto D, Santini P, Di Gregorio F (1997) Transvalvular impedance (TVI) sensing: a new way toward the hemodynamic control of cardiac pacing. In: Vardas PE (ed) Europace '97. Monduzzi, Bologna, pp529–533

16. Gasparini M, Curnis A, Mantica M et al (2001) Hemodynamic sensors: what clinical value do they have in heart failure? In: Raviele A (ed) Cardiac arrhythmias 2001. Springer, Milan, pp 576–585

17. Di Gregorio F, Curnis A, Pettini A et al (2002) Trans-valvular impedance (TVI) in the hemodynamic regulation of cardiac pacing. In: Mitro P, Pella D, Rybár R, Valočik G (eds) Cardiovascular diseases 2002. Monduzzi, Bologna, pp 53–57
18. Gasparini G, Curnis A, Gulizia M et al (2003) Can hemodynamic sensors ensure physiological rate control? In: Raviele A (ed) Cardiac arrhythmias 2003. Springer, Milan, pp 725–731

Initial Experience of Implanted Pacemakers with Intracardiac Haemodynamic Sensor: Evaluation of Sensor Safety

N. Galizio[1], J. Gonzalez[1], R. Chirife[2], H. Fraguas[1], J. Barra[1], S. Graf[1], E. De Forteza[1], F. Di Gregorio[3]

Introduction

The autonomic nervous system stimulation of the heart affects, simultaneously, chronotropism, dromotropism, and inotropism. Intracardiac haemodynamic sensors detect changes in the performance of the heart, which depends on the inotropic regulation of myocardial fibres. Intracardiac haemodynamic sensors include:
- Intraventricular pressure
- Peak endocardial acceleration
- Ventricular impedance
- Transvalvular impedance

Transvalvular impedance (TVI) is a measure of blood impedance derived between the right atrium and ventricle. With conventional electrodes, the low-amplitude, constant-current is driven from the source to the atrial ring and ventricular ring or tip. This configuration has the least wall motion artefact and the best correlation with intracardiac volumes (Fig. 1). Combining more than two poles offers better rendering of volume changes and gives a better signal-to-noise ratio than intraventricular impedance [1].

Figure 2 shows TVI and volume waveforms, ECG, and atrial electrograms. TVI increases during ventricular systole and throughout the QT period, and decreases during passive and active ventricular filling.

TVI is the opposite of volume waveform: atrial contraction produces an increase in volume (atrial kick) followed by a rapid volume decrease (ventricular ejection). After ejection, the rapid-filling (RFW) and slow-filling waves (SFW) are seen. The minimum TVI is sensitive to all conditions known to modify the preload. The maximum TVI corresponds to end-sys-

[1]Electrophysiology Division, Institute of Cardiology and Cardiovascular Surgery, Favaloro Foundation and Rene G. Favaloro University, Buenos Aires; [2]J. A. Fernandez Hospital, Buenos Aires Argentina; [3]Medico Clinical Research, Rubano (Padua), Italy

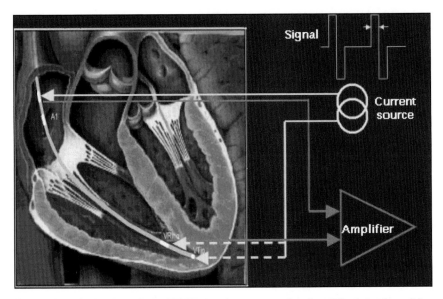

Fig. 1. Transvalvular impedance (TVI). Current source, signal and the injection of the low-voltage pulsed carrier signal between the pacing electrodes

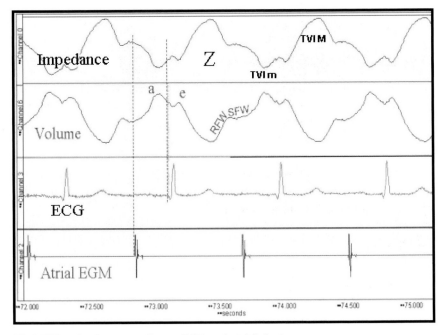

Fig. 2. TVI and volume waveforms, ECG, and atrial electrograms

tolic volume (ESV), which is sensitive to changes in cardiac contractility [2–5]. Relative variations in end-diastolic volume, end-systolic volume, stroke volume, and ejection fraction define a cardiac inotropic index, completely independent of preload effects, which is a direct expression of the autonomic nervous system's regulation of the heart [6–9].

Study Objective

Measurement of intracardiac impedance requires the injection of a low-voltage pulsed carrier signal between the pacing electrodes. The aim of the study was to evaluate whether these pulses interfere with standard functions of the Sophòs (Medico-SpA) pacemaker.

Methods

The experimental protocol was approved by the Institutional Animal Care and Use Committee of Favaloro University, and the study was conducted in three castrated adult male sheep according to the Guide for the Care and Use of Laboratory Animals published by the United States National Research Council (1996). Five days before surgery, three pairs of subcutaneous electrodes were implanted for Holter monitoring. Cables were tunnelled subcutaneously to emerge at the interscapular space.

Anaesthesia and Intraoperative Monitoring

After 24 h starvation and 12 h without drinking water, general anaesthesia was induced in the animals with sodium thiopental and maintained with 1.5–2% halothane carried in pure oxygen (2.5 l/min) under assisted ventilation. Ventilation was performed using positive pressure ventilation at a rate of 12 breaths per minute and a tidal volume of 600 ml adjusted to maintain an end-tidal CO_2 of approximately 25–30 mmHg. Surface ECG and PCO_2 were continuously displayed on a monitor. Heart rate and blood oxygen saturation were measured by pulse oximetry.

Data Acquisition

Blood pressure was measured using a pressure transducer (Gould 6600 SeriesTransducer). Aortic pressure and ECG signals were registered on a six-channel signal conditioner (Gould 5900) and simultaneously on a chart recorder which allowed the signals to be displayed on a PC monitor. Instantaneous pressure and/or ECG signals were sampled and analysed off-line on a computer equipped with a multi-channel 12-bit analogue-to-digital converter. Signals were digitised every 4 ms and stored as ASCII text files using specific software developed in the Biomedical Engineering Department of Favaloro University.

Surgery

With the animals in right lateral decubitus, pacing leads (Oscor HT52 PSBV atrial screw-in and Medico 340 tined ventricular leads) were inserted via the jugular vein guided by fluoroscopy using a C-arm angiography apparatus. Atrial and ventricular pacing and sensing thresholds were measured with TVI on and off. Then, the pacemaker was placed subcutaneously in the lateral surface of the neck. After implantation, recording of arterial pressure and ECG were performed under baseline conditions and during intravenous infusion of isoproterenol (2 µg/ml). Holter monitoring was performed 2 weeks and 4 weeks after implantation to look for pacemaker malfunctions (undersensing or oversensing).

Results

Figure 3 shows ventricular capture and sensing threshold at implantation and 2 and 4 weeks after implantation. Ventricular capture thresholds had increased a little after 2 weeks, as usual, but there was no difference between measurements with TVI on or TVI off. There was no difference in ventricular sensing thresholds either. The same result was obtained for measurements of atrial capture and sensing thresholds with TVI on or off (Fig. 4).

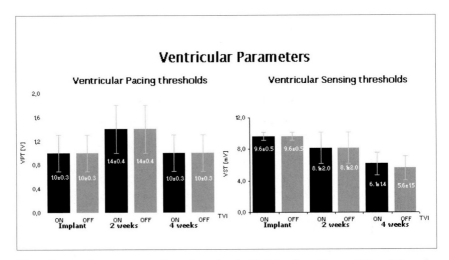

Fig. 3. Ventricular capture and sensing threshold at implantation and 2 and 4 weeks after implantation

In Figure 5 we can see normal sinus rhythm (a) before pacemaker implantation and normal pacemaker function after implantation (b). Sporadic atrial undersensing was found after 2 weeks (c). This was corrected by reprogramming the atrial pacemaker sensitivity.

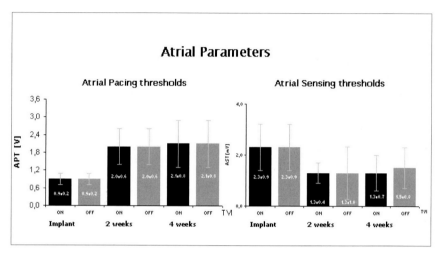

Fig. 4. Atrial capture and sensing thresholds at implantation and 2 and 4 weeks after implantation

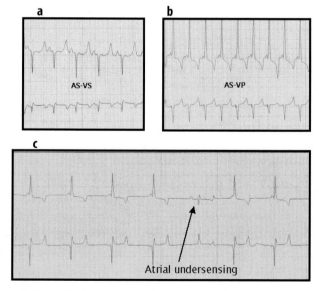

Fig. 5. a Normal sinus rhythm. **b** Normal pacemaker function after implantation. **c** Sporadic atrial undersensing

Conclusions

In the present animal model study, TVI sensor operation did not interfere with conventional pacemaker functions of implanted Sophòs pacemakers. These results look promising since this sensor could play an important part in haemodynamic monitoring: for physiological rate adaptation, for beat-to-beat capture confirmation, in patients with neurocardiogenic syncope, for the follow-up of patients with heart failure, to indicate the best interventricular delay in CRT, and to identify arrhythmias and their haemodynamic impact in implantable cardioverter–defibrillators [10–12].

References

1. Chirife R (2003) Haemodynamic assessment with implantable pacemakers. How feasible and reliable is it? In: Raviele A (ed) Cardiac arrhythmias 2003. Springer, Milan pp 705–712
2. Di Gregorio F, Morra A, Finesso M et al (1996) Transvalvular impedance (TVI) recording under electrical and pharmacological cardiac stimulation. Pacing Clin Electrocardiol 19(II):1689–1693
3. Bongiorni MG, Soldati E, Arena G et al (1997) Transvalvular impedance as a marker of cardiac activity. In: Vardas PE (ed) Europace '97. Monduzzi, Bologna, pp 525–528
4. Morra A, Panarotto D, Santini P et al (1997) Transvalvular impedance (TVI) sensing: a new way toward the haemodynamic control of cardiac pacing. In: Vardas PE (ed) Europace '97. Monduzzi, Bologna, pp 529–533
5. Bongiorni MG, Soldati E, Arena G et al (2003) Transvalvular impedance: does it allow automatic capture detection? In: Raviele A (ed) Cardiac arrhythmias 2003. Springer, Milan, pp 733–739
6. Chirife R, Ortega DF, Salazar A (1993) Feasibility of measuring relative right ventricular volumes and ejection fraction with implantable rhythm control devices. Pacing Clin Electrophysiol 16:1673–1683
7. Gasparini M, Curnis A, Mantica M et al (2002) Hemodynamic sensors: what clinical value do they have in heart failure? In: Raviele A (ed) Cardiac arrhythmias 2001. Springer, Milan, pp 576–585
8. Bongiorni MG, Soldati E, Arena G et al (2001) Hemodynamic sensors: what clinical value do they have in chronotropic incompetence? In: Raviele A (ed) Cardiac arrhythmias 2001. Springer, Milan, pp 595–601
9. Di Gregorio F, Curnis A, Pettini A et al (2002) Trans-valvular impedance (TVI) in the hemodynamic regulation of cardiac pacing. In: Mitro P, Pella Rybár R, Valo?ik G (eds) Cardiovascular diseases 2002. Monduzzi, Bologna, pp 53–57
10. Gasparini G, Curnis A, Mascioli G et al (2003) Clinical test of a pacing device driven by trans-valvular impedance. XII World Congress on Cardiac Pacing and Electrophysiology. Hong Kong, 19–22 February 2003. Pacing Clin Electrophysiol 26(II):S204 (abstract)
11. Gasparini G, Curnis A, Gulizia M et al (2003) Can hemodynamic sensors ensure physiological rate control? In: Raviele A (ed) Cardiac arrhythmias 2003. Springer, Milan, pp 725–731

12. Gulizia M, Gasparini G, Curnis A et al (2003) Hemodynamic rate-responsive pacing by trans-valvular impedance detection. Europace Supplements 4:B96 (abstract)

Transvalvular Impedance in the Autoregulation of a Cardiac Pacemaker

F. Dorticós[1], M.A. Quiñones[1], F. Tornes[1], Y. Fayad[1], R. Zayas[1], J. Castro[1], A. Barbetta[2], F. Di Gregorio[2]

Introduction

Self-adaptation of the main pacing parameters to changing conditions in daily life is a major challenge in pacemaker technology, which started with the development of devices designed to regulate the stimulation rate according to the patient's metabolic needs. A variety of rate-responsive sensors have been applied to this purpose [1]. The most widely used system relies on the detection of body movement by means of an accelerometer mounted in the pacemaker circuit, which is known to ensure high sensitivity and quick rate adaptation to the walking speed. However, the accelerometric sensor cannot discriminate between active and passive motion, thus producing overpacing whenever the patient is shaken or trembling. Furthermore, the accelerometric signal immediately returns to baseline when a physical activity is stopped; in consequence, the pacing rate is not regulated during the recovery period. To prevent such inconveniences, dual-sensor pacemakers have been developed by coupling the accelerometer with a physiological sensor, such as the minute ventilation or the Q–T interval [2, 3]. A combined sensing system provides different indications which complement each other and are usually averaged in programmable proportion by a blending algorithm to derive the most suitable pacing rate.

In principle, a haemodynamic sensor would be the most appropriate physiological counterpart of the accelerometer. Haemodynamic sensors are designed to record changes in cardiac inotropic regulation, which are expected to be faster and more specific than the modifications in respiratory activity or Q–T duration [4, 5]. In recent years, a new haemodynamic sensor based on transvalvular impedance (TVI) has been proposed to monitor both

[1]Institute of Cardiology and Cardiovascular Surgery, La Havana, Cuba; [2]Medico Clinical Research, Rubano (Padua), Italy

stroke volume (SV) and preload at the same time, in order to infer an estimate of myocardial contractility devoid of the intrinsic regulation, which is independent of the autonomic nervous system and therefore unrelated to the sinus rate [6–9]. We report the preliminary results of a pilot study which is testing in human patients the general properties and the rate-responsive function of the first implantable pacemaker featuring the TVI sensor.

Materials and Methods

The study was approved by the local Ethical Committee and all enrolled patients gave their written informed consent. Six patients presenting with sick sinus syndrome with marked bradycardia and depressed chronotropic response have been implanted with the Sophòs 100 DDD-R pacemaker (Medico, Padua, Italy), which is equipped with a dual-sensor rate-responsive system including an accelerometer and the TVI recorder. The stimulator was connected with bipolar, passive fixation, atrial and ventricular pacing leads (Medico models 366 and 340, respectively) provided with porous Ti electrodes coated with Pt. The atrial lead was positioned in the right appendage and the ventricular lead in the apex.

The patients were checked before discharge and at 1 and 2 months after the implantation. During this initial follow-up period, the TVI sensor was enabled only to collect data to test the response during postural changes and controlled physical activity. The regulation of the rate-responsive function was totally entrusted to the accelerometer, the reliability of which was assessed during fast walking as well as by 24-h Holter monitoring. The rate-response profile of the accelerometric sensor consists in a dual-slope linear increase in pacing rate as a function of the acceleration detected: the first slope is defined by the difference between the programmable 'snap rate' and the basic rate, while the second slope results from the difference between the sensor upper rate and the snap rate.

TVI is the electric impedance recorded between right atrium and ventricle along the cardiac cycle. The Sophòs 100 pacemaker measures TVI by applying square subthreshold current pulses of 125-μs duration and amplitude automatically adapted to the detected impedance, up to a maximum of 45 μA. Although several combinations between current injecting and voltage sampling electrodes are allowed, the present study focused on two alternative TVI configurations: impedance recording between the atrial ring and the ventricular ring (Ar–Vr), or between the atrial ring and the ventricular tip electrodes (Ar–Vt). The minimum (edTVI) and maximum (esTVI) values detected in each cardiac cycle within two rate-adaptive time windows, corresponding to the maximum predictable duration of the isometric systole and the ejection period, respectively, are stored in the memory and processed by the pacemaker in order to derive the inotropic index and the corresponding TVI-indicated pacing rate.

The TVI waveform transmitted by real-time telemetry and the trends of edTVI and esTVI were recorded with the patient resting in the supine position, right lateral decubitus, left lateral decubitus, and standing upright, as well as during physical exercise of various degrees (slow and fast walking, stair climbing, leg bending), with the aim of evaluating TVI sensitivity and specificity to the cardiovascular challenge induced by common activities of daily living. In addition, the sensitivity of the pacemaker to intrinsic electrical activity was assessed in the presence or absence of TVI sampling current. Mean data are reported ± 1 standard deviation. The significance of differences was evaluated by the paired Student's t-test and the Wilcoxon signed rank test, respectively, for parametric and non-parametric data.

Results

The implantations were carried out by the standard procedure. Acute atrial and ventricular pacing thresholds were, respectively, 0.46 ± 0.22 V and 0.39 ± 0.22 V (0.5-ms pulses, unipolar mode). The corresponding pacing impedance at 5 V averaged 695 ± 132 Ω and 768 ± 201 Ω. The A wave amplitude on implantation was 4.4 ± 1.3 mV in unipolar and 4.1 ± 1.9 mV in bipolar mode. The R wave was 8.0 ± 2.6 and 9.3 ± 3.2 mV in unipolar and bipolar mode, respectively.

The first follow-up check was performed within the first 2 days after the implantation. In each patient, TVI was assessed in both the Ar–Vr and the Ar–Vt configuration, after individual tuning of the sampling current. The former TVI configuration was preferred in three cases, while the latter was chosen in the other three patients. An example of the recorded TVI waveform is illustrated in Figure 1. The TVI signal regularly showed the expected general properties, with minimum and maximum peaks falling within the respective detection windows. In order to check whether the application of the TVI sampling current might affect the pacemaker sensing function, the upper value of bipolar atrial and ventricular sensitivity allowing 100% detection of intrinsic A and R waves was determined with the TVI sensor either enabled or turned *off*. The upper limit of fully effective atrial sensitivity (averaging 1.12 ± 0.85 mV and 1.13 ± 0.93 mV with the TVI sensor *off* and *on*, respectively) was not affected by TVI sensor activation in four out of six cases, while it was decreased by one programming step in one case and increased by one programming step in a second case. Similarly, the upper limit of fully effective ventricular sensitivity (averaging 5.17 ± 2.82 mV and

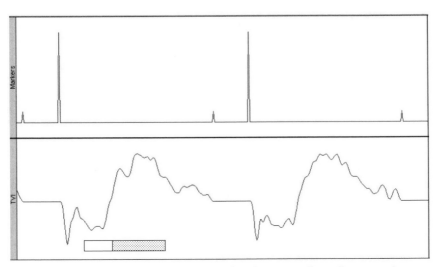

Fig. 1. Pacemaker event markers (*upper trace*) and TVI waveform (*lower trace*) transmitted in real time by pacemaker telemetry and recorded by the programmer. The markers indicate sequential atrial and ventricular pacing at 60 bpm. TVI was measured in the Ar–Vt configuration; the *open* and *shaded bars* correspond to the detection windows of the minimum and maximum TVI, which averaged 768 ± 1 and 808 ± 1 Ω, respectively. The TVI sampling is suspended throughout the atrioventricular delay

5.00 ± 2.49 mV with the TVI sensor *off* and *on*, respectively) was not affected by the TVI sensor activation in five out of six cases and was decreased by one programming step in one case. Such small differences have no statistical significance.

The TVI signal response to exercise and postural changes was evaluated at 1 and 2 months from the implantation. The absolute values of both edTVI and esTVI could be affected by posture, even in the absence of relevant modifications in the patient's activity and metabolic demand (Fig. 2). On the other hand, the TVI signal was modulated by the cardiovascular adaptation to physical activity. The inotropic index derived from TVI increased during stress exercise and remained elevated for a while in the recovery phase (Fig. 3). The maximum values of the inotropic index at rest, at peak exercise, and after 5 min recovery averaged 0.14 ± 0.10, 0.85 ± 0.52 and 0.51 ± 0.23, respectively, in the whole patient group. The increase with respect to baseline was statistically significant for both exercise and recovery conditions ($P < 0.05$).

The pacing rate dynamics indicated by the accelerometric sensor in standard configuration was tested during fast walking (Fig. 4) and proved adequate in all the patients, with a maximum rate increase of 38 ± 9 bpm above the basic rate. No episode of sensor-induced tachycardia was noticed in daily life by 24-h Holter recording.

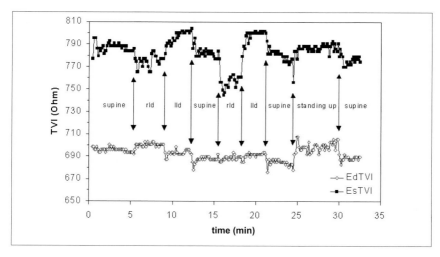

Fig. 2. Effects of postural changes on end-diastolic (*open symbols*) and end-systolic TVI (*filled symbols*), recorded in the Ar–Vt configuration. The patient was resting in the supine position, then moved to right lateral decubitus (*rld*), left lateral decubitus (*lld*), supine, right lateral decubitus, left lateral decubitus, supine, standing up, and supine again. The *arrows* mark the time of each transition

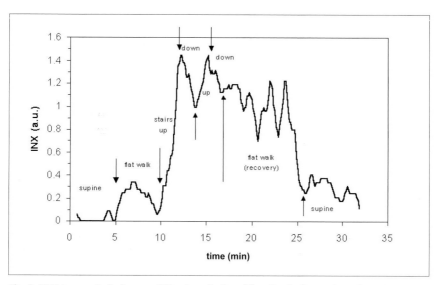

Fig. 3. TVI inotropic index modifications induced by physical exercise. The patient was initially lying in the supine position, then walked slowly on the flat with little or no effort. Thereafter, he was asked to climb and descend the stairs for three storeys twice as fast as he was able, to walk slowly on the flat again in the recovery phase after the stress, and finally to lie down in the supine position. The *arrows* mark the time of each transition. Note the increase in the inotropic index during exercise, followed by a delayed decrease in the recovery period

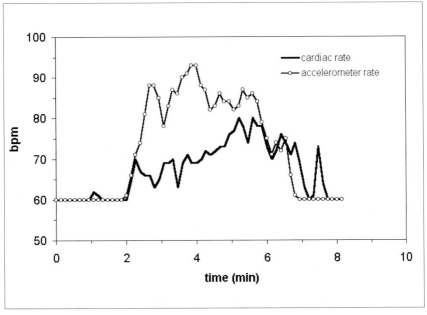

Fig. 4. Cardiac rate (*thicker curve*) and accelerometer-indicated rate (*lighter curve with open circles*) during fast walking. The accelerometric sensor was enabled in passive mode, so the pacemaker worked out the accelerometer-indicated rate and stored it in the memory without actually increasing the pacing rate. This allowed comparison of the sensor-indicated rate and the sinus rate, whenever the latter exceeded the basic rate (60 bpm)

Discussion

A rate-responsive algorithm based upon two complementary sensors is expected to be sensitive to a wider range of physiological conditions and more specific than a single sensor system, as a result of sensor cross-check [3]. All currently available sensors feature advantages and disadvantages. The accelerometer is a sensitive tool, but can be erroneously activated by passive motion imposed on the patient's body or even on the pacemaker alone. Physiological sensors are generally more specific, but less sensitive and slowly activated [10]. Haemodynamic sensors can be affected by preload and afterload modifications [7, 9] and may require the use of special leads including dedicated hardware, as is the case for the dP/dt and the peak endocardial acceleration (PEA) sensors [4, 11]. As an alternative, information on the inotropic state of the heart can be derived from electric impedance measurements obtained with standard pacing leads. The heart mechanical activity entails impedance changes at every beat that can reflect the contraction strength [12–14]. Rate-responsive systems based upon impedance recording proved generally effective in clinical practice [15, 16], although some cases of overpacing associated with the orthostatic position were reported [17].

The TVI sensor is quite different from the tools used so far to record cardiac impedance. The TVI waveform is a stable periodic signal which allows impedance measurement with DC coupling. The information on the absolute values of edTVI and esTVI, measured independently of each other with respect to zero, is applied to monitor preload changes and protect the system from the influence of the intrinsic heart regulation on the inotropic performance [7–9]. Our preliminary experience confirms the good sensitivity of TVI to the increased demand for blood supply induced by physical exercise. The sensor response was also evident in the recovery phase following the stress, when the patient was still or performing minimal activity. However, TVI measurements could be affected by postural changes as well, even in the absence of physiological modifications in either preload or myocardial contractility. Although it is conceivable that the postural effects are more pronounced in the early post-implant stages than in chronic conditions, when the electrode fixation is expected to improve, a close interaction between TVI and the accelerometer is mandatory to prevent possible false activations caused by any of the two sensors. The Sophòs 100 pacemaker is provided with special algorithms designed for this purpose, which will be tested in the next steps of our study.

In conclusion, our results demonstrate that the Sophòs 100 pacemaker is a reliable device that ensures precise pacing and sensing performance whether the TVI sensor is enabled or not. Suitable rate regulation can be achieved even by means of the accelerometer alone, which is properly tuned for pacemaker patients who show normal motility. The TVI sensor can extend the sensitivity of the rate-responsive system to isometric activities, can drive the pacing rate in the recovery phase, and must integrate the accelerometer in sensor cross-checking. In addition, TVI could play a pivotal role in the autoregulation of a pacing device, providing permanent haemodynamic validation of pacing and sensing effectiveness at every beat [18].

References

1. Lau CP (1993) Rate adaptive cardiac pacing: single and dual chamber. Futura Publishing Company, Inc., Mount Kisco, NY
2. Leung SK, Lau CP, Tang MO et al (1996) New integrated sensor pacemaker: comparison of rate responses between an integrated minute ventilation and activity sensor and single sensor modes during exercise and daily activities and nonphysiological interference. Pacing Clin Electrophysiol 19[Pt II]:1664–1671
3. Barold SS, Clémenty J (1997) The promise of improved exercise performance by dual sensor rate adaptive pacemakers. Pacing Clin Electrophysiol 20[Pt I]:607–609

4. Bennett T, Sharma A, Sutton R et al (1992) Development of a rate adaptive pacemaker based on the maximum rate-of-rise of right ventricular pressure (RV dP/dt$_{max}$). Pacing Clin Electrophysiol 15:219–234

5. Pichlmaier AM, Braile D, Ebner E et al (1992) Autonomic nervous system controlled closed loop cardiac pacing. Pacing Clin Electrophysiol 15:1787–1791

6. Di Gregorio F, Morra A, Finesso M et al (1996) Transvalvular impedance (TVI) recording under electrical and pharmacological cardiac stimulation. Pacing Clin Electrophysiol 19[Pt II]:1689–1693

7. Chirife R, Tentori MC, Mazzetti H et al (2001) Hemodynamic sensors: are they all the same? In: Raviele A (ed) Cardiac arrhythmias 2001. Springer, Milan, pp 566–575

8. Di Gregorio F, Curnis A, Pettini A et al (2002) Trans-valvular impedance (TVI) in the hemodynamic regulation of cardiac pacing. In: Mitro P, Pella D, Rybár R, Valočik G (eds) Cardiovascular diseases 2002. Monduzzi, Bologna, pp 53–57

9. Chirife R (2003) Hemodynamic assessment with implantable pacemakers. How feasible and reliable is it? In: Raviele A (ed) Cardiac arrhythmias 2003. Springer, Milan, pp 705–712

10. Barold SS (1993) Limitations and adverse effects of rate-adaptive pacemakers. In: Benditt DG (ed) Rate-adaptive cardiac pacing. Current technologies and clinical applications. Blackwell, Boston, pp 233–263

11. Rickards AF, Bombardini T, Corbucci G et al (1996) An implantable intracardiac accelerometer for monitoring myocardial contractility. Pacing Clin Electrophysiol 19:2066–2071

12. Chirife R (1991) Acquisition of hemodynamic data and sensor signals for rate control from standard pacing electrodes. Pacing Clin Electrophysiol 14:1563–1565

13. Chirife R, Ortega DF, Salazar A (1993) Feasibility of measuring relative right ventricular volumes and ejection fraction with implantable rhythm control devices. Pacing Clin Electrophysiol 16:1673–1683

14. Osswald S, Cron T, Gradel C et al (2000) Closed-loop stimulation using intracardiac impedance as a sensor principle: correlation of right ventricular dP/dt max and intracardiac impedance during dobutamine stress test. Pacing Clin Electrophysiol 23:1502–1508

15. Griesbach L, Gestrich B, Wojciechowski D et al (2003) Clinical performance of automatic closed-loop stimulation systems. Pacing Clin Electrophysiol 26[Pt I]:1432–1437

16. Santini M, Ricci R, Pignalberi C et al (2004) Effect of autonomic stressors on rate control in pacemakers using ventricular impedance signal. Pacing Clin Electrophysiol 27:24–32

17. Cron TA, Hilti P, Schächinger H et al (2003) Rate response of a closed-loop stimulation pacing system to changing preload and afterload conditions. Pacing Clin Electrophysiol 26[Pt I]:1504–1510

18. Bongiorni MG, Soldati E, Arena G et al (2003) Transvalvular impedance: does it allow automatic capture detection? In: Raviele A (ed) Cardiac arrhythmias 2003. Springer, Milan, pp 733–739

SYNCOPE: PRACTICAL ISSUES
OF DIAGNOSIS AND TREATMENT

Guidelines for the Management of Syncope

M. Brignole

Syncope is a transient, self-limited loss of consciousness usually leading to a fall, due to transient global cerebral hypoperfusion. Causes of syncope are:
- Neurally mediated (reflex) syncopal syndromes
- Orthostatic
- Cardiac arrhythmias (as primary cause)
- Structural cardiac or cardiopulmonary disease

First of all, syncope must be differentiated from other 'non-syncopal' conditions associated with real or apparent transient loss of consciousness such as, for example, metabolic disorders, epilepsy, intoxication, transient ischaemic attacks (TIA), and psychogenic 'syncope'.

Initial Evaluation

The initial evaluation is based on a careful history and physical examination including orthostatic blood pressure measurements. Other than in young patients without heart disease, a 12-lead ECG should usually be part of the general evaluation. Three key questions are:
- Is loss of consciousness attributable to syncope or not?
- Is heart disease present or absent?
- Are there important clinical features in the history that suggest the diagnosis?

History and Physical Examination

Questions should be asked about:
- *Circumstances just prior to the attack:* body position, activity, predisposing factors, and precipitating events

Department of Cardiology and Arrythmologic Centre, Ospedali del Tigullio, Lavagna (Genua), Italy

- *Onset of the attack:* nausea, vomiting, abdominal discomfort, feeling of cold, sweating, aura, pain in neck or shoulders, blurred vision
- *Attack* (eyewitness): manner of the fall, skin colour, duration of loss of consciousness, breathing pattern, movements and their duration, onset of movement in relation to fall, tongue biting
- *End of attack:* nausea, vomiting, sweating, feeling of cold, confusion, muscle aches, skin colour, injury, chest pain, palpitations, urinary or faecal incontinence
- *Background:* family history, cardiac and neurological history, metabolic disorders, medication, information about previous syncope

Physical findings that are useful in diagnosing syncope include cardiovascular and neurological signs and orthostatic hypotension. The presence of a murmur or severe dyspnoea is indicative of structural heart disease and of a cardiac cause of syncope.

Baseline Electrocardiogram

A normal ECG (most common finding) is associated with a low probability of cardiac syncope as the cause. When abnormal, the ECG may disclose an arrhythmia associated with a high likelihood of syncope, or an abnormality which may predispose to arrhythmia development and syncope.

Abnormalities suggesting an arrhythmic syncope are:
- Bifascicular block or other intraventricular conduction abnormalities (QRS duration > 0.12 s)
- Mobitz I second-degree atrioventricular block
- Asymptomatic sinus bradycardia (< 50 beats/min) or sinoatrial block
- Pre-excited QRS complexes
- Prolonged QT interval
- Right bundle branch block pattern with ST elevation in leads V1-V3 (Brugada syndrome)
- Negative T waves in right precordial leads, epsilon waves, and ventricular late potentials suggestive of arrhythmogenic right ventricular dysplasia
- Q waves suggesting myocardial infarction

Definitive Diagnosis

Initial evaluation may lead to a definite diagnosis (no further evaluation may be needed and treatment can be planed), in the following situations:
- *Vasovagal syncope:* if precipitating events such as fear, severe pain, emotional distress, instrumentation or prolonged standing are associated with typical prodromal symptoms

- *Situational syncope:* if syncope occurs during or immediately after urination, defecation, cough, or swallowing
- *Orthostatic syncope:* when there is documentation of orthostatic hypotension associated with syncope or presyncope. A decrease in systolic blood pressure > 20 mmHg or a decrease of systolic blood pressure to < 90 mmHg measured after 1 or 3 min of standing is defined as orthostatic hypotension regardless of whether or not symptoms occur
- *Cardiac ischaemia-related syncope:* when symptoms are present with ECG evidence of acute ischaemia with or without myocardial infarction, independently of its mechanism
- *Arrhythmia-related syncope* in presence of the following ECG abnormalities:
  - Sinus bradycardia < 40 beats/min or repetitive sinoatrial blocks or sinus pauses > 3 s in the absence of negatively chronotropic medications
  - Mobitz II second- or third-degree atrioventricular block
  - Alternating left and right bundle branch block
  - Rapid paroxysmal supraventricular tachycardia or ventricular tachycardia
  - Pacemaker malfunction with cardiac pauses

Unexplained Syncope

In the presence of structural heart disease or an abnormal ECG, cardiac evaluation consisting of echocardiography, stress testing, and tests for arrhythmia detection such as prolonged electrocardiographic and loop monitoring or electrophysiological study is recommended.

If cardiac evaluation does not show evidence of arrhythmia as a cause of syncope, evaluation for neurally mediated syndromes is recommended in patients with recurrent or severe syncope.

In patients without structural heart disease and a normal ECG, evaluation for neurally mediated syncope is recommended for those with recurrent or severe syncope.

Reappraisal

When no cause of syncope can be determined, reappraisal of the work-up is needed since subtle findings or new historical information may change the entire differential diagnosis.

Role of Anamnesis: Is It a Complete Tool?

P. Alboni, M. Dinelli, F. Pacchioni

Syncope is a symptom, defined as transient, self-limited loss of consciousness, usually leading to a fall. The onset of syncope is relatively rapid, and the subsequent recovery is spontaneous, complete, and usually prompt. The underlying mechanism is a transient global cerebral hypoperfusion. The subdivision of syncope is based on the pathophysiology as follows [1]:
- Neurally mediated reflex syncope
- Orthostatic hypotension
- Cardiac arrhythmias as a primary cause
- Structural cardiac or cardiopulmonary disease and steal syndromes (when a blood vessel has to supply both parts of the brain)

Syncope must be differentiated from other 'non-syncopal' conditions (i.e. those not secondary to global cerebral hypoperfusion) associated with real or apparent loss of consciousness, such as epilepsy, hypoglycaemia, hypoxia, vertebrobasilar transient ischaemic attack, fall, cataplexy, drop attack, and psychogenic pseudo-syncope.

It is commonly accepted that taking the history is an essential part of the work-up of patients with transient loss of consciousness. The historical findings per se may be diagnostic of the cause of syncope, or may suggest a strategy of evaluation. The clinical features of the presentation are most important, especially factors that might predispose to syncope and its sequelae. Some attempts have been made to validate the diagnostic value of the history in prospective and case-control studies [2–6]. When taking a history, all the items listed in Table 1 should be carefully investigated [1]. Moreover, three key questions should be addressed during the initial evaluation: (1) Is the loss of consciousness attributable to syncope or not? (2) Is heart disease present or absent ? (3) Are there important clinical features in the history that suggest the diagnosis?

Division of Cardiology and Arrhythmologic Centre, Ospedale Civile, Cento (Ferrara), Italy

Table 1. Important features in the history

Questions about circumstances just prior to attack
  Position (supine, sitting, or standing)
  Activity (rest, change in posture, during or after exercise, during or immediately after urination, defecation, coughing, or swallowing)
  Predisposing factors (e.g. crowded or warm places, prolonged standing, postprandial period)
  Precipitating events (e.g. fear, intense pain, neck movements)

Questions about onset of attack
  Nausea, vomiting, abdominal discomfort, feeling cold, sweating, aura, pain in neck or shoulders, blurred vision, chest pain, palpitations

Questions about the attack (eye witness)
  Manner of fall (slumping or keeling over), skin colour (pallor, cyanosis, flushing), duration of loss of consciousness, breathing pattern (snoring), movements (tonic, clonic, tonic-clonic or minimal myoclonus, automatism) and their duration, onset of movement in relation to fall, tongue biting

Questions about the end of the attack
  Nausea, vomiting, feeling cold, sweating, confusion, muscle aches, skin colour, injury, chest pain, palpitations, urinary or faecal incontinence

Questions about the background
  Family history of sudden death
  Previous cardiac disease
  Neurological history (parkinsonism, epilepsy, narcolepsy)
  Metabolic disorders (diabetes, etc.)
  Medication (antihypertensive, anti-anginal, antidepressant agent, anti-arrhythmic, diuretics, and QT prolonging agents)
  (In the case of recurrent syncope:) Information on recurrences such as the time from the first syncopal episode and the number of spells

---

With regard to the first question, the most frequent cause of non-syncopal loss of consciousness appears to be epilepsy. The diagnosis of the latter is generally easy if loss of consciousness is observed by an eyewitness. Clinical features suggesting epilepsy are as follows: tonic-clonic movements which are usually prolonged (> 15 s) and whose onset coincides with loss of consciousness, hemilateral clonic movements, tongue biting, blue face, typical aura, prolonged confusion, aching muscles, and 'pins and needles' before the event.

With regard to the second question, it is important to evaluate the presence of heart disease, not only because of its prognostic significance, but because with few exceptions its absence excludes a cardiac cause of syncope.

In fact, in a recent study [5], heart disease was an independent predictor of cardiac cause of syncope, with a sensitivity of 95% and a specificity of 45%; by contrast, the absence of heart disease allowed exclusion of a cardiac cause of syncope in 97% of the patients.

Finally, accurate history taking alone may allow diagnosis of the cause of syncope or may suggest an evaluation strategy. The results of the initial evaluation are diagnostic of the cause of syncope in the following situations [1]:

- Vasovagal syncope is diagnosed if precipitating events such as fear, severe pain, emotional distress, instrumentation, or prolonged standing are associated with typical prodromal symptoms.
- Situational syncope is diagnosed if syncope occurs during or immediately after urination, defecation, cough, or swallowing.
- Orthostatic syncope is diagnosed when there is documentation of orthostatic hypotension associated with syncope or presyncope. Orthostatic blood pressure measurements are recommended after 5 min of lying supine, followed by measurements each minute, or more often, after standing for 3 min. Measurements may be continued for longer, if blood pressure is still falling at 3 min. If the patient does not tolerate standing for this period, the lowest systolic blood pressure during the upright posture should be recorded. A decrease in systolic blood pressure ≥ 20 mmHg or a decrease of systolic blood pressure to < 90 mmHg is defined as orthostatic hypotension regardless of whether or not symptoms occur.
- Cardiac-ischaemia-related syncope is diagnosed when symptoms are present with electrocardiographic evidence of acute ischaemia with or without myocardial infarction, whatever its mechanism.

Under these circumstances, no further evaluation of the disease or disorder may be needed and treatment, if any, can planned. More commonly, the initial evaluation leads to a suspected diagnosis, when one or more of the following features are present:

- *Neurally mediated syncope:* absence of cardiological disease; long history of syncope after sudden unpleasant sight, sound, smell, or pain; prolonged standing or crowded, hot places; nausea, vomiting associated with syncope during the meal or in the absorptive state after a meal; with head rotation; pressure on carotid sinus; after exertion.
- *Syncope due to orthostatic hypotension:* after standing up, temporal relationship with start of medication leading to hypotension, prolonged standing especially in crowded, hot places, presence of autonomic neuropathy or parkinsonism, after exertion.
- *Cardiac syncope:* presence of definite structural heart disease, during exertion or supine, preceded by palpitation, family history of sudden death.

- *Cerebrovascular syncope:* with arm exercise, differences in blood pressure or pulse in the two arms.

It should be underlined that neurally mediated syncopes (tilt-induced, carotid sinus) show very similar clinical features, apart from classical vaso-vagal syncope [7]. In the presence of clinical features suggesting a cardiac cause of syncope, the first examinations to be performed are the cardiological ones (echocardiography, prolonged electrocardiographic monitoring, etc.), whereas in the presence of features suggesting a neurally mediated syncope, the first examinations to be performed are the autonomic tests (tilt testing, carotid sinus massage). Therefore, a careful history can optimise the work-up of syncope, avoiding useless tests and reducing the high diagnostic costs in patients with syncope.

Data from seven population-based studies showed that the history and physical examination identified a potential cause of syncope in 726 of 1607 patients (45%) whose primary disorder can be diagnosed [1]. However, the diagnostic criteria for vasovagal syncope, which represents the most frequent cause of loss of consciousness, have been varied among studies and, probably, too extensive criteria have been used. In more recent studies [5, 8], history and physical examination identified a potential cause of syncope in 15–20% of patients.

History appears more useful in the younger than in the elderly (≥ 65 years); in fact a possible cause of syncope was suggested on the basis of the history in 32% of the former and in only 6% of the latter [8]. The clinical manifestations of syncope change significantly in elderly patients, since during the prodromal and recovery phase the frequency of symptoms (predominantly the autonomic ones) decreases in older patients, thus reducing the utility of the history.

References

1. Brignole M, Alboni P, Benditt DG et al (2004) Guidelines on management (diagnosis and treatment) of syncope. Update 2004. Europace 6:467–537
2. Kapoor WN, Karf M, Wieand S et al (1983) A prospective evaluation and follow-up of patients with syncope. N Engl J Med 309:197–204
3. Martin GJ, Adams SL, Martin HG et al (1984) Prospective evaluation of syncope. Ann Emerg Med 3:499–504
4. Calkins H, Shyr Y, Frumin H et al (1995) The value of clinical history in the differentiation of syncope due to ventricular tachycardia, atrioventricular block and neurocardiogenic syncope. Am J Med 98:365–373
5. Alboni P, Brignole M, Menozzi C et al (2001) Diagnostic value of history in patients with syncope with or without heart disease. J Am Coll Cardiol 37:1921–1928

6. Sheldon R, Rose S, Ritchie D et al (2002) Historical criteria that distinguish syncope from seizures. J Am Coll Cardiol 40:142–148

7. Alboni P, Brignole M, Menozzi C et al (2004) Clinical spectrum of neurally mediated reflex syncopes. Europace 6:52–56

8. Del Rosso A, Alboni P, Brignole M et al (2004) The clinical presentation of syncope depends on the age of the patients (submitted for publication)

Is There Still a Role for Drug Therapy in Vasovagal Syncope?

M. Gulizia, G.M. Francese

By definition, syncope is not a disease, but a symptom clinically characterised by transient loss of consciousness, which generally leads to falling, followed by spontaneous recovery [1]. It can be due to neuromediated mechanisms as well as to cardiac or cerebrovascular causes. The Framingham study [2], which investigated 5209 patients with 26 years' follow-up, indicated that syncope occurring in patients without cardiovascular or neurological pathology is likely to be neuromediated in nature, with a proportion ranging from 0.8% in the age group between 35 and 44 years to 4% in the oldest patients (age > 75 years). No increase in the incidence of sudden death, acute myocardial infarction, or cerebral stroke was noticed with respect to the syncope-free group throughout the follow-up. Nevertheless, some authors [3] define particular forms of vasovagal syncope as 'malignant', not because they carry an increased likelihood of sudden death, but because they can result in severe trauma, especially when the syncope is not preceded by relevant prodromes, as frequently happens in the elderly. Therefore, therapy against neuromediated syncope should essentially be aimed at preventing trauma and improving quality of life, especially in patients involved in risky professional activities, such as public transport drivers and aircraft pilots.

All patients should be reassured as to the benign nature of the disorder and receive behavioural advice. They should be trained to avoid syncope-triggering conditions (such as over-warm or crowded environments, or prolonged standing up) and to recognise possible prodromes and all signs and symptoms preceding the event, in order to react with appropriate manoeuvres to abort the syncope and prevent any injury. A volume increase is necessary, which can be achieved by liquid (2–3 l water) [4] and salt injection (up

Cardiology Department, San Luigi - S. Currò Hospital, Catania, Italy

to 120 mmol/day NaCl) [5]. Regular light physical exercise is recommended. Alcohol drinking and other addictions should be avoided or strongly reduced.

Several drugs with various mechanisms of action have been proposed for the prevention of syncopal events: e.g. clonidine, scopolamine, domperidone, ethylephrine, beta-blockers, dihydroergotamine, enalapril, disopyramide, theophylline, paroxetine, fludrocortisone, and midodrine. The wide spectrum of drugs reflects both the variability of and the limited knowledge about the pathophysiological mechanisms of neuromediated syncope in different patients. Generally, while results from uncontrolled or short-term controlled studies were satisfactory [6], with few exceptions, all but one studies with control versus placebo design were disappointing. Beta-blockers have been used for their negative inotropic effects, with the aim of reducing the mechanoreceptor activation associated with decreased venous return, as well as to counteract the rate increase induced by high levels of circulating adrenaline, which precedes the loss of consciousness [7]. Studies performed by Scott et al. [8] and Ventura et al. [9], with follow-up longer than 6 months, demonstrated a reduction in recurrences with respect to untreated patients, while Brignole et al. [10] and Madrid et al. [11], who studied the effects of atenolol–ergotamine–domperidone and atenolol alone, respectively, did not confirm the drug benefit. Data from Ventura et al. [9] indicate that lipophilic beta-blockers, like propranolol and methoprolol, which can cross the blood–brain barrier, show a greater effect (29% recurrences versus 79% in non-treated patients; $P = 0.004$). Nevertheless, a placebo mechanism cannot be excluded. At present, it is not clear whether beta-blockers are effective in reducing syncopal recurrences. An arm of the randomised controlled versus placebo study VASIS, designed to analyse the effects of ethylephrine, was closed after 10 months because the drug proved ineffective [12]. Similarly, controlled studies performed with domperidone [10], disopyramide [13], and dihydroergotamine [10] did not demonstrate significant drug effects. The main limitations of these studies are short follow-up and the lack of placebo-treated control groups. Ward et al. [14] performed a prospective controlled study on the short-term effects of midodrine in severely symptomatic aged patients affected by vasodepressive vasovagal syndrome with frequent syncopal episodes. Positive results were reported, but the study was not controlled versus placebo. Another study from Natale et al. [15] investigated the effectiveness of midodrine in 6 months follow-up, showing a reduction in the number of syncopal events, but this study also had a short follow-up and no placebo administration in the control group. Di Girolamo et al. [16] demonstrated positive effects of paroxetine, a serotonin reuptake inhibitor, in a large controlled versus placebo study with a follow-up of 25 months. A reduction of syncope prevalence from 53% to 17% was reported, but the results were not confirmed in other investigations and the drug is not indicated at present. Enalapril, an ACE inhibitor, was used in a study by Zeng et al. [17] with positive results, which were likely due to the inhibition of the sympathetic nervous system (Table 1).

Available clinical information does not show clearly whether drug treatment is advisable in patients affected by vasovagal syncope and what drug could be selectively indicated. The usually benign course of the disorder, often showing long periods without symptoms, together with the possible therapeutic effects of tilt testing and increased self-confidence in the patient, which can be helped by reassurances from the physician, can produce a false impression of efficacy for any drug treatment under evaluation. In the past, an expected drug action had to be confirmed by the tilt test, since lack of syncope in previously tilt-test-positive patients was considered a marker of therapeutic effectiveness. This technique is no longer used, however, since some trials have reported equal reduction in the occurrence of syncope in treated and untreated patients [10, 12, 13, 18].

In conclusion, no drug has proved clearly effective in syncope prevention so far, and further randomised placebo-controlled studies are required to ascertain the real effectiveness of any pharmacological treatment.

Table 1. Effects of different drugs in the prevention of vasovagal syncope recurrences

Author	Year	Drug	Dosage	No. pts	Follow-up (months)	Results
Madrid et al. [11]	2001	Atenolol	50	50	12	N.S.
Scott et al. [8]	1995	Atenolol	25–100	29	6	Effective
Brignole et al. [10]	1992	Atenolol	100	15	10	N.S.
Ventura et al. [9]	2002	Propranolol	80–100	56	12	Effective
Ventura et al. [9]	2002	Metoprolol	50–100	56	12	Effective
Moya et al. [18]	1995	Ethylephrine	30	60	12	N.S.
Raviele et al. [12]	1999	Ethylephrine	75	126	12	N.S.
Morillo et al. [13]	1993	Diisopyramide	800	21	29	N.S.
Brignole et al. [10]	1992	Dihydroergotamine	18	4	10	N.S.
Brignole et al. [10]	1992	Domperidone	60	4	10	N.S.
Natale et al. [15]	1999	Midodrina	15–45	61	6	Effective
Zeng et al. [17]	1998	Enalapril	10	30	13	Effective
Di Girolamo et al. [16]	1999	Paroexetine	20	68	25	Effective
Scott et al. [8]	1995	Fludrocortisone	100–200	29	6	Effective

References

1. Brignole M, Alboni P, Benedict L et (2001) Guidelines on management (diagnosis and treatment) of syncope. Eur Heart J 22:1256–1306

2. Savage DD, Corwin L, Mc Gee DL et al (1985) Epidemiologic features of isolated syncope: the Framingham study. Stroke 16:626–629

3. Fitzpatrick A, Theodorakis G, Travill C et al (1991) Incidence of malignant vasovagal syndrome in patients with recurrent syncope. Eur Heart J 12:389–394

4. Younoszai AK, Franklin WH, Chan DP et al (1998) Oral fluid therapy. A promising treatment for vasodepressor syncope. Arch Pediatr Adolesc Med 152:165–168

5. El-Sayed H, Hainsworth R (1996) Salt supplement increases plasma volume and orthostatic tolerance in patients with unexplained syncope. Heart 75:114–115

6. Raviele A, Themistoclakis S, Gasparini G (1996) Drug treatment of vasovagal syncope. In: Blanc JJ, Beneditt D, Sutton R (eds) Neurally mediated syncope: pathophysiology, investigations, and treatment, Futura, Armonk, NY, pp 113–121

7. Klingenheben T, Kalusche D, Li Y-G et al (1996) Changes in plasma epinephrine concentration and in heart rate during head-up tilt testing in patients with neurocardiogenic syncope: correlation with successful therapy with B-receptor antagonist. J Cardiovasc Electrophysiol 7:802–808

8. Scott WA, Giacomo P, Bromberg BI et al (1995) Randomized comparison of atenolol and fludrocortisone acetate in the treatment of pediatric neurally mediated syncope. Am J Cardiol 76:400–402

9. Ventura R, Maas R, Zeidler D et al (2002) A randomized and controlled pilot trial of beta-blockers for the treatment of recurrent syncope in patients a positive or negative response to head-up tilt test. Pacing Clin Electrophysiol 25:816–821

10. Brignole M, Menozzi C, Gianfranchi L et al (1992) A controlled trial of acute and long-term medical therapy in tilt-induced neurally mediated syncope. Am J Cardiol 70:339–342

11. Madrid AH, Ortega J, Rebollo RG et al (2001) Lack of efficacy of atenolol for the prevention of neurally mediated syncope in a highly symptomatic population: a prospective double blind, randomised and placebo controlled study. J Am Coll Cardiol 37:554–559

12. Raviele A, Brignole M, Sutton R et al (1999) Effect of etilefrine in preventing syncopal recurrence in patients with vasovagal syncope: a double-blind, randomized, placebo-controlled trial. The Vasovagal Syncope International Study. Circulation 99:1452–1457

13. Morillo C, Leitch J, Yee R et al (1993) A placebo-controlled trial of intravenous and oral disopyramide for prevention of neurally mediated syncope induced by head-up tilt test. J Am Coll Cardiol 22:1843–1848

14. Ward CR, Gray JC, Gilroy JJ et al (1998) Mididrine: a role in the management of neurocardiogenic syncope. Heart 79:45–49

15. Natale A, Beheiry S, Tomassoni GF et al (1999) Randomized placebo control assessment of midodrine in the treatment of neurocardiogenic syncope. J Am Coll Cardiol 33:269 (abs)

16. Di Girolamo E, Di Forio C, Sabatini O et al (1999) Effects of paroxetine hydrochloride, a selective serotonin reuptake inhibitor, on refractory vasovagal sincope: a randomized, double-blind, placebo-controlled study. J Am Coll Cardiol 33:1227–1230

17. Zeng C, Zhu Z, Liu G et al (1998) A randomized, double-blind, placebo-controlled trial of oral enalapril in patients with neurally-mediated sincope. Am Heart J 136:852–858

18. Moya A, Permanyer-Miralda G, Sagrista-Sauleda J et al (1995) Limitations of head-up tilt test for evaluating the efficacy of therapeutic interventions in patients with vasovagal syncope: results of a controlled study of etilefrine versus placebo. J Am Coll Cardiol 25:65–69

When Do We Need a Permanent Pacemaker in Neuromediated Syncope?

F. Giada, A. Raviele

Introduction

Syncope is a very frequent clinical disease [1]. About 30% of the general population undergo one syncopal episode in their lifetime, while at least 3% faint more than once. Moreover, it is the cause of about 3% of visits to hospital emergency rooms. In most cases, the aetiology of syncope is neuromediated.

Neuromediated syncope is related to bradycardia and hypotension caused by an abnormal cardiac activation of baroreceptors and of major vessels. Baroreceptor activation produces a vagal overtone and a decrease in sympathetic efferents, thus leading to bradycardia, vasodilation, and hypotension. Though neuromediated syncope does not directly cause death, it is often associated with severe trauma and, when recurrent, significantly impairs the patient's quality of life [2–4].

In most cases, neuromediated syncope is an isolated event and patients improve after tilt testing and specialist reassurance regarding their condition [1]. However, some patients continue to have frequent fainting fits and suffer severe functional and psychological limitations which significantly undermine their quality of life. Such patients need specific treatment.

The treatment of neuromediated syncope involves behavioural measures for all patients, drug therapy for those who are most symptomatic, and pacemaker implantation in very selected cases [1].

Studies on drugs for the treatment of neuromediated syncope have yielded disappointing results [5–11]. In only two brief small-scale investigations [12, 13] did the drug used prove to be more effective than placebo. Thus, drug therapy for neuromediated syncope is still controversial and remains under examination.

Cardiovascular Department, Umberto I Hospital, Mestre-Venice, Italy

Role of Pacing in the Treatment of Neuromediated Syncope

While single-chamber VVI mode pacing has proved to be ineffective in the treatment of neuromediated syncope [14], several non-randomised studies [15–17] have shown a significant decrease in syncope recurrence in patients who had undergone dual-chamber pacing. In the last few years, three randomised non-controlled studies revealed the efficacy of dual-chamber pacemaker implantation in reducing recurrences in patients with recurrent neuromediated syncope. The VPS study [18] demonstrated the effectiveness of DDD with rate-drop-response pacemakers in patients affected by neuromediated syncope who had a positive result on head-up tilt testing and presented a variable cardioinhibitory component. The VASIS study [19], on the other hand, showed the effectiveness of a DDI mode pacemaker with hysteresis in patients with vasovagal syncope and positive head-up tilt testing with a marked cardioinhibitory component. Finally, the SYDIT study demonstrated the superiority of DDD with rate-drop-response pacemakers with respect to drug therapy [20].

However, since the above-mentioned studies were non-controlled (patients randomised to the control arm did not receive a pacemaker), the benefits observed might have been due to the placebo effect of the pacemaker. Indeed, the very recently published VPS II trial [21] and SYNPACE trial [22], two randomised, double-blind, placebo-controlled studies in which all enrolled patients underwent pacemaker implantation and were afterwards randomised to active pacing or inactive pacing, were unable to show any statistically significant superiority of pacemaker treatment over placebo. The main finding of the SYNPACE study [22] is that active cardiac pacing is not more effective than inactive pacing in preventing syncopal recurrences in patients with severe neuromediated syncope: neither the number of patients with syncopal recurrence nor the time to the first syncopal recurrence significantly differed between pacemaker *on* and pacemaker *off* patients. Moreover, the incidence and number of presyncopes were similar between patients with active pacing and those with inactive pacing. Furthermore, in the SYNPACE study the presence of a marked cardioinhibitory component during tilt-induced syncope did not identify patients who were likely to benefit from permanent pacing. These results confirm previous observations regarding the poor value of head-up tilt testing in predicting the efficacy of a given therapeutic intervention [5].

Thus, at the present time, we have insufficiently compelling data on the real efficacy of electrical therapy for the treatment of neuromediated syncope.

Future Perspectives

A crucial point in the use of permanent cardiac pacing in the treatment of neuromediated syncope is the right selection of patients. Perhaps the documentation of severe bradycardia/asystole during spontaneous syncope by means of an implanted loop recorder, and not the observation of a cardioinhibitory response during tilt-induced syncope, will identify patients who will benefit most from pacemaker implantation.

One of the most important limitations of pacing in neuromediated syncope is timely detection of the onset of the neuromediated reaction and triggering of pacing. Rate-drop response, like the other algorithms utilised in the studies mentioned above, is a sensing modality based on a reduction in the heart rate. It is possible that the use of different sensing modalities, such as those based on cardiac contractility [23] or respiratory changes [24], might yield better results in preventing syncopal relapse.

Finally, the combination of a dual-chamber pacemaker with an implantable drug delivery system using vasoactive drugs able to counteract both bradycardia and vasodilation could be proposed for very symptomatic patients [25].

References

1. Brignole M, Alboni P, Benditt L et al (2001) Guidelines on management (diagnosis and treatment) of syncope. Eur Heart J 22:1256–1306
2. Linzer M, Pontinen M, Gold DT et al (1991) Impairment of physical and psychosocial function in recurrent syncope. J Clin Epidemiol 44:1037–1043
3. Linzer M, Gold DT, Pontinen M et al (1994) Recurrent syncope as a chronic disease: preliminary validation of disease-specific measure of functional impairment. J Gen Intern Med 9:181–186
4. Rose S, Koshman ML, McDonald S et al (1996) Health-related quality of life in patients with neuromediated syncope (abstract). Can J Cardiol 12:131E
5. Moya A, Permanyer-Miralda G, Sagrista-Sauleda J et al (1995) Limitations of head-up tilt test for evaluating the efficacy of therapeutic interventions in patients with vasovagal syncope: results of a controlled study of ethylephrine versus placebo. J Am Coll Cardiol 25:65–69
6. Brignole M, Menozzi C, Gianfranchi L et al (1992) A controlled trial of acute and long-term medical therapy in tilt-induced neurally mediated syncope. Am J Cardiol 70:339–342
7. Morillo CA, Leicht JW, Yee R et al (1993) A placebo-controlled trial of intravenous and oral disopyramide for prevention of neurally mediated syncope induced by head-up tilt. J Am Coll Cardiol 22:1843–1848
8. Raviele A, Brignole M, Sutton R et al (1999) Effect of ethylephrine in preventing syncopal recurrence in patients with vasovagal syncope. A double-blind, randomized, placebo-controlled trial. Circulation 99:1452–1457

9. Madrid AH, Ortega J, Rebollo JG et al (2001) Lack of efficacy of atenolol for the prevention of neurally mediated syncope in a highly symptomatic population: a prospective, double-blind, randomized and placebo-controlled study. J Am Coll Cardiol 37:554–559

10. Ventura R, Maas R, Zeidler D et al (2002) A randomized and controlled pilot trial of β-blockers for the treatment of recurrent syncope in patients with positive or negative response to head-up tilt test. Pacing Clin Electrophysiol 25: 816–821

11. Flevari P, Livanis EG, Theodorakis GN et al (2002) Vasovagal syncope: a prospective, randomized, crossover evaluation of the effect of propranolol, nadolol and placebo on syncope recurrence and patient's well-being. J Am Coll Cardiol 40:499–504

12. Ward CR, Grey JC, Gilroy JJ et al (1998) Midodrine: a role in the management of neurocardiogenic syncope. Heart 79:45–49

13. Di Girolamo E, Di Iorio C, Sabatini P et al (1999) Effects of paroxetine hydrochloride, a selective serotonin re-uptake inhibitor, on refractory vasovagal syncope: a randomized, double-blind, placebo-controlled study. J Am Coll Cardiol 33:1227–1230

14. Benditt DG, Petersen M, Lurie KG et al (1995) Cardiac pacing for the prevention of recurrent vasovagal syncope. Ann Intern Med 122:204–209

15. Petersen MEV, Chamberlain-Webber R, Fitzpatrick AP et al (1994) Permanent pacing for cardioinhibitory malignant vasovagal syndrome. Br Heart J 71:274–281

16. Benditt DG, Sutton R, Gammage M et al for the Rate-drop Response Investigators (1997) Clinical experience with Thera DR rate drop response pacing algorithm in carotid sinus syndrome and vasovagal syncope. Pacing Clin Electrophysiol 20:832–839

17. Sheldon R, Koshman ML, Wilson W (1998) Effect of dual-chamber pacing with automatic rate-drop sensing on recurrent neurally mediated syncope. Am J Cardiol 81:158–162

18. Connolly SJ, Sheldon R, Roberts RS et al (1999) The North American Vasovagal Pacemaker Study (VPS). A randomized trial of permanent cardiac pacing for the prevention of vasovagal syncope. J Am Coll Cardiol 33:16–20

19. Sutton R, Brignole M, Menozzi C et al on behalf of the Vasovagal Syncope International Study (VASIS) Investigators (2000) Dual-chamber pacing is efficacious in treatment of neurally-mediated tilt-positive cardioinhibitory syncope. Pacemaker versus no therapy: a multicentre, randomized study. Circulation 102:294–299

20. Ammirati F, Colivicchi F, Santini M et al (2001) Permanent cardiac pacing versus medical treatment for the prevention of recurrent vasovagal syncope. Circulation 104:52–57

21. Connolly SJ, Sheldon R, Thorpe KE et al (2003) Pacemaker therapy for prevention of syncope in patients with recurrent severe vasovagal syncope. Second Vasovagal Pacemaker Study (VPS II): a randomized trial. JAMA 289:2224–2229

22. Raviele A, Giada F, Menozzi C et al (2004) A randomised, double-blind, placebo-controlled study of permanent cardiac pacing for the treatment of recurrent tilt-induced vasovagal syncope. The vasovagal syncope and pacing trial (synpace). Eur Heart J 6:1–8

23. Deharo JC, Peyre JP, Chalvidian T et al (2000) Continuous monitoring of an endocardial index of myocardial contractility during head-up tilt test. Am Heart J 139:1022–1030
24. Kurbaan AS, Erikson M, Petersen MEV et al (2000) Respiratory changes in vaso-vagal syncope. J Cardiovasc Electrophysiol 11:607–611
25. Raviele A, Giada F, Gasparini G et al (2005) Efficacy of a patient-activated pharmacological pump using phenylephrine as active drug and prodromal symptoms as a marker of imminent loss of consiousness to abort tilt-induced syncope. J Am Coll Cardiol 2:320-321

LATEST TECHNOLOGIES IN CARDIOVASCULAR IMAGING: AN UPDATE FOR THE CLINICAL CARDIOLOGIST

CT Coronary Angiography with 16-Row Multi-slice Scanner: Do We Still Need Conventional Coronary Angiography?

F. Cademartiri, G. Runza, M. Belgrano, P. Malagutti, N. Mollet, P. de Feyter

Background

Coronary artery disease (CAD) remains globally the leading cause of death and long-term morbidity. Among the many manifestations of CAD, acute coronary syndrome, ranging from unstable angina to acute myocardial infarction, is the most catastrophic event due to our inability to predict its occurrence. Despite improved treatments for CAD, acute coronary syndrome results in sudden death or permanent disability in a substantial percentage of patients. In patients who have an acute coronary syndrome, rapid and accurate risk stratification is crucial. If we could predict the timing of acute coronary syndrome or, better yet, prevent its occurrence, we could alter the otherwise unfavourable course of CAD.

Non-invasive visualisation of the heart is a demanding application for any imaging modality [1, 2]. The use of multi-slice CT (MSCT) for the evaluation of the heart and coronary arteries was born in 1999 with the introduction of four-row MSCT scanners [3]. The results of that generation of scanners were encouraging but still insufficient to ensure diagnostic confidence because of the high percentage of segments that could not be assessed [4]. The subsequent introduction of 16-row MSCT scanners significantly enhanced the spatial and temporal resolution, allowing the evaluation of almost all the coronary segments [4].

Technique

High temporal resolution is required to freeze cardiac motion and avoid motion artefacts due to the heart beat [4]. High spatial resolution is also

Department of Cardiology and Radiology, Erasmus Medical Centre, Rotterdam, The Netherlands

needed for the depiction of small structures and the complex anatomy of the coronary arteries [4].

The heart volume must be examined within one breath-hold to avoid motion artefacts. Two different methods were developed to acquire motionless images of the coronary vessels, depending respectively on prospective triggering of the acquisition or retrospective reconstruction of a static image. With prospective ECG triggering, the heart volume is covered by single axial scans acquired after a selectable delay following the onset of an R wave. With retrospective ECG gating, the heart volume is covered continuously by a spiral scan. The patient's ECG signal is acquired simultaneously to allow retrospective selection of data segments for image reconstruction. It became immediately evident that retrospective ECG reconstruction was the winning technique for the study of the coronary vessels by CT angiography, because of its ability to overcome technical difficulties caused by the patient's hearth rate irregularities.

Cardiac scanning is characterised by spiral geometry with a very low pitch, generally 0.25, that implies an oversampling of the information throughout the cardiac cycle. Simultaneously the ECG is recorded [4]. During the acquisition a bolus of contrast medium is administered. A high flow rate (usually 5 ml/s) is necessary to obtain optimal coronary opacification during the acquisition [5–7]. After the scan is performed, the raw data are retrospectively reconstructed in the diastolic phase of the heart cycle using the ECG track as the reference point. Within the ECG, the R wave is widely used as a triggering point, because it is an easy wave for the software to recognise.

At this point the operator has to carry out the reconstructions to obtain a motionless dataset. Based on this dataset the radiologist performs the image reconstructions of the entire coronary tract. Sometimes motion artefacts due to irregularities of the heart rhythm necessitate additional reconstructions in order to obtain an image of the coronary artery that is diagnostic. To obtain diagnostic images the operator uses all the tools that the console will allow: multiplanar reformatting (MPR), curved multiplanar reformatting (cMPR), maximum intensity projection (MIP), 3D volume rendering, and 4D volume rendering [8–10]. The width of the temporal window that is used for the reconstruction is linked to the temporal resolution of the scanner. Modern scanners have high gantry rotation speed (0.4 s for the 16-row MSCT, Siemens Sensation 16) that allows high temporal resolution and a shorter temporal window. One image can be reconstructed using the information derived from 180° of gantry rotation. Therefore, if the gantry rotation time is 400 ms, the temporal resolution for a single image will be 200 ms [4]. This level of resolution is still far from the 50- to 100-ms range that characterises Electron Beam CT (EBCT) and magnetic resonance imaging.

Nevertheless, 16-row MSCT can provide high spatial resolution (< 0.5 mm) and retrospective reconstruction algorithms.

An important parameter that affects image quality is the patient's heart rate. The development of faster scanners has reduced the rotation time and increased the temporal resolution, but a high heart rate reduces the width of the temporal window available to the software to perform the reconstruction of a single fixed image. For these reasons, optimal motion-free cardiac phase can always be found in patients with heart rates below 65 bpm. When the heart rate is higher than 65 bpm, premedication based on beta-blockers is needed. Despite this, however, coronary imaging with MSCT appears promising and will probably soon come into clinical use in selected patient populations who have fewer limitations.

Results

MSCT coronary angiography (MSCT-CA) has been a reliable non-invasive tool for the detection of CAD in selected populations of patients since the introduction of 16-slice CT scanners (Table 1). High spatial and temporal resolution allows the evaluation of coronary segments down to 1.5 mm in diameter. Aggressive heart rate control remains of paramount importance for reliable results. Sensitivity and specificity for the detection of significant coronary artery stenosis (> 50% lumen reduction) have been reported in the range of around 94% and around 90%, respectively [11–18].

Clinical Applications

One of the main indications for MSCT is non-invasive coronary artery imaging. Although at the moment only selected populations of patients are suitable candidates for this method, there are many of them and they only partly overlap with the population traditionally selected to undergo conventional coronary angiography. In particular, they include young asymptomatic patients at high risk of cardiovascular disease, symptomatic patients with inconclusive conventional tests (e.g. ECG, ultrasound, stress echocardiography), and patients being followed for coronary stent and graft patency (Table 2).

With this new approach we can scan patients with unclear symptoms and inconclusive tests in a very short time: the patient preparation for the scan, if the heart rate is below 65 bpm, is the same as for a normal CT angiography scan and requires only few minutes; the image reconstruction and evaluation by a trained radiologist require about 15–30 min. The advantages of this technique are obvious in view of the vascular wall and plaque characterisation, which allows plaque morphology to be studied via a non-invasive exam

Table 1. Diagnostic performance of MSCT to detect coronary stenosis, with conventional angiography as the standard of reference (16-slice CT)

Reference	Study population (n)	Assessment[a]	Diameter reduction[b] (%)	Stenoses per patient[c] (n)	Excluded[d] (%)	Sensitivity (%)	Specificity (%)	PPV (%)	NPV (%)	Overall sensivity[e] (%)
[11]	58	> 2.0-mm branches	50	1.1	-	95	86	80	97	95
[12]	77	> 1.5-mm branches	50	1.0	12	92	93	79	97	73
[16]	60	Segments	50	1.2	6	72	97	72	97	NR
[13]	128	Segments	50	1.6	-	92	95	79	98	92

PPV, positive predictive value, and NPV, negative predictive value, regarding the assessable segments or branches; NR, not reported

[a] Branch- or segment-based assessment

[b] Diameter reduction considered significant

[c] Mean number of stenosed vessels or segments per patient

[d] Percentage of excluded segments or branches

[e] Overall sensitivity including missed lesions in non-assessable segments or branches

Table 2. Potential applications of CT coronary angiography

Early detection of stenosis:
  Non-symptomatic high-risk patients

Exclusion of stenosis:
  High-risk patients [14, 17, 18]
  Prior to major (non-cardiac) surgery

Detection and/or exclusion of stenoses:
  Atypical (unstable) chest pain [17]
  Refractory chest pain of doubtful coronary origin
  Non-conclusive stress tests

Substitution for conventional coronary angiography:
  Prior to percutaneous coronary intervention [21]
  High-risk patients: aortic disease

Adjuvant to coronary angiography:
  Plaque characterisation [19, 20, 22, 23]
  Complicated coronary catheterisation
  Total coronary occlusion [21]

Follow-up:
  Percutaneous coronary intervention
  Bypass surgery [24, 25]

that takes only a short time to perform and does not require admission of the patient for 1 day.

A new approach to the unstable patient is now possible. Usually when a patient presents with atypical chest pain and non diriment ECG and blood marker results, the normal approach is to admit the patient to a semi-intensive coronary unit to monitor the development of the situation and to collect enough data to make a correct diagnosis and perhaps eventually to treat the coronary stenoses or occlusion. Multi-slice CT in the emergency department could be useful in this setting in order to exclude an acute coronary syndrome immediately (without needing to await cardiac enzyme confirmation) and allow the patient to be discharged directly or the referring doctor to be pointed in another direction. If, on the other hand, the MSCT is positive, the patient can undergo the proper treatment sooner.

Role of MSCT in Acute Coronary Syndrome

Several studies have demonstrated that most acute coronary syndromes develop from previously mild to moderate stenoses. Based on these and autopsy studies, sudden disruption or rupture of the non-obstructive 'vulnerable' atherosclerotic lesion is currently considered to be the cause of acute coronary syndrome [19, 20].

MSCT can display coronary arteries – both lumen and wall – non-invasively with good performance. It has been shown that good results can be obtained in stable and unstable patients. Plaque visualisation, quantification, and sometimes characterisation appear feasible in preliminary reports. The potential role of MSCT coronary angiography in acute coronary syndrome could be in anticipating and extending the ability to visualise the coronary tree and, in particular, the coronary wall in those groups of patients with intermediate probability to develop an acute myocardial infarction and/or more atypical findings and symptoms. The use of MSCT coronary angiography prior to conventional coronary angiography could be of help in identifying subtle lesions causing atypical chest pain or typical chest pain with normal coronary artery tree. In addition, MSCT coronary angiography could be used to target sub-groups of patients defined as 'vulnerable' in whom the likelihood of acute coronary syndrome is higher.

Other Applications

Other applications of MSCT are non-invasive evaluation of the supra-aortic trunks for suspected cerebrovascular diseases: CT for this application is robust, easy to perform, patient-friendly, and operator-independent. With the implementation of brain perfusion assessment, it could be applied in the acute settings. In non-invasive peripheral artery evaluation, too, MSCT can rely on robustness and ease of application.

Conclusions

MSCT coronary angiography is a promising technique for the non-invasive visualisation of coronary arteries. Based on the current literature, it is expected to have a role in the diagnosis of acute coronary syndrome. Its capability to visualise coronary artery plaques will play a role in the targeting of culprit/vulnerable plaques.

References

1. Flohr T, Ohnesorge B, Bruder H et al (2003) Image reconstruction and performance evaluation for ECG-gated spiral scanning with a 16-slice CT system. Med Phys 30:2650–2662

2. Flohr T, Stierstorfer K, Bruder H et al (2002) New technical developments in multi-slice CT – Part 1: Approaching isotropic resolution with sub-millimeter 16-slice scanning. Rofo Fortschr Geb Rontgenstr Neuen Bildgeb Verfahr 174:839–845

3. Nieman K, Oudkerk M, Rensig BJ et al (2001) Coronary angiography with multislice computed tomography. Lancet 357:599–603

4. Flohr TG, Schoepf UJ, Kuettner A et al (2003) Advances in cardiac imaging with 16-section CT systems. Acad Radiol 10:386–401

5. Cademartiri F, Luccichenti G, Marano R et al (2004) Use of saline chaser in the intravenous administration of contrast material in non-invasive coronary angiography with 16-row multislice computed tomography. Radiol Med 107:497–505

6. Cademartiri F, Nieman K, van der Lugt A et al (2004) IV contrast administration for CT coronary angiography on a 16-multidetector-row helical CT scanner: test bolus vs. bolus tracking. Radiology 233:817–823

7. Cademartiri F, van der Lugt A, Luccichenti G et al (2002) Parameters affecting bolus geometry in CTA: a review. J Comput Assist Tomogr 26:598–607

8. Cademartiri C, Torelli P, Cologno D et al (2002) Upper and lower cluster headache: clinical and pathogenetic observations in 608 patients. Headache 42:630–637

9. Cademartiri F, Mollet NR, Lemos PA et al (2004) Standard vs. user-interactive assessment of significant coronary stenoses with multislice computed tomography coronary angiography. Am J Cardiol 94:1590–1593

10. Vogl TJ, Abolmaali ND, Diebold T et al (2002) Techniques for the detection of coronary atherosclerosis: multi-detector row CT coronary angiography. Radiology 223:212–220

11. Nieman K, Cademartiri F, Lemos PA et al (2002) Reliable noninvasive coronary angiography with fast submillimeter multislice spiral computed tomography. Circulation 106:2051–2054

12. Ropers D, Baum U, Pohle K et al (2003) Detection of coronary artery stenoses with thin-slice multi-detector row spiral computed tomography and multiplanar reconstruction. Circulation 107:664–666

13. Mollet NR, Cademartiri F, Nieman K et al (2004) Multislice spiral computed tomography coronary angiography in patients with stable angina pectoris. J Am Coll Cardiol 43:2265–2270

14. Martuscelli E, Romagnoli A, D'Eliseo A et al (2004) Accuracy of thin-slice computed tomography in the detection of coronary stenoses. Eur Heart J 25:1043–1048

15. Hoffmann U, Moselewski F, Cury RC et al (2004) Predictive value of 16-slice multidetector spiral computed tomography to detect significant obstructive coronary artery disease in patients at high risk for coronary artery disease: patient- versus segment-based analysis. Circulation 110:2638–2643

16. Kuettner A, Trabold T, Schroeder S et al (2004) Noninvasive detection of coronary lesions using 16-detector multislice spiral computed tomography technology: initial clinical results. J Am Coll Cardiol 44:1230–1237

17. Mollet NR, Cademartiri F, Krestin GP et al (2005) Improved diagnostic accuracy with 16-row multi-slice computed tomography coronary angiography. J Am Coll Cardiol 45:128–132

18. Kuettner A, Beck T, Drosch T et al (2005) Diagnostic accuracy of noninvasive coronary imaging using 16-detector slice spiral computed tomography with 188 ms temporal resolution. J Am Coll Cardiol 45:123–127

19. Leber AW, Knez A, Becker A et al (2004) Accuracy of multidetector spiral computed tomography in identifying and differentiating the composition of coronary atherosclerotic plaques: a comparative study with intracoronary ultrasound. J Am Coll Cardiol 43:1241–1247

20. Achenbach S, Moselewski F, Ropers D et al (2004) Detection of calcified and non-calcified coronary atherosclerotic plaque by contrast-enhanced, submillimeter multidetector spiral computed tomography: a segment-based comparison with intravascular ultrasound. Circulation 109:14–17

21. Mollet NR, Hoye A, Lemos PA et al (2005) Value of preprocedure multislice computed tomographic coronary angiography to predict the outcome of percutaneous recanalization of chronic total occlusions. Am J Cardiol 95:240–243

22. Schroeder S, Kopp AF, Baumbach A et al (2001) Noninvasive detection and evaluation of atherosclerotic coronary plaques with multislice computed tomography. J Am Coll Cardiol 37:1430–1435

23. Achenbach S, Ropers D, Hoffmann U et al (2004) Assessment of coronary remodeling in stenotic and nonstenotic coronary atherosclerotic lesions by multidetector spiral computed tomography. J Am Coll Cardiol 43:842–847

24. Nieman K, Pattynama PM, Rensing BJ et al (2003) Evaluation of patients after coronary artery bypass surgery: CT angiographic assessment of grafts and coronary arteries. Radiology 229:749–756

25. Martuscelli E, Romagnoli A, D'Eliseo A et al (2004) Evaluation of venous and arterial conduit patency by 16-slice spiral computed tomography. Circulation 110:3234–3238

Multislice CT for the Study of Aortic Aneurysms

V. Magnano San Lio, E.M. Di Maggio

Introduction and Technical Principles

In 1988 Siemens Medical Systems introduced the first single-section helical (spiral) computed tomography (SSCT). In 1992, Elscint introduced a dual-section helical scanner that is considered to be the first multisection CT. This technology was improved in 1998 with the advent of quad-section technology. This technology was up to four times faster than conventional SSCT. The next step was to increase the rotation speed to two revolutions per second. This enabled multi-detector-row CT scanners to operate up to eight times faster than SSCT. Nowadays the principal equipment manufacturers are able to produce multi-detector-row CT scanners (MDCT) carrying out 32 or 64 slices per second. These two improvements have combined to increase scanning speed by a factor of 30 or 60 over most conventional SSCT scanners [1]. The benefits of MDCT in comparison with SSCT are evident: (a) the volume scan can be performed much faster, resulting in improved temporal resolution (time to cover the entire volume) and consequently in reduced motion artefacts caused by voluntary and involuntary movement; (b) breath-holding times are reduced; (c) volume coverage is increased, permitting imaging of the entire aorta or the aortoiliac arteries and the peripheral vessels of the lower extremity within one acquisition [2]; and (d) spatial resolution along the longitudinal axis of the patient (z-axis) is improved, as is guaranteed by the thinner sections (1 mm). All these factors concur to improve the temporal, spatial, and contrast resolution of the images and significantly increase the diagnostic accuracy of the examination. MDCT technique is applied to a wide spectrum of clinical indications which require long coverage and or multiphase studies. Another important application of MDCT is the multipla-

Struttura Complessa di Radiologia Diagnostica ed Interventistica, Azienda Ospedaliera Garibaldi-Nesima, Catania, Italy

nar reformation (postprocessing) in selected pathology and virtual endoscopy. Cardiac imaging is currently considered the most technologically advanced application of MDCT. With modern MDCT it is possible to obtain a near-isotropic resolution along the z-axis. These significant improvements in z-axis resolution are obtained on condition that the sections are acquired at a fine thickness and reconstructed at fine intervals (less than the section). A true isotropic spatial resolution obtained by MDCT means that we can obtain a cubic voxel, so that the image has equal resolution in any plane of the scanned volume. This development has facilitated three-dimensional (3D) image reconstruction [3]. Shaded surface display (SSD), maximum intensity projection (MIP), volume rendering (VR), and virtual angioscopy (Fig. 1) are the most commonly used 3D reconstruction techniques. In vascular imaging, MIP and VR obtained from MDCT angiography can enable visualisation that is equal or superior to that obtained with catheter angiography. Postprocessing can be performed quickly and easily to obtain a two-dimensional MIP image. A 3D effect can be achieved with stepwise rotation of the object. VR has a high diagnostic accuracy and is the method most often used for reconstruction of CT angiographic image data. These techniques therefore are becoming the initial or the only imaging methods used for surgical planning in emergency vascular conditions. CT angiography, which was limited to a small volume with SSCT, can be applied extensively to all areas with MDCT. The two-dimensional multiplanar reconstruction (MPR) images and 3D image quality are improved with reduced image artefacts.

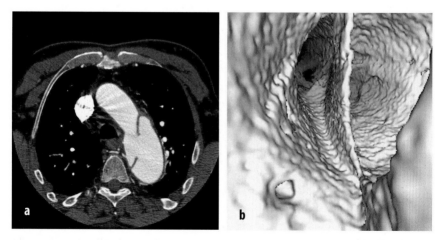

Fig. 1. a Stanford type B aorta dissection. Axial scan at the level of aortic arch shows the intimal flap tear that characterises communicating dissections. **b** Virtual angioscopy in Stanford type B aorta dissection. Virtual angioscopy shows the true lumen on the left side and the false lumen on the right, separated by the intimal flap that shows a large tear

Clinical Applications

SSCT has been used for evaluation of the aortic aneurysms since its debut. This technique provides all row data during a single breathhold, minimising motion artefacts due to respiratory activity and reducing those due to cardiac activity. Moreover, all images are obtained during optimal contrast enhancement. In large prospective studies regarding the evaluation of aortic dissections, which are considered the most difficult diagnosis within acute aortic pathology, an overall sensitivity better than 95% has been reported, with an overall accuracy of 96% [4]. However, SSCT has some limitations: it cannot cover a large volume in a short time and has a lower longitudinal spatial resolution [5]. This problem is particularly felt in the case of aortic dissection in the assessment of the real extent of the dissection (supra-aortic branches, iliac arteries). These limitations have been overcome with the introduction of MDCT, which has the capability of rapidly scanning large longitudinal volume with high z-axis resolution. MDCT angiography can be performed more efficiently because scanning is done more quickly and vascular contrast enhancement is improved. The diagnostic approach for patients with suspected thoracic or abdominal aortic aneurysms has changed substantially in the last few years. Digital subtraction angiography for the evaluation of the thoracic and abdominal aorta has given way to sonography, MR angiography, and CT angiography. Both preoperative planning and postoperative evaluation can be performed with a non-invasive technique like MDCT.

Thoracic Aortic Dissection

Thoracic aortic dissection (AD) is the most frequent cause of aortic emergency and requires immediate diagnosis and treatment. It may be described as acute or chronic, depending on the timing of its clinical manifestation. In addition, dissection is classified according to the extent of involvement of the thoracic aorta, determined using the Stanford system into type A, involving the ascending aorta or the aortic arch, or type B, involving the descending aorta distal to the left subclavian artery. Acute type A dissection should be repaired immediately, as any delay in diagnosis and treatment can be fatal. In contrast, type B dissection is normally treated medically, except in the case of abdominal organ ischaemia, which can require surgery. About one-third of patients with aortic dissection show signs indicative of systemic involvement [6]. In this group of patients it is important to evaluate the entire aorta so as to determine the distal extent of the dissection.

Ischaemic complications related to the main abdominal arterial branches are best detected with arterial phase imaging.

SSCT and MDCT permit differentiation between proximal aortic dissec-tion (type A) and distal aortic dissection (type B) with a sensitivity and specificity of nearly 100% [4]. Limited to the thoracic aorta, the examination begins with an unenhanced CT scan, useful for diagnosing intramural haematoma, displacement of intimal calcifications, or acute haemorrhage. The intravenous contrast CT scan is performed to include an area from the supra-aortic branches to iliac arteries. With the new generation of 16-section MDCT it is possible to cover the entire volume with a collimation of 1 mm, in a single continuous acquisition and in a single breathhold. A classic diag-nosis of aortic dissection is based on the detection of an intimal flap in the thoracic aorta due to displacement of the intima (Fig. 2); however, atypical dissections caused by intramural haematoma and penetrating atherosclerot-ic ulcer may manifest similar signs.

The most important diagnostic gain deriving from the clinical introduc-tion of MDCT is the high quality of MPR (Fig 3). This is particularly true in the presence of aortic dissection type B, or in extension along the descend-ing aorta of a type A dissection. In these cases only a high quality, sagittal oblique reformatted image of the thoracic aorta obtained with a MDCT scanner can identify the origin of the intimal flap, proximal or distal to the left subclavian artery (Fig. 4). Batra et al. [7] have described a variety of pit-falls and artefacts that mimic aortic dissection at SSCT angiography, poten-

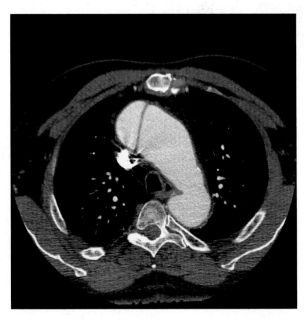

Fig. 2. Stanford type A aortic dissection. MDCT shows the intimal flap in the ascending aorta

tially leading to confusion with flap dissection. They conclude that CT angiography of the thoracic aorta remains the imaging technique of choice for evaluating patients with suspected or known aortic dissection. One of the causes of artefacts in ascending thoracic aorta is related to the aortic wall motion. The recent introduction of prospective and retrospective electrocardiographically (ECG) assisted imaging, normally used in cardiac imaging, has been used by Roos et al. [8] to determine the influence of ECG-assisted MDCT to reduce motion artefact of the ascending aorta. Their results showed a significant reduction of motion-related artefacts for the entire thoracic aorta, especially the ascending portion.

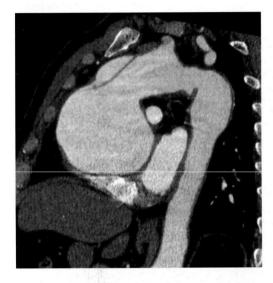

Fig. 3. Stanford type A aortic dissection. MPR shows aneurysm in the ascending aorta with aortic dissection. The intimal flap is proximal to the anonymous trunk

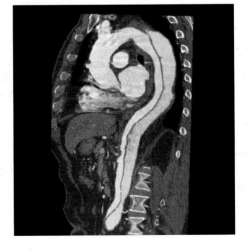

Fig. 4. Stanford type B aorta dissection. MPR shows intimal flap between true and false lumen, involving the descending aorta distal to the left subclavian artery

Abdominal Aortic Aneurysm

Aneurysmal dilatation of the infrarenal aorta is defined as a diameter of more than 29 mm. By this criterion, 9% of all people older than 65 have an abdominal aortic aneurysm (AAA) [9]. Rupture of an AAA is one of the most urgent vascular conditions and requires rapid intervention. In autopsy studies reported by Lederle et al. [10], the 1-year incidence of AAA rupture according to initial diameter was 9.4% for diameters of 5.5–5.9 cm, 10.2% for diameters of 6.0–6.9 cm, and 32.5% for diameters of 7.0 cm or more. A diagnosis of ruptured AAA may be made on the basis of a non-enhanced CT scan that shows an AAA with adjacent periaortic haemorrhage that extends into the perirenal and pararenal spaces of the retroperitoneum. Open surgical repair is increasingly being replaced by endovascular repair, which is more efficient and has lower associated morbidity and mortality [11]. Lee et al. [12] found that patient eligibility for endovascular repair depends on the anatomy of the proximal aneurysm neck. Great effort has been put into the development of specialised software MDCT for planning endoluminal treatment of AAA. Most of the measurements required for determination of the optimal dimensions and type of aortic stent-graft are now obtained with MDCT image reconstruction.

Endovascular Stent-Graft Evaluation and Assessment of Complication

The current standard treatment for AAA is open surgical repair, which is associated with a low overall risk. The reported mortality rate associated with elective surgical repair ranges from 1.4% to 6.5% [13]. However, in high-risk patients with a comorbid medical condition such as severe cardiovascular, pulmonary, or renal disease, the risk of death during surgical repair of AAA is considerably higher (5.7–31%) [14]. In an attempt to reduce risk in these patients, less invasive methods of repair have been considered. Treatment of AAA with transfemoral placement of an endovascular stent-graft is increasingly being used as an alternative to surgical repair [15]. In 1991, Parodi et al. [16] reported the transfemoral placement of non-bifurcated stent-grafts for treatment of AAA in a series of human patients. Although conventional arteriography has long been considered the modality of choice for arterial imaging, there are several reasons why helical CT angiography may be superior in the assessment of the abdominal arteries. First, the acquisition of volumetric data with helical CT allows clear delineation of the tortuous aorta and branch vessels and of adjacent aneurysms and pseudoaneurysms. Second, blood pool imaging with the intravenous administration of contrast material allows visualisation of true and false luminal flow channels, intramural haematomas communicating with the aortic lumen, and slow perigraft flow around aortic stent-grafts. Finally, the aortic wall and non-communicating intramural collections can be directly visualised with CT angiography. These advantages of SSCT with the fast and high quality of MDCT angiography images today confine conventional angiography to interventional procedures only. Pre-procedural assessment of endoluminal stent-graft therapy with MDCT of the length and tortuosity of the proximal neck of the aneurysm, mural thrombus irregularity, and inferior mesenteric artery patency may help predict complications such as endoleak, shower embolism, and colonic ischaemia. Use of high quality MIP images often clarifies the complex anatomy of the tortuous aorta and branch vessels by showing the precise intravascular position and configuration of the stent-graft, whilst axial source images accurately demonstrate leaks and the patency of the stent-graft. Various complications may occur after treatment with endovascular stent-graft, and MDCT is fast, minimally invasive, and is considered the gold standard procedure for the assessment of such common (endoleak, graft thrombosis, graft kinking; Fig. 5) and rare complications (pseudo-aneurysm caused by graft infection, graft occlusion, shower embolism, perforation of mural thrombus by means of inadvertent penetration of the delivery system, colon necrosis, aortic dissection, or haematoma at the arteriotomy site).

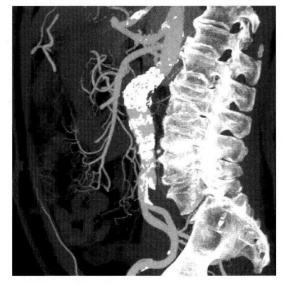

Fig. 5. Aortic aneurysm treated by stent-graft. Sagittal MIP image 6 months after therapy shows severe angulation of the aortic stent-graft

References

1. Klingenbeck-Regn K, Schaller S, Flohr T et al (1999) Subsecond multi-slice computed tomography: basics and applications. Eur J Radiol 31:110–124
2. Rubin GD, Shiau MC, Leung AN et al (2000) Aorta and iliac arteries: single versus multiple detector-row helical CT angiography. Radiology 215:670–676
3. Calhoun PS, Kuszyk BS, Heath DG et al (1999) Three-dimensional volume rendering of spiral CT data: theory and method. Radiographics 19:745–764
4. Sommer T, Fehske W, Holzknecht N et al (1996) Aortic dissection: a comparative study of diagnosis with spiral CT, multiplanar transesphageal echocardiography, and RM imaging. Radiology 199:347–52
5. Rubin GD, Shiau MC, Schmidt AJ et al (1999) Computed tomographic angiography: historical perspective and new state-of-the-art using multi detector-row helical computed tomography. J Comput Assist Tomogr 23(Suppl 1):S83-S90
6. Cambria RP, Brewster DC, Gertler J et al (1988) Vascular complications associated with spontaneous aortic dissection. J Vasc Surg 7:199–209
7. Batra P, Bigoni B, Manning J et al (2000) Pitfalls in the diagnosis of thoracic aortic dissection at CT angiography. Radiographics 20:309–320
8. Roos J, Willmann J, Weishaupt D et al (2002) Thoracic aorta: motion artifact reduction with retrospective and prospective electrocardiography-assisted multi–detector row CT. Radiology 222:271–277
9. Alcorn HG, Wolfson SK Jr, Sutton-Tyrrell K et al (1996) Risk factors for abdominal aortic aneurysms in older adults enrolled in the Cardiovascular Health Study. Arterioscler Thromb Vasc Biol 16:963–970
10. Lederle FA, Johnson GR, Wilson SE et al (2002) Rupture rate of large abdominal aortic aneurysms in patients refusing or unfit for elective repair. JAMA 287:2968–2972
11. Moore WS, Kashyap VS, Vescera CL et al (1999) Abdominal aortic aneurysm: a 6-year comparison of endovascular versus transabdominal repair. Ann Surg 230:298–308
12. Lee WA, Huber TS, Hirneise CM et al (2002) Eligibility rates of ruptured and symptomatic AAA for endovascular repair. J Endovasc Ther 9:436–442
13. Ernst CB (1993) Abdominal aortic aneurysm. N Engl J Med 328:1167–1172
14. Hollier LH, Reigel MM, Kazmier FJ et al (1986) Conventional repair of abdominal aortic aneurysm in the high-risk patient: a plea for abandonment of nonresective treatment. J Vasc Surg 3:712–717
15. Dorffner R, Thurnher S, Polterauer P et al (1997) Treatment of abdominal aortic aneurysms with transfemoral placement of stent-grafts: complications and secondary radiologic intervention. Radiology 204:79–86
16. Parodi JC, Palmaz JC, Barone HD (1991) Transfemoral intraluminal graft implantation for abdominal aortic aneurysms. Ann Vasc Surg 5:491–499

MRI in the Diagnosis of Right Ventricular Dysplasia

M. Midiri, M. Galia, T.V. Bartolotta

Introduction

Arrhythmogenic right ventricular dysplasia (ARVD) is a form of cardiomyopathy that is characterised clinically by ventricular arrhythmias with left bundle branch block (LBBB) that may lead to cardiac arrest and morphologically by fatty or fibrofatty infiltration of the right ventricular myocardium [1–5]. Although the incidence and prevalence of ARVD are unknown, ARVD is recognised as a major cause of sudden death in young adolescents; in one series it accounted for 20% of sudden deaths in all individuals younger than 35 years and 22% of sudden deaths in young athletes [6]. Therefore, an early and accurate diagnosis followed by appropriate therapy for this condition is increasingly important, for it may prevent lethal arrhythmias.

Aetiology

ARVD must be considered as a part of the group of idiopathic cardiomyopathies, based on its nature of progressive heart muscle disease with unclear pathogenesis and aetiology. The male-to-female ratio is 2.7:1.0.

Basso et al. [1] addressed the aetiology and pathogenesis and proposed four hypotheses as possible explanations. The first hypothesis concerns *apoptosis*, that is, programmed cell death, which leads to progressive myocardial muscle loss followed by fibrofatty replacement and enhances the electrical vulnerability of the right ventricle, which in turn can cause potentially life-threatening arrhythmias [7]. According to the *dysontogenetic* theory, ARVD should be regarded as a congenital heart disease in which abnormal

Dipartimento di Biotecnologie Mediche e Medicina Legale, Sezione di Scienze Radiologiche, University of Palermo, Italy

development of the right ventricle may lead to dysplasia. In the *degenerative* theory, a metabolic disorder may affect the right ventricle and result in progressive replacement of myocardial cells by fat and fibrous tissue. In the *inflammatory* theory, the fibrofatty replacement is viewed as a healing process in the context of myocarditis [8].

Several reports suggest that there is a familial occurrence of ARVD of about 30–50% [2, 9–12], with mainly autosomal dominant inheritance, variable penetrance, and polymorphic phenotypic expression. Several genetic disorders responsible for ARVD have been identified on chromosome 14 and, recently, on chromosome 3 [9, 11, 12]. The diagnosis of ARVD may have important consequences for direct relatives, because they have an increased chance of having the disease, and therefore an increased risk of sudden death. Gene mapping may open new avenues for cloning the defective gene, identifying the encoded protein, and potentially instituting gene therapy. Four loci have been mapped, but none of the genes have been identified yet, and the findings of polymorphism in ARVD currently preclude gene therapy [5, 9, 11].

Pathological Features

Two morphological variants of ARVD have been reported: fatty and fibrofatty [6, 13–16]. The fatty form is characterised by almost complete replacement of the myocardium without thinning of the ventricular wall, and it occurs exclusively in the right ventricle. The fibrofatty variant is associated with significant thinning of the right ventricular wall, and the left ventricular myocardial wall may also be involved. Other anatomic malformations of the right ventricle associated with ARVD consist of mild to severe global dilatation of the ventricle, ventricular aneurysms, and segmental hypokinesia. The sites of involvement of anatomic abnormalities are found in the so-called triangle of dysplasia, namely, the right ventricular subtricuspid areas, the apex, and the infundibulum [14].

Clinical Characteristics

The clinical manifestations of ARVD may vary widely, but the disorder is classically characterised by ventricular tachycardia with LBBB, originating from the right ventricle. ARVD probably represents a spectrum of different abnormalities rather than a single identity, and ranges from an asymptomatic form consisting of ventricular ectopic beats to biventricular heart failure with or without arrhythmias and sudden death in young patients and athletes [5, 15]. Furthermore, ARVD is a disease that may have a temporal progression, and the disease may manifest differently according to the time of patient presentation.

Prognosis and Therapy

Although the prognosis of ARVD is considerably better than that of sustained ventricular tachycardia with left ventricular heart disease, ARVD is a progressive disease and will probably lead to right ventricular failure in the long term unless sudden cardiac death occurs first. The death rate for patients with ARVD has been estimated at 2.5% per year [17]. The disease certainly cannot be considered as a benign condition in patients with symptoms of syncope, episodes of recurrent ventricular tachycardia, and anatomic or functional abnormalities of the right ventricle [18].

Fortunately, patients with recurrences of ventricular tachycardia have a favourable outcome when they are treated medically. The four therapeutic options in patients with ARVD are antiarrhythmic agents, catheter ablation, implantable cardioverter defibrillators, and surgery [19]. Pharmacological treatment is the first choice, the antiarrhythmic agents being sotalol, verapamil, beta-receptor-blocking agents, amiodarone, and flecainide. Catheter ablation is an alternative in patients who do not respond to drug treatment and who have localised disease. In addition, catheter ablation has been shown to improve the effectiveness of pharmacological treatment: 70% of patients may respond to antiarrhythmic agents to which they were unresponsive prior to ablation therapy [20]. Implantation of cardioverter defibrillators is indicated in patients who are intolerant of antiarrhythmic therapy and who are at serious risk of sudden death. Surgery should be considered only as a very last resort, and treatment consists initially of ventriculotomy, followed by total disconnection of the right ventricular free wall. In the case of progressive or intractable right ventricular failure, cardiac transplantation may be the ultimate option for treating patients with ARVD. Currently, drug treatment, ablation, and cardioverter defibrillator therapy are the most suitable therapeutic approaches in patients with ARVD.

MR Imaging Assessment

ARVD is being diagnosed with increasing frequency, mostly because MR imaging allows improved recognition of myocardial fatty and fibrofatty replacement [13]. Several studies have reported on the use of MR imaging to detect the characteristic high signal intensity of fat in the right ventricular myocardium on T_1-weighted images [1, 6, 21–24]. However recent studies demonstrated that significant fatty infiltration of the right ventricle occurs in more than 50% of normal hearts in elderly people [25, 26]. Mehta et al. [27] found signs of fatty replacement in only 22% of 27 patients with ventricular tachycardia with LBBB (as diagnosed with endomyocardial biopsy). Menghetti et al. [21] reported a sensitivity and specificity of 67% and 100%, respectively, with the use of spin echo MR imaging. Basso et al. [1], however, found that among nine patients with the pathological diagnosis of ARVD (based on gross or histological evidence of regional or diffuse transmural fatty or fibrofatty replacement), MR imaging revealed abnormally high signal intensity in all cases [1]. Although these findings indicate that the presence of some fat in the right ventricular myocardium may not be specific enough for the diagnosis of ARVD, the presence of transmural fatty replacement or diffuse thinning of the right ventricular myocardium as demonstrated with MR imaging should be considered in the overall clinical context to be a major criterion for the diagnosis of ARVD.

Several studies examined the value of using MR imaging in patients for whom the first manifestation of right ventricular disease was right ventricular outflow tract tachycardia [28–34]. Carlson et al. [30] showed that right ventricular outflow tract tachycardia was associated with local structural and wall motion abnormalities of the right ventricular outflow tract, and that the structural abnormalities observed with MR imaging were often not detected with echocardiography. Proclemer et al. [34] investigated 19 patients who had frequent ventricular extrasystoles (100/h) with LBBB pattern (minor criterion). In all 19 patients, results from two-dimensional echocardiography were normal; however, MR imaging showed significantly greater dimensions of the right ventricular outflow tract than those seen in the control group of 10 volunteers. The similarity of these findings to those previously obtained in patients with right ventricular tachycardia suggests a similar underlying mechanism of the right ventricular outflow tract arrhythmias.

MR imaging can also be used to assess both systolic and diastolic function in great detail. Several studies have addressed the presence of right ventricular diastolic dysfunction as an early marker of disease, even when systolic function is still preserved [35]. In a previous study, we showed that diastolic function of the right ventricle was significantly altered in 15 patients with non-ischaemic tachyarrhythmias of right ventricular origin, even though systolic function was normal [31]. Of the 15 patients in that study, 5 (33%) had a clinical diagnosis of ARVD, indicating that ARVD may be associated with diastolic function abnormalities preceding systolic function abnormalities. Therefore, it could be suggested that diastolic dysfunction might be considered as an additional feature or criterion of ARVD. The typical criteria that can be demonstrated with MR imaging are (a) fatty infil-tration of the right ventricular myocardium with high signal intensity on T_1-weighted images (major criterion); (b) fibrofatty replacement, which leads to diffuse thinning of the right ventricular myocardium (major criterion); (c) aneurysms of the right ventricle and right ventricular outflow tract (major criterion); (d) dilatation of the right ventricle and right ventricular outflow tract (when severe, major criterion; when mild, minor criterion); (e) regional contraction abnormalities (minor criterion); and (f) global systolic dysfunc-tion (major criterion) and global diastolic dysfunction (minor criterion).

In summary, MR imaging is useful for evaluating not only fatty replace-ment of the right ventricular myocardium, but also global and regional func-tional abnormalities of the right ventricle and right ventricular outflow tract. The demonstration of right ventricular abnormalities should be con-sidered in the overall clinical context.

MR Imaging Protocol

For all examinations, a phased array cardiac synergy coil with five elements has to be used. For the evaluation of right ventricular anatomy, we perform a multisection inversion-recovery ('black blood') segmented turbo spin echo pulse sequence to obtain images with section thicknesses of 4 mm or less in transverse and sagittal planes. 'Black blood' in MR images can be achieved by using a non-selective 180° pulse to invert all spins. This inversion pulse is directly followed by a selective 180° pulse, which resets the signal of the sec-tion under investigation. This technique causes the blood with inverted sig-nal to flow into the selected section. After a delay (inversion time), the blood signal is nulled (inversion time depends on heart rate) and the imaging pulse sequence (e.g. a fast spin echo during patient breath-hold) is started [36, 37]. For the evaluation of right ventricular global and regional systolic function, we use a multisection, multiphase, balanced fast-field-echo pulse sequence [38] to obtain images with section thicknesses of 8–9 mm in the transverse plane. Balanced fast-field-echo pulse sequences belong to the group of 'steady state free precession' sequences and are characterised by the applica-tion of time-balanced gradients for all gradient directions: section selection, frequency readout, and phase encoding. Together with the alternating phase of the excitation pulse, this technique ensures that both signals (free induc-tion decay and echo) are obtained. The sequence produces a very high signal for tissues with a high T_2:T_1 ratio, independent of the repetition time. The balanced gradients contribute to a low sensitivity for flow disturbances. Because the field homogeneity is very important, balanced fast field echo requires the use of shimming before each study. For the evaluation of right ventricular diastolic function, MR velocity mapping is performed to measure flow across the tricuspid valve [39]. The number of time frames used to sample the cardiac cycle is set to 30, resulting in a temporal resolution of less than 30 ms per cardiac frame. Peak velocity is set at 100 cm/s to avoid aliasing. Flow measurements are performed in double oblique planes, identified from a coronal spin echo image and a transverse gradient echo image. End-diastolic and end-systolic positions of the tricuspid valve are determined, and the imaging plane is selected between these positions perpendicular to transtricuspid flow direction.

Summary

ARVD is part of the group of cardiomyopathies characterised pathologically by fibrofatty replacement of the right ventricular myocardium and clinically by right ventricular arrhythmias of the LBBB pattern. Pathogenesis, prevalence, and aetiology are yet not fully known. The diagnosis of ARVD is based on the presence of structural, histological, electrocardiographic, and genetic factors. Therapeutic options include antiarrhythmic medication, catheter ablation, implantable cardioverter defibrillation, and surgery. Angiography and echocardiography lack sensitivity and specificity in the diagnosis of ARVD. MR imaging allows a three-dimensional evaluation of especially the right ventricle, and provides the most important anatomical, functional, and morphological criteria for diagnosis of ARVD within one single study. Although demonstration of morphological/functional abnormalities of the right ventricle, especially fat in the right ventricular myocardium, shows high specificity but low sensitivity, MR imaging appears to be the optimal imaging technique for detection and follow-up of clinically suspected ARVD. Positive MR imaging findings, based on the criteria of McKenna et al. [16], should be used as important additional criteria in the clinical diagnosis of ARVD, although negative MR imaging findings do not rule out ARVD.

References

1. Basso C, Thiene G, Corrado D et al (1996) Arrhythmogenic right ventricular cardiomyopathy: dysplasia, dystrophy, or myocarditis? Circulation 94:983–991
2. Corrado D, Fontaine G, Marcus FI et al (2000) Arrhythmogenic right ventricular dysplasia/cardiomyopathy: need for an international registry. Circulation 101:E101–E106
3. Metzger J, de Chillou C, Cheriex E et al (1993) Value of the 12-lead electrocardiogram in arrhythmogenic right ventricular dysplasia, and absence of correlation with electrocardiographic findings. Am J Cardiol 72:964–967

4. Pinamonti B, Sinagra G, Camerini F (2000) Clinical relevance of right ventricular dysplasia/cardiomyopathy (editorial). Heart 83:9–11

5. van der Wall EE, Kayser HW, Bootsma MM et al (2000) Arrhythmogenic right ventricular dysplasia: MRI findings. Herz 4:356–364

6. Thiene G, Nava A, Corrado D et al (1988) Right ventricular cardiomyopathy and sudden death in young people. N Engl J Med 318:129–133

7. James T (1994) Normal and abnormal consequences of apoptosis in the human heart: from postnatal morphogenesis to paroxysmal arrhythmias. Circulation 90:556–573

8. Hofmann R, Trappe HJ, Klein H et al (1993) Chronic (or healed) myocarditis mimicking arrhythmogenic right ventricular dysplasia. Eur Heart J 14:717–720

9. Ahmad F, Li D, Karibe A et al (1998) Localization of a gene responsible for arrhythmogenic right ventricular dysplasia to chromosome 3p23. Circulation 98:2791–2795

10. Nava A, Thiene G, Canciani B et al (1998) Familial occurrence of right ventricular dysplasia: a study involving nine families. J Am Coll Cardiol 12:1222–1228

11. Rampazzo A, Nava A, Danieli GA et al (1994) The gene for arrhythmogenic right ventricular cardiomyopathy maps to chromosome 14q23-q24. Hum Mol Genet 3:959–962

12. Rampazzo A, Nava A, Erne P et al (1995) A new locus for arrhythmogenic right ventricular cardiomyopathy (ARVD2) maps to chromosome 1q42-q43. Hum Mol Genet 4:2151–2154

13. Corrado D, Basso C, Thiene G (2000) Arrhythmogenic right ventricular cardiomyopathy: diagnosis, prognosis, and treatment. Heart 83:588–595

14. Fontaine G, Fontaliran F, Frank R (1998) Arrhythmogenic right ventricular cardiomyopathies: clinical forms and main differential diagnoses (editorial). Circulation 97:1532–1535

15. Pinamonti B, Pagnan L, Bussani R et al (1998) Right ventricular dysplasia with biventricular involvement. Circulation 98:1943–1945

16. McKenna WJ, Thiene G, Nava A et al (1994) Diagnosis of arrhythmogenic right ventricular dysplasia/cardiomyopathy. Br Heart J 71:215–218

17. Fontaine G, Fontaliran F, Hebert J et al (1999) Arrhythmogenic right ventricular dysplasia. Annu Rev Med 1999; 50:17–35

18. Marcus FI, Fontaine GH, Guirodon G et al (1982) Right ventricular dysplasia: a report of 24 adult cases. Circulation 65:384–398

19. Leclercq JF, Coumel P (1989) Characteristics, prognosis and treatment of the ventricular arrhythmias of right ventricular dysplasia. Eur Heart J 10:D61–D67

20. Movsowitz C, Schwartzman D, Callans DJ et al (1996) Idiopathic right ventricular outflow tract tachycardia: narrowing the anatomic location for successful ablation. Am Heart J 131:930–936

21. Menghetti L, Basso C, Nava A et al (1996) Spin-echo nuclear magnetic resonance for tissue characterisation in arrhythmogenic right ventricular cardiomyopathy. Heart 76:467–470

22. Marcus FI, Fontaine G (1995) Arrhythmogenic right ventricular dysplasia/cardiomyopathy: a review. Pacing Clin Electrophysiol 18:1298–1314

23. Auffermann W, Wichter T, Breithardt G et al (1993) Arrhythmogenic right ventricular disease: MR imaging vs angiography. AJR Am J Roentgenol 161:549–555

24. Globits S, Kreiner G, Frank H et al (1997) Significance of morphological abnormalities detected by MRI in patients undergoing successful ablation of right ventricular outflow tract tachycardia. Circulation 96:2633–2640

25. Burke A, Farb A, Tashko G et al (1998) Arrhythmogenic right ventricular cardiomyopathy and fatty replacement of the right ventricular myocardium: are they different diseases? Circulation 97:1571–1580

26. Fontaliran F, Fontaine G, Fillette F et al (1991) Nosologic frontiers of arrhythmogenic dysplasia: quantitative variations of normal adipose tissue of the right heart ventricle. Arch Mal Coeur Vaiss 84:33–38

27. Mehta D, Davies MJ, Ward DE et al (1994) Ventricular tachycardias of right ventricular origin: markers of subclinical right ventricular disease. Am Heart J 127:360–366

28. White RD, Trohman RG, Flamm SD et al (1998) Right ventricular arrhythmia in the absence of arrhythmogenic dysplasia: MR imaging of myocardial abnormalities. Radiology 207:743–751

29. Markowitz SM, Litvak BL, Ramirez de Arellano EA et al (1997) Adenosine-sensitive ventricular tachycardia: right ventricular abnormalities delineated by magnetic resonance imaging. Circulation 96:1192–1200

30. Carlson MD, White RD, Trohman RG et al (1994) Right ventricular outflow tract ventricular tachycardia: detection of previously unrecognized anatomic abnormalities using cine magnetic resonance imaging. J Am Coll Cardiol 24:720–727

31. Kayser H, Schalij M, van der Wall E et al (1997) Biventricular function in patients with nonischaemic right ventricular tachyarrhythmias assessed with MR imaging. AJR Am J Roentgenol 159:995–999

32. Kayser H, de Roos A, van der Wall E (1998) Diagnosis of cardiac abnormalities in patients with nonischaemic tachyarrhythmias: additional value of MR imaging. Int J Card Imaging 14:279–285

33. Midiri M, Finazzo M, Brancato M et al (1997) Arrhythmogenic right ventricular dysplasia: MR features. Eur Radiol 7:307–312

34. Proclemer A, Basadonna PT, Slavich GA et al (1997) Cardiac magnetic resonance imaging findings in patients with right ventricular outflow tract premature contractions. Eur Heart J 18:2002–2010

35. Appleton CP, Hatle LK, Popp RL (1988) Relation of transmitral flow velocity patterns to left ventricular diastolic function: new insights from a combined haemodynamic and Doppler echocardiographic study. J Am Coll Cardiol 12:426–440

36. Simonetti O, Kim R, Fieno D et al (2001) An improved MR imaging technique for the visualization of myocardial infarction. Radiology 218:215–223

37. Simonetti O, Finn J, White RD et al (1996) 'Black blood' T2-weighted inversion-recovery MR imaging of the heart. Radiology 199:49–57

38. Steenbeck J, Pruessmann K (2001) Technical developments in cardiac MRI: 2000 update. Rays 26:15–34

39. Kayser H, Stoel B, van der Wall E et al (1997) MR velocity mapping of tricuspid flow: correction for through-plane motion. J Magn Reson Imaging 7:669–673

Subject Index